Psychosocial Interventions for Cardiopulmonary Patients

A Guide for Health Professionals

Wayne M. Sotile, PhD
Wake Forest University Cardiac Rehabilitation Program

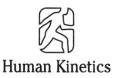

Human Kinetics

Library of Congress Cataloging-in-Publication Data

Sotile, Wayne M., 1951-
  Psychosocial interventions for cardiopulmonary patients : a guide
for health professionals / Wayne M. Sotile.
    p. cm.
  Includes bibliographical references and index.
  ISBN 0-87322-766-2 (case text)
  1. Cardiopulmonary system--Diseases--Psychological aspects.
  2. Adjustment (Psychology)   I. Title.
  RC702.S67   1996
  616.1'203--dc20   95-35146
                                                                 CIP

ISBN: 0-87322-766-2

Acquisitions Editor: Richard A. Washburn; **Developmental Editor**: Elaine Mustain; **Assistant Editors**: Erin Cler, Dawn Barker, and Susan Moore; **Copyeditor**: Barbara Fields; **Proofreader**: Dawn Barker; **Indexer**: Barbara E. Cohen; **Production Manager**: Kris Ding; **Typesetter and Layout Artist**: Sandra Meier; **Text Designer**: Stuart Cartwright; **Photo Editor**: Boyd LaFoon; **Cover Designer**: Jack Davis; **Illustrator**: Tim Stiles; **Mac Artist**: Jennifer Delmotte; **Printer**: BookCrafters

Printed in the United States of America

10   9   8   7   6   5   4   3   2   1

Human Kinetics
P.O. Box 5076, Champaign, IL 61825-5076
1-800-747-4457

Canada: Human Kinetics, Box 24040, Windsor, ON N8Y 4Y9
1-800-465-7301 (in Canada only)

Europe: Human Kinetics, P.O. Box IW14, Leeds LS16 6TR, United Kingdom
(44) 1132 781708

Australia: Human Kinetics, 2 Ingrid Street, Clapham 5062, South Australia
(08) 371 3755

New Zealand: Human Kinetics, P.O. Box 105-231, Auckland 1
(09) 523 3462

To my wife, Mary,
the most courageous truth-teller I know
and the reason so many of my dreams come true.

∎ ACKNOWLEDGMENTS ∎

Publishing a book of this magnitude is only done with the support and tolerance of an army of caring people. To each of the following I offer my sincere appreciation and thanks:

- First and foremost, Mary, my wife, for your help with research and writing, for your endless patience and tolerance, for reminding me of what is true, and for being there to take up the slack in our life that my obsessions create. You are my only one.

- Rebecca and Julia, our daughters, for the many Saturdays you helped me in the library, for making me laugh, for laughing at me, and for being the special people you are. I love each of you the most.

- Kathy Hall, my administrative assistant and office manager, for your endless energy, endless loyalty, and painstaking attention to the details that make my *big life* run.
- Lynn Swaim, for typing my words—even when I don't speak them clearly—and for your gentle reminders to not forget who I am.
- The Wake Forest University cardiac rehabilitation program staff—Andrea Shutt, Sue Casey, and, especially, Sherry Steele—for your cheerful help and for tolerating me and my travel schedule.
- Esteemed colleagues of many years—Henry Miller, MD; Paul Ribisl, PhD; A.C. Hillman, MA; Jack Rejeski, PhD; Julie Ellis, MPH; Don Bergey, MA; JoAnn Tuttle, RN; Peter Brubaker, PhD; and Bill Pollock, MS—for teaching me what caring collaboration and lasting working friendships are all about.
- Patricia Farrell, MD, for your friendship and generous help in shaping my comments regarding psychotropic medications.
- My friend Barry Franklin, PhD, former editor-in-chief of the *Journal of Cardiopulmonary Rehabilitation*, for encouraging me to put my thoughts and experiences on paper. Our conversations during our travels through Australia were the catalyst for the writing of this book.
- The nice people of the American Association of Cardiovascular and Pulmonary Rehabilitation, for your mission of promoting the best of care for cardiac and pulmonary patients, and for letting me belong.
- The many pharmaceutical and medical equipment companies who, in challenging times, have continued to invest money in the education of health professionals.
- Linda Hall, PhD, my friend, for your endorsement of my work and for steering me to Human Kinetics.

I give special thanks to the nice and competent people at Human Kinetics, especially to

- Rik Washburn, PhD, for your enthusiasm and support as we expanded the original design of this project,
- Rainer Martens, publisher and president, for your interest in my work,
- And, most of all, to Elaine Mustain, editor. Every author knows from painful experience that editors can be a brutally honest lot. I sincerely thank you for your tact, compassion, and enthusiasm as you so astutely helped me to reshape my original manuscript.

Finally, my thanks and admiration go to the many colleagues throughout the country with whom I have the privilege of consulting. Your days fill with quiet acts of heroism as you care for your patients. You inspire me.

■ CONTENTS ■

■ PREFACE ■

More people are living with heart or lung illnesses today than at any time in history, placing tremendous burdens on contemporary medical, economic, and family systems. These burdens challenge us to help heart and lung patients not only survive but also thrive while living with illness. To meet this challenge, we must deliver medical and rehabilitation care that promotes overall biopsychosocial functioning of both the patients we serve and their loved ones. While we appear to be meeting this challenge in the biological realm, much remains to be done in addressing the psychosocial issues of recovering heart and lung patients. This book is offered as a guide for reengineering the ways in which the psychosocial needs of recovering heart and lung patients are addressed.

The first step in this reengineering is to sanction the delivery of psychosocial care by professionals who may not be formally trained in the behavioral sciences but who (a) are involved on the front lines of delivery of care, and (b) have received at least brief training in how to recognize and address psychosocial issues important in rehabilitation. Included here might be nurses, exercise physiologists, respiratory therapists, pharmacists, dieticians, physical therapists, occupational therapists, and those involved in vocational rehabilitation, home health care, and nonpsychiatric medicine.

I believe this sanctioning is vital for two reasons. First, it validates what is already happening. In practice, psychosocial services to recovering cardiopulmonary patients typically are not being delivered by mental health specialists. A survey of European cardiac services (Maes, 1992) found that, with the exception of Italy, Austria, the Netherlands, and Finland, mental health professionals are largely unrepresented on cardiac rehabilitation teams. A survey of 1,628 U.S. coronary care units (Sikes & Rodenhauser, 1987) found that psychosocial counseling is typically provided by nurses (in 95% of the programs surveyed), followed by social workers (47%), nonpsychiatric physicians (30%), and dieticians (23%). In only 12% of the surveyed programs did patients consult with a psychologist, and in even fewer (9%) did patients consult with a psychiatrist.

The second reason for sanctioning the delivery of psychosocial interventions by health care providers who are not experts in mental health comes from my personal experiences as a clinical psychologist, consultant, and researcher. Over the past 17 years, I have assessed and/or treated over 3,000 recovering cardiopulmonary patients or their families. In addition, I have had the privilege of consulting with over 200 hospitals and health care organizations and thousands of health care providers throughout the United States and Australia. These clinical and consulting experiences, coupled with the broad research literature cited in this book, led me to the undeniable conclusion that psychosocial intervention with heart and lung patients does not need to be elaborate for it to be effective. To serve our patients well, then, those of us who are mental health specialists must recognize where their care is coming from and assist these providers with appropriate training. That is what *Psychosocial Interventions for Cardiopulmonary Patients* seeks to do.

I am not arguing against the value that experts in mental health specialties can bring to the overall treatment of cardiopulmonary patients. As will be discussed, I believe strongly that there is a place for the mental health expert in delivering care to cardiopulmonary patients. But there are not enough mental health experts in place to satisfy the treatment needs of the millions of cardiopulmonary patients being seen each day in hospital, outpatient, and rehabilitation settings.

Psychosocial services in medical settings should be sensitive both to the coping challenges that come with particular illnesses and to the stresses caused by our treatments. The pages that follow are filled with practical recommendations for soothing these stresses in inpatient, office, and formal rehabilitation settings.

AN OVERVIEW OF WHAT IS TO FOLLOW

Part I consists of three chapters that create a backdrop for designing and implementing effective psychosocial interventions. Chapter 1 presents an overview of the importance of providing psychosocial services to recovering heart and lung patients. Chapter 2 presents several frames of reference for understanding the psychosocial experiences of cardiopulmonary patients and specific advice for conducting psychosocial assessments and for offering feedback to heart and lung patients. This chapter also presents guidelines for recognizing and managing serious maladjustments, including postoperative delirium, organic mental disorders, alcohol and substance abuse, and psychosomatic invalidism. Chapter 3 describes the psychosocial adjustment patterns evidenced by recovering cardiopulmonary patients and general strategies for structuring psychosocial interventions across treatment settings and patient populations.

Part II is devoted to my Effective Emotional Management (EEM) model for practical psychosocial interventions with medical patients. Chapter 4 provides an overview of the EEM model and descriptions of various levels of psychosocial intervention in medical settings. Subsequent chapters offer practical advice regarding the various core components of EEM: understanding and controlling stress (chapter 5); promoting relaxation (chapter 6); managing personality-based coping patterns (chapter 7); addressing marital and family issues (chapter 8); controlling cognitions (chapter 9); and keys for promoting positive living (chapter 10).

Part III discusses several topics that deserve special attention in treating cardiopulmonary patients. Sexual aspects of living with heart and lung illnesses are discussed in chapter 11. Chapter 12 presents a comprehensive discussion of smoking cessation. The unique psychosocial challenges faced by chronic obstructive pulmonary disease (COPD) patients and by aged patients are discussed in chapter 13. An integrative discussion of ways to improve adherence and structure psychosocial interventions across treatment settings is presented in chapter 14.

I hope that this information will prove useful to a multidisciplinary audience of health care professionals. The mental health professional experienced in working with cardiopulmonary patients will find practical treatment strategies and a guide for expanding existing clinical services. In addition, I hope that the information to follow will appeal to the health care provider not professionally trained in mental health but who wants to become better at recognizing and responding to the psychosocial needs of recovering cardiopulmonary patients.

The pages that follow are filled with practical recommendations regarding how this can be done in inpatient, office, and formal rehabilitation settings. I hope that this book will spur an expansion of existing psychosocial interventions in the reader's clinical practice and stimulate interest in further controlled investigations of the effectiveness of such interventions.

CAVEATS REGARDING THIS LITERATURE

For the most part, the scientific literature on cardiac and pulmonary psychosocial issues is limited in terms of both experimental design and clinical creativity. Most of the investigations that have addressed risk factor or psychosocial concerns of recovering heart patients have suffered from methodological shortcomings or problems in reporting (Hill, Kelleher, & Shumaker, 1992). Relatively few studies have addressed the value of psychosocial interventions in patients with chronic lung diseases, but the studies that do exist share numerous methodologic problems with the investigations of cardiac populations (Blake, Vandiver, Braun, Bertuso, & Straub, 1990).

From an experimental design perspective, this literature can generally be criticized in many ways. For example, many of these investigations employed inadequate evaluation designs, including small sample sizes and inadequate controls. Many have failed to randomize samples or to compare effects of various treatment strategies. Often, investigations have used measures of psychosocial functioning that either have not been validated or have been validated on inadequately described subject populations. Furthermore, this literature typically contains reports that have employed only general interventions based on educational rather than behavioral approaches (Blumenthal & Emery, 1988; Godin, 1989; Hill et al., 1992; Houston-Miller, Taylor, Davidson, Hill, & Krantz, 1990; Razin, 1982).

Given the shortcomings mentioned above, presenting a summary of interventions limited to the cardiopulmonary literature would be of little clinical value. To do so would run the risk of narrowing rather than broadening awareness of potentially effective psychosocial care. However, an integration of suggestions from the cardiopulmonary literature with those from the broad literatures of health psychology, family systems medicine, behavior modification, behavioral medicine, psychosomatic medicine, and nursing can shed light on many psychosocial interventions that have proven effective with various medical populations and that logically might be helpful for recovering cardiopulmonary patients. The information in this book focuses primarily, but not exclusively, on practical applications of findings from over 1,000 selected research studies from this combined literature.

This is not intended to be an exhaustive, critical review of this literature. Rather, the implications of relevant research and my own clinical experiences in treating a wide range of medical patients for psychosocial concerns in both inpatient and outpatient settings will be presented. My goal is to organize this information into a model for structuring clinical efforts to promote psychosocial adjustments for heart and lung patients. The efficacy of these interventions remains to be evaluated in controlled clinical trials.

Finally, a word about the methodology that resulted in the integration of information contained in this book. In their summary of research regarding the behavioral perspectives of coronary heart disease, Smith and Leon (1992) concluded that "although some differences exist . . . emotional, social, and vocational functioning among post-myocardial infarction (MI), angioplasty, and bypass patients is generally similar . . . Therefore, [discussion of psychological aspects of] these groups of patients [can be] considered together" (p. 116). This same sentiment applies to many of the psychosocial adjustments faced by patients who suffer from various chronic lung illnesses (especially COPD, asthma, and cystic fibrosis) and to both cardiac and pulmonary patients, as groups. This fact is echoed by a number of experts in the field of pulmonary rehabilitation (e.g., Connors & Hilling, 1993; Foster & Thomas, 1990; Squires, Allison, Miller, & Gan, 1991).

In the pages to follow, information relevant to the psychosocial aspects of living with various cardiac and pulmonary illnesses will be freely integrated. Where appropriate, issues that are specific to a given medical population (e.g., asthmatics, COPD patients, those suffering from myocardial infarction, coronary heart disease, or coronary artery bypass graft surgery) will be noted. The term *cardiopulmonary* will be used with reference to information that is generally applicable to both heart and lung patients. As will be seen, most of the concepts in this book can be used to structure psychosocial interventions with patients suffering from any illness.

A logistical dilemma in writing this book was the treatment of more than 1,000 references, given that lengthy strings of references detract from a text's readability. Certainly, this text could have cited fewer reference works. However, because I want this book to provide not only a clinical guide, but also a comprehensive listing of outstanding or seminal research efforts relevant to psychosocial issues, I resolved the dilemma by limiting the number of citations in the text proper and by creating the two bibliographies that close this work. Text citations are restricted to the most noteworthy and recent publications. The References and General Bibliography provides an alphabetized listing of these text citations in addition to other useful background materials. The Indexed Bibliography groups still more sources of information, first by chapter and then under headings appropriate to specific topics covered in *Psychosocial Interventions for Cardiopulmonary Patients*. The serious researcher or clinician should review both the relevant text citations and the Indexed Bibliography for a comprehensive listing of publications that address a given issue.

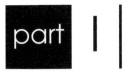

part I

INTRODUCTION

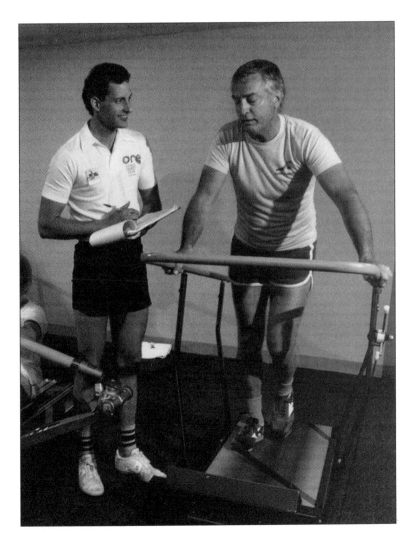

THE IMPORTANCE OF PSYCHOSOCIAL INTERVENTIONS IN THE TREATMENT OF CARDIOPULMONARY PATIENTS

Contemporary statistics regarding the prevalence and consequences of heart and lung illnesses are staggering:

- Each day in America, 4,000 people suffer a myocardial infarction (MI), and one of five Americans has an MI before age 60 (American Heart Association, 1989).

- Five million Americans have clinically apparent coronary heart disease (CHD) of some form, including myocardial ischemia, angina pectoris, unstable angina, and acute MI. Of these, approximately 400,000 suffer heart failure each year in the United States.

- More than 25,000 coronary artery bypass graft (CABG) surgeries and over 300,000 percutaneous transluminal coronary angioplasty (PTCA) or other transcatheter procedures for detecting heart disease are performed annually in the United States alone (American Heart Association, 1989).

- Although nearly 80% of patients with uncomplicated MI do return to work, nearly 2.5 million Americans have some degree of vocational disability or limitation caused by heart illness. In fact, in the United States, CHD is the leading problem for which patients receive premature disability benefits. In Canada, heart diseases constitute the second largest disability group, accounting for $3 billion in annual disability costs, excluding physician costs (Dafoe, Franklin, & Cupper, 1993).

- Over 14 million Americans currently suffer from chronic obstructive pulmonary disease (COPD) including emphysema and chronic bronchitis (American Lung Association, 1994). As of 1993, nearly 26 million Americans were living with COPD or some form of chronic lung disease, most of which are so slow in their progression that they create lifelong health problems and health care costs.

- In the United States alone, the number of COPD sufferers increased 41.5% from 1982 to 1993 (American Lung Association, 1994). In fact, COPD represents the most rapidly growing health problem in America (U.S. Government Task Force, 1979).

- Although the death rates from heart illness decreased nearly 30% between 1979 and 1989, deaths from COPD increased more than 60% (American Lung Association, 1994). Worldwide, death rates from COPD are increasing, especially in women in developed countries and in individuals age 65 or older (Neish & Hopp, 1988; S.J. Williams, 1989).

- COPD patients experience exceptionally high rates of hospitalization, and the lengths of stay for COPD patients are typically twice as long as those for patients with other respiratory diseases (Rabinowitz & Florian, 1992).

- Lung diseases also account for a significant percentage of the time and money spent on outpatient medical care. Data from the National Ambulatory Medical Care Survey (Higgins, 1989) indicated that COPD and allied conditions accounted for 16.4% of physician office visits for men and 12.5% for women in 1985. In Great Britain, chronic lung disease accounts for 25% of consultations with general practitioners (Holland, 1989).

- Lung disease is the leading cause of disability among the working population of the United States and ranks as a major medical problem worldwide. Symptoms of COPD are the most common reasons for absence from work in the United Kingdom, accounting for 10% of recorded working days lost due to sickness and 10% of hospital bed occupancy in Great Britain (Ries, 1990; S.J. Williams, 1989). Similar findings have been reported in studies from Israel (Rabinowitz & Florian, 1992).

- In the late 1970s, the economic costs of COPD were estimated to be as high as $15 billion per year for disability, health care cost, and time lost from work. This figure increased to an estimated $26 billion as of 1982 (Lenfant, 1982; U.S. Government Task Force, 1979).

Fortunately, the survival rates for both cardiac and pulmonary illnesses are quite high. Seventy percent of victims of an initial MI and 50% of individuals who suffer a recurrent MI survive, as do 80%-88% of MI patients who reach a well-equipped coronary care unit (CCU). A growing number of survivors of MI are younger than 65 (Gillum, 1989; Smith & Leon, 1992). Although the eventual consequences of COPD are devastating, the progression of impairment is typically very slow, spanning 20 to 40 years. Even though COPD is often not diagnosed until its advanced stages, the survival rate is over 50% at 5 years and 25% at 10 years (Ries, 1990).

WHAT IS BEING DONE TO HELP PATIENTS COPE?

Because the survival rates for cardiopulmonary illnesses are quite high, and the vast majority of people who suffer these illnesses live for a number of years after onset, the need to provide both immediate and rehabilitative services for this population is obvious. How can such patients be helped during medical crisis and throughout the rehabilitation period? Since the 1970s, the practice of medicine and the study of illness and health have been influenced by the biopsychosocial model originally proposed by George Engel (1977). This model serves as a cornerstone for the contemporary, comprehensive treatment of cardiopulmonary patients. Regarding heart and lung patients, the biopsychosocial model emphasizes research and intervention in a number of areas:

- Smoking cessation
- Reduction of blood cholesterol
- Obesity/weight reduction
- Behavioral control of hypertension
- Modification of Type A behavior pattern (TYABP) with emphasis on reducing hostility and managing stress
- Concerns regarding adherence to medication prescriptions and to risk-reduction behaviors
- Well-being (quality of life)
- Social support
- Stress management and psychophysiological research regarding stress
- Control of depression and anxiety
- Return to work
- Control of alcohol/substance abuse
- Marital and sexual aspects of rehabilitation

The advisability of bolstering the psychosocial aspect of cardiopulmonary care is being increasingly underscored in the professional literature. The American Thoracic Society (1981), the American Association of Cardiovascular and Pulmonary Rehabilitation (AACVPR), and the World Health Organization have all strongly recommended integrating psychosocial services into overall rehabilitation efforts (Connors & Hilling, 1993; Ries, 1990).

Contradictory information is available on whether or not the psychosocial needs of recovering cardiopulmonary patients are being met. On one hand, there is evidence that, worldwide, the psychosocial aspects of recovery are too often ignored or undertreated in both inpatient and outpatient settings. In the United States, Berra (1991) reported that only 4% of the 558 cardiac rehabilitation programs polled incorporated support groups or group counseling of patients. Another survey of 202 cardiac rehabilitation programs indicated that they rarely included extended psychosocial intervention (Southard & Broyden, 1990).

A glimpse at cardiac care in Europe suggests that such deficits in providing psychosocial intervention exist on a global level. Maes (1992) polled representatives of cardiac rehabilitation in 16 European countries and found that only 4 of them routinely offer psychosocial care. The range of delivery of psychosocial services noted in this survey was remarkable. Virtually all heart patients receive some form of psychosocial care in Italy and Finland, and in Switzerland and Austria, psychosocial services are provided to between 40% and 60% of recovering patients. On the other hand, the remaining countries polled provide psychosocial intervention to less than 20% of recovering heart patients.

Although more encouraging data emerge from an examination of inpatient settings, we have yet to approach our potential for integrating psychosocial interventions into ongoing rehabilitation efforts spanning both inpatient and outpatient medical and rehabilitation settings. A recent survey of 1628 coronary care units in U.S. hospitals (Sikes & Rodenhausen, 1987) found widespread availability of inpatient psychosocial services, mainly consisting of individual counseling. This survey found that family members of hospitalized heart patients were included in counseling sessions approximately half the time; however, only about half of the facilities routinely referred recovering MI patients for further psychosocial intervention after hospital discharge.

Even when psychosocial intervention is provided, it is most often offered without respect to the contexts within which the patient is living and recovering. Only recently have attempts been made to integrate what is known about the importance of social support, family systems, behavior modification, and psychological adjustment to illness into comprehensive clinical models for helping patients and their loved ones work cooperatively in coping with illness (e.g., Sotile, 1992).

IS PSYCHOSOCIAL INTERVENTION REALLY NECESSARY?

Early studies of the psychological effects of medical procedures called attention to the need for preoperative psychosocial intervention geared toward facilitating postsurgery coping (Kendall et al., 1979). Egbert, Battit, Welch, and Bartlett (1964) set the stage for the use of psychosocial interventions with nonpsychiatric patients in medical settings by demonstrating the effectiveness of providing anticipatory guidance to surgical patients. Compared to controls, patients who were given specific information about what to expect during the postoperative period and were coached in deep-breathing relaxation and movement control strategies for coping with postoperative pain and discomfort required less pain medication during their hospital stays and were discharged from the hospital 2 days earlier.

Mumford, Schlesinger, and Glass (1982) reviewed 34 studies of psychological intervention with surgery patients and found that patients provided with simple psychosocial interventions (e.g., information or emotional support to help them master the crisis of surgery) evidenced better physical and emotional adjustments postsurgery than did patients who received only ordinary care. A variety of researchers (e.g., Andrew, 1970; Kendall et al., 1979) have documented a wealth of postoperative benefits of preoperative psychosocial interventions, including: increased patient cooperation and satisfaction; fewer requests for pain medications; fewer reported and observed symptoms of anxiety; and more willingness to return to the hospital, if needed, but decreased medical need for rehospitalization.

Throughout the last two decades, several intervention strategies have been shown to be effective in promoting overall psychosocial adjustment in various populations treated in various medical settings (Smith & Leon, 1992). Many of these interventions have been quite simple; most have been brief. Although some critics (e.g., Anderson & Masur, 1983) argue that this literature is filled with relatively poorly controlled investigations, it has also been argued that research to date has, at minimum, demonstrated the efficacy of a number of clinical guidelines for structuring psychosocial interventions with medical patients and their families (e.g., Anderson & Masur, 1983; Kendall et al., 1979; Sotile, Sotile, Ewen, & Sotile, 1993; Sotile, Sotile, Sotile, & Ewen, 1993).

The recommendation that patients with little health knowledge should receive intensive in-hospital patient education and follow-up is seldom questioned (Havik & Maeland, 1990); however, debate does exist about whether or not psychosocial interventions should be incorporated into the routine delivery of medical care to cardiopulmonary patients. This controversy hinges on the fact that research has yet to determine how to identify cardiopulmonary patients who need psychosocial intervention to facilitate positive long-range adjustment. Research has clearly established that many cardiopulmonary patients cope quite well without receiving special psychosocial treatment. For example, Mayou (1990) pointed out that only 20%-30% of recovering heart patients evidence long-term symptoms of psychosocial struggle, and even the most vocal proponents of aggressive psychosocial services must acknowledge that no more than 50% of recovering heart patients become psychosocially symptomatic (e.g., Lloyd & Cawley, 1983).

On the other hand, a growing legion of researchers are calling for aggressive expansion of the psychosocial component of traditional medical care. For example, Lewin and colleagues recently demonstrated the cost-effectiveness of a simple home-based self-help program for enhancing post-MI adjustment (Lewin, Robertson, Cay, Irving, & Campbell, 1992). They pointed out that the cost and difficulty of screening patients to determine intervention needs should be weighed against two factors: (a) the relative cost-effectiveness of brief, simple psychosocial interventions; and (b) the notion that "to restrict help to those clearly having problems would be to ignore those who are coping but who could cope even better with a little additional help" (Lewin, Robertson, Cay, Irving, & Campbell, p. 1039).

In my opinion, to exclude psychosocial intervention because of statistics from traditional psychosocial research literature would be foolhardy and shortsighted. To do so would be to ignore three important perspectives on this issue.

THE MIND-BODY CONNECTION

Although the importance of controlling traditional risk factors to preserve health or promote rehabilitation is not questioned, in truth, the standard biological risk factors (i.e., smoking, serum cholesterol levels, and high blood pressure) do not identify the majority of new cases of CHD (Jenkins, 1983). This awareness has lead to both a refinement of traditional risk factors (e.g., the fractionization of cholesterol) and a closer examination of the importance of psychosocial variables that might affect health (Howell & Krantz, 1994). The emerging field of psychoneuroimmunology calls attention to the intimate interplay between mind and body, underscoring the importance of delivering medical care that is not constrained by the antiquated, Descartian notion that mind and body function independently of each other. This school of thought argues strongly for sensible incorporation of psychosocial interventions into traditional medical care.

A burgeoning literature is lending support to the tenets of psychoneuroimmunology. Creative researchers have documented the integral relationship between psychosocial adjustment and various important physical processes, including:

- the functioning of the immunological system (Kiecolt-Glaser & Glaser, 1988);
- cardiovascular reactivity (Lynch, 1977); and
- pulmonary functioning (Moran, 1991; S.J. Williams, 1989).

Psychosocial coping patterns have also been found to affect incidences of morbidity and mortality (Levy, Lee, Bagley, & Lippman, 1988; Pennebaker, Kiecolt-Glaser, & Glaser, 1988).

PRAGMATISM

The mainstream medical literature, too, offers empirical support for not only including but also expanding existing levels of psychosocial care for cardiopulmonary patients. Treatment programs that have reported regression in heart illness (Ornish et al., 1990) and metastatic breast cancer (Spiegel, Bloom, Kraemer, & Gottheil, 1989) have hinged on extensive psychosocial components. The massive literature summarized in this book—drawn from psychosomatic medicine, health psychology, medical psychology, behavioral medicine, and family systems medicine—argues strongly that psychosocial factors are crucial in determining outcomes such as decreased incidence of morbidity and mortality in the wake of illness and enhanced adherence to medical prescriptions.

Dangers of Ignoring Psychosocial Issues

The fact that many recovering cardiopulmonary patients and their loved ones do adapt in the long run should not obscure several universal facts. First, the very act of going to the hospital has been shown to be a significant stressor that fuels numerous physical and psychological changes, both for patients and for their loved ones. Between 50% and 60% of all cardiac patients who enter CCUs experience elevated levels of depression, anxiety, or fear, and similar statistics apply to family members (Kurosawa, Shimizu, Nishimatsu, Hiruse, & Takano, 1980). The majority of COPD patients experience pronounced periods of anxiety associated with episodes of dyspnea, and it is estimated that over 40% suffer from clinical depression (Gift & McCrone, 1993; Gift, Moore, & Soeken, 1992).

Recovering cardiopulmonary patients and their loved ones also struggle with changing their behavior after hospitalization. It has been estimated that between 30% and 50% of the general cardiac population experiences anxiety, depression, and/or impairments in marital, family, and vocational functioning for up to 3 years postevent (Rose & Robbins, 1993). It has also been reported that well over 50% of COPD patients have little faith in the efficacy of treatment—yet another contributor to depression levels (Borak, Silwinski, Piasecki, & Zielinski, 1991).

Furthermore, it appears that psychosocial factors sometimes predict recurrent episodes of CHD events, rehospitalization, and the continuation of anginal pain and the management of this syndrome (Havik & Maeland, 1990). Evidence that mental, emotional, and behavioral events can trigger MI and sudden cardiac death is also accumulating (Howell & Krantz, 1994).

For COPD patients, emotional factors (e.g., level of anxiety or depression) have been found to be even more crucial than physical factors (e.g., respiratory functions measured by spirometry testing) for determining response to treatment. Affected are such crucial areas as

- the patient's perception and tolerance of breathlessness (dyspnea);
- the number of pulmonary symptoms;
- the ability to perform activities of daily living;
- the numbers of outpatient health care consultations;
- exercise tolerance; and
- responses to rehabilitation (Dales, Spitzer, Schechter, & Suisa, 1989).

Positive Effects of Psychosocial Intervention

Pychosocial adjustment has also been shown to have a positive effect on morbidity for CHD and MI patients (Cooper, Faragher, Bray, & Ramsdale, 1985; Prince, Frasure-Smith, & Rolicz-Woloszyk, 1982), as well as for recovering CABG (Pimm & Feist, 1984) and COPD patients (S.J. Williams, 1989). Finally, the fact that various psychosocial factors may predict mortality from heart illness has been convincingly argued in a number of landmark epidemiological investigations (e.g., Case, Moss, Case, McDermott, & Eberly, 1992; Williams et al., 1992) and strongly suggested in a number of investigations employing COPD patients (e.g., Pattison, Rhodes, & Dudley, 1971).

An international literature has documented that simple, hospital-based psychosocial interventions such as relaxation training and brief counseling during acute stages of hospitalization can enhance patient adjustments both during and after hospitalization and for up to 5 years (e.g., Frasure-Smith, 1991). Attending to psychosocial factors during hospitalization has also been shown to improve crucial medical outcomes such as

- adherence to medical interventions (Oldridge & Pashkow, 1993);
- lengths of hospital stays (Schindler, Shook, & Schwartz, 1989); and
- long-term levels of mortality and morbidity for recovering cardiopulmonary patients (Blake et al., 1990; Frasure-Smith, 1991).

As has been noted, it also appears that many effective psychosocial interventions can be delivered by health care providers who are not trained mental health experts. For example, trained technicians have been found to be as competent as mental health professionals in identifying patients in need of treatment for depression after MI (Taylor, DeBusk, Davidson, Houston, & Burnett, 1981). In fact, relatively simple nursing interventions that involved screening, education, and home-based components have promoted positive psychosocial functioning, diminished episodes of rehospitalization, lessened morbidity, shortened hospital stays, and deterred visits to outpatient medical providers in both cardiac and pulmonary populations (Blake et al., 1990; Dracup, Moser, Marsden, Taylor, & Guzy, 1991; Frasure-Smith, 1991; Lewin et al., 1992; Rabinowitz & Florian, 1992).

Controlled investigations have also shown that as few as 4 to 12 sessions of outpatient cardiopulmonary rehabilitation incorporating exercise instructions and basic psychosocial counseling can significantly improve medical, psychological, and social recovery (e.g., Kallio, Hamalainen, Hakkila, & Laurila, 1979). Without question, attending to psychosocial factors in outpatient settings modifies cardiac risk factors and promotes physical, emotional, and family adjustments to CHD (Dracup et al., 1991). With COPD patients, such programs lead to a wealth of benefits:

- Improved exercise tolerance (Belman, 1986)
- Decreased anxiety and depression (Mall & Medeiros, 1988; Prigatano, Wright & Levin, 1984)

- Elevated patient self-esteem (Kersten, 1990a, 1990b)

- Improved functional ability (American Thoracic Society, 1987)

Perhaps most noteworthy, for both cardiac and pulmonary patients, such improvements have consistently been shown to persist for 6 to 12 months (Kersten 1990a, 1990b; Lovibond, Birrell, & Langeluddecke, 1985).

It seems clear that attending to psychosocial concerns is a crucial factor in providing comprehensive care across treatment venues.

A LARGE NUMBER OF PATIENTS COULD BE HELPED

The third—and perhaps most compelling—argument for incorporating a solid psychosocial component into cardiopulmonary treatment is the vast number of patients who would benefit from such a change. Only 30% of the people living with cardiopulmonary illness and struggling with psychosocial adjustment would translate into millions of patients in need of help. Few studies (i.e., Dracup, Guzy, Taylor, & Barry, 1986) have reported any harmful effects from psychosocial interventions. A marked need for psychosocial intervention has not been correlated with the effects of psychosocial intervention or nonintervention. This fact, coupled with the evidence of positive effects of psychosocial interventions with recovering cardiopulmonary patients, suggests that even those patients who are not identified as needing such intervention are not harmed by it. Even those interventions that lead to no apparent immediate outcome may ultimately nudge the patient along a continuum of making needed changes in health behaviors (Prochaska & DiClemente, 1992).

FURTHER CONSIDERATIONS

These diverse research findings, coupled with a wealth of clinical experiences and observations, lead to the firm conclusion that psychosocial intervention in treating recovering cardiopulmonary patients is well justified, safe, and wise. Health care providers should take advantage of the opportunities for psychosocial treatment that are created by the crises of illness or entry into rehabilitation.

Even if only minimal psychosocial intervention is actually provided, the importance of psychosocial factors in coping with cardiopulmonary illness should be recognized. Doing so paves the way for patients and their loved ones to develop a sensible, healing context within which they can view their psychosocial struggles and opens doors of communication between the patient and future health care providers that can enhance patient responses to treatment.

A FRIENDLY WARNING

In the emerging health care system, the importance of attending to psychosocial factors in treating cardiopulmonary patients goes beyond humanistic concern. Worldwide, health care providers and the facilities in which they work are being faced with increasing demands for accountability and with increasing competition in the marketplace. We have been warned that the hospitals, practitioners, and rehabilitation programs that are to remain in business are likely to be those that can document cost-effective, positive results from their treatment interventions (Hall, 1994a).

Because psychosocial adjustments by cardiopulmonary patients and their loved ones greatly affect medical outcomes, bolstering the psychosocial components of care is imperative. Psychosocial adjustment may function as the factor that differentiates patients who adhere to rehabilitation advice from those who do not and, among adherent patients, as the factor that differentiates those who thrive from those who merely survive. The economic implications of this possibility are enormous in the changing health care market. As will be discussed throughout this book, collaborative family health care that involves even brief psychosocial interventions coordinated by multidisciplinary teams of health care providers working closely with each other, with patients, and with the family members of patients can be remarkably cost-effective in the treatment of recovering cardiopulmonary patients. We can no longer afford *not* to attend to the psychosocial needs of this population.

SUMMARY

Cardiopulmonary illnesses pose significant threats to the well-being of millions of people worldwide. Effective psychosocial functioning is a crucial aspect of the promotion of recovery from these illnesses. Existent psychosocial services are sadly lacking, especially in outpatient settings. This is an unfortunate and unnecessary situation, given that research has shown that even brief psychosocial intervention delivered by caring health care providers who are not mental health specialists can significantly enhance overall psychosocial functioning of recovering cardiac and pulmonary patients and thereby positively affect both mortality and morbidity subsequent to these illnesses. In the newly developing health care system, we can no longer afford not to attend to the psychosocial aspects of cardiopulmonary care. Such attention starts with providing astute assessment of psychosocial issues, the topic of the following chapter.

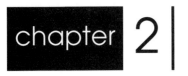

ASSESSMENT

Helping patients and their loved ones deal with the stresses and crises that face them starts with recognizing their strengths and their struggles. The specific skills and needs of each individual we serve will vary. The first step in leading a person into more adaptive coping is to assess these factors. The tools and strategies for psychosocial assessment can be helpful in this regard.

It is important to recognize that a patient's psychosocial status can be most accurately assessed by combining clinical interviewing with the use of objective psychometric assessment instruments. Such combinations provide infinitely richer and more accurate psychosocial diagnostic data than solo assessment techniques, which have actually been shown to be risky. For example, Rapp, Parisi, Walsh, and Wallace (1988) pointed out that using clinical interviewing alone for diagnosis of psychosocial concerns often results in failure to detect depression in many medical patients. On the other hand, in an excellent discussion of methods for assessing and treating depression in COPD patients, Gift and McCrone (1993) argued that psychometric tests used alone often result in misdiagnosis of conditions such as depression in aged and medically ill populations. This chapter will outline a number of practical, commonsense guidelines for conducting clinical interviews and will list a wealth of psychosocial test instruments currently available.

CONTEXTS TO CONSIDER DURING ASSESSMENT

Three frames of reference can be invaluable in understanding the psychosocial experiences of the people we treat:

- The family system of the patient
- The stress and crisis caused by illness and treatment
- The psychological reactions to the crises of illness and rehabilitation

These are the contexts that are created and affected when illness strikes. These are also the contexts into which our interventions are delivered: the cognitive, emotional, interpersonal, and behavioral fields that determine whether or not our interventions promote desired changes or fizzle into

13

ineffectiveness. Understanding patients and their loved ones from these perspectives sheds light on what needs to be matched in establishing and maintaining rapport.

SEEING FAMILIES AS TEAMS: IN SICKNESS AND IN HEALTH

Traditionally, psychological assessment and intervention in cardiopulmonary rehabilitation has focused on the examination and treatment of the individual patient; however, the burgeoning field of family systems medicine reminds us that, in reality, patients and their loved ones function as teams. Accordingly, health care providers should consider how the challenges of illness and rehabilitation impact the family and how family patterns affect the course of rehabilitation for a given patient. Extensive discussion of marital and family issues will be presented in chapter 8.

THE CRISES OF ILLNESS AND REHABILITATION

A second crucial frame of reference to consider during psychosocial assessment is that both acute medical treatment and outpatient rehabilitation confront the patient and his or her loved ones with stress and crisis. Stress occurs when perceived coping demands exceed perceived abilities to cope (Lazarus & Folkman, 1984). And what is crisis? Crisis occurs in response to any stressor that (a) overloads the individual's capacity to cope; (b) reactivates a previously unresolved conflict; (c) triggers previously learned maladaptive responses; and/or (d) is not soothed by use of one's most familiar coping strategies (Caplan, 1964; Pimm & Feist, 1984).

During such crisis, a range of stress responses, varying from transient episodes of anxiety or depression to psychotic reactions, can be expected in patients, even those with no known prior history of psychiatric disturbance (Soloff, 1977). Such symptoms should subside relatively quickly once the crisis is over. For example, according to crisis theory, cardiopulmonary patients should show a calming of this symptomatology during the first months after hospitalization or entry into rehabilitation (Havik & Maeland, 1990).

PSYCHOLOGICAL REACTIONS TO ILLNESS AND REHABILITATION: WHO ARE THE PEOPLE WE TREAT?

The crisis model argues that the patient and his or her family should be viewed as emotionally healthy individuals who are simply facing a frightening and unusual situation (Rose & Robbins, 1993). Although this is often the case, it is also true that many individuals struggle in their efforts to cope long before the shock of illness is added to their list of stressors (Pancheri et al., 1978; Rosen & Bibring, 1966).

Even a cursory glance at relevant research in this area illuminates the importance of being aware of this final context into which cardiopulmonary care is delivered—the psychological frame of reference of the individual patient and his or her loved ones. For example, both longitudinal and cross-sectional studies have found that depression often predates MI (e.g., Crisp, Desouza, & Queenan, 1981; Dreyfuss, Dasberg, & Cassaell, 1969). Retrospective studies of MI patients have also documented that as many as 50% of the patients show symptoms of pre-MI psychiatric illness (e.g., Lloyd & Cawley, 1983).

Preexisting psychological and psychosocial problems can seriously complicate the long-range course of rehabilitation. For example, Havik and Maeland (1990) prospectively studied 283 MI patients for 3-5 years and found that those who evidenced the most problematic adjustments during rehabilitation were characterized by high levels of pre-MI marital conflict, premorbid psychiatric treatment, emotional problems, and unemployed status. Similar studies with COPD patients have found that those who suffer the greatest levels of irritability, anxiety, helplessness, and alienation also show more morbidity (e.g., Traver, 1988).

Finally, it is important to remember that many factors can cause emotional reactions to wax and wane during the recovery process. Independent of preillness psychological status, stressors such as failure to return to work when work return is desired, medical complications, adjustment difficulties of loved ones, or the simple wear-and-tear effects of life's stresses can contribute to emotional problems (Havik & Maeland, 1990; Lloyd & Cawley, 1983). I propose that the question of whether an individual's modes of coping are normal or abnormal is of less clinical importance than the question of whether that individual's reactions are adaptive (i.e., promotive of positive coping outcomes) or maladaptive (i.e., promotive of negative coping outcomes).

In this chapter, ways to recognize and manage specific syndromes of maladjustment will be discussed. Included are discussions of postoperative delirium, organic mental disorders, alcoholism, psychosomatic invalidism, various depressive disorders, and various anxiety disorders. The first four conditions will be discussed relatively briefly, followed by a more detailed discussion of depressive and anxiety disorders. A list of assessment instruments and a summary of cogent assessment questions will close this discussion.

RECOGNIZING AND MANAGING SERIOUS MALADJUSTMENT PATTERNS

Any professional who works in a health care setting is sometimes confronted with unusual behavior exhibited by recovering patients. Four specific patterns of serious maladjustment that can occur in cardiopulmonary treatment settings are postoperative delirium, organic mental disorders, alcoholism, and psychosomatic invalidism.

POSTOPERATIVE DELIRIUM

Postoperative delirium, also referred to as ICU or CCU psychosis, mimics severe psychiatric disorders. Symptoms can vary from a slight clouding of consciousness to global cognitive impairment signaled by confusion, disorientation, and hallucinations or delusions (Inaba-Roland & Maricle, 1992). Because a delirious patient has difficulty maintaining attention to external stimuli, attempts at conversation are likely to be filled with perseveration, missed information, and non sequiturs. Impaired short- and long-term memory may be present, along with increased or decreased psychomotor activity and disturbed sleep-wake cycles that can lead to insomnia and/or daytime sleepiness (American Psychiatric Association [APA], DSMIII-R, 1987).

Delirium is often first noted when nursing staff or visiting relatives become aware of periods of confused thinking, suspiciousness, and irritability. Patients in the early stages of delirium are often misdiagnosed as simply being obnoxious or "difficult," as their slipping cognitive functions lead to poor impulse control, agitation, and emotional lability (Inaba-Roland & Maricle, 1992). The symptoms of delirium can fluctuate rapidly and often occur intermingled with periods of lucidity and normality. Symptoms may worsen at night, after a move to a new bed, or in the presence of novel stimuli, and may not begin until several days into hospitalization (Knapp & Blackwell, 1985).

A patient's premorbid personality tendencies may combine with certain elements of treatment to influence the nature of the delirium syndrome. For example, Mackenzie and Popkin (1980) presented the case study of a patient suffering from rheumatic heart disease who was hospitalized for mitral valve replacement. She was described as a typically private person who was cautious about relationships with others. Following surgery, she experienced delirium that was manifested by a combination of paranoid delusions, including accusing one of her physicians of raping her and the conviction that walrus tusks had been grown in her throat. Postdelirium discussions with the patient indicated that her rape delusion may have been derived from the fact that during her recovery period she had been catheterized and given a rectal examination. The walrus tusk delusion was thought to have been spurred by the physical discomfort associated with her respiratory and gastrointestinal care.

In the general hospital population, postoperative delirium is seen in approximately one out of every three patients. Even higher incidences have been reported for open heart surgery patients (22% to 57%) and for CABG patients (13% to 28%) (Volow, 1972). Postoperative delirium is especially prevalent in populations of patients exceeding 60 years of age, patients with severe chronic diseases, or patients with preoperative central nervous system problems such as dementia (Smith & Leon, 1992).

The exact etiology of postoperative delirium is unclear. Postsurgical metabolic imbalances, medication effects, cardiogenic hypoxia, impaired cerebral perfusion, brain or other neurologic lesions resulting from disease, trauma, or illness have all been implicated as significant etiological factors (Inaba-Roland & Maricle, 1992; Razin, 1982). Many researchers claim that the uniquely strange ICU environments promote delirium through a combination of both understimulation and overstimulation, a lack of familiar figures, minimized communication, and minimized environmental cues of diurnal sequence. Such confusing and disorienting conditions may result in the gross disruption in brain physiology that characterizes delirium (e.g., Kimball, 1978; Kornfeld, Zimberg, & Malm, 1965).

Clinical experience indicates that this syndrome often progresses in this way: symptoms of anxiety lead to agitation, which progresses to delirium. Early recognition and management of this process can prove crucial in preventing a full-blown bout of delirium. A number of treatment strategies can be used effectively to prevent or treat delirium.

Most important is to remember that delirium can be successfully disrupted using preventive measures. For example, research has documented that forewarning patients and their loved ones of the possibility of postsurgery delirium, reassuring them of the normal and transient nature of this condition, can effectively enhance both the patient's and the family's comfort and control when confronted with such experiences (Owens & Hutelmyer, 1982).

During presurgical counseling, warn patients and their loved ones of the possibility of postoperative delirium and reassure them that if delirium does occur, the symptoms will be brief and benign (Smith & Leon, 1992). Presurgical training in relaxation techniques can be a way of providing an adaptive coping tool to counter the progression of anxiety, agitation, and delirium.

In clinical practice, the most frequently used treatment for delirium—both prophylactically and secondarily—is psychotropic medications. These include antianxiety medications such as lorazepam, diazepam, or chlordiazepoxide and the major tranquilizers such as haloperidol or droperidol. Even mild doses of such medications tend to prove effective in lessening symptoms of delirium within 24 to 48 hr (Goldman & Kimball, 1985; Inaba-Roland & Maricle, 1992; Knapp & Blackwell, 1985).

Helping the patient remain oriented to time and place should be a routine aspect of delivering ICU and CCU care. This can be done in several ways: taking time to introduce yourself repeatedly; providing cues that are reality-orienting, such as familiar objects or pictures of loved ones; and coaching loved ones to help orient the patient to time and place. Showing patients videos of family, friends, and home environment can be especially effective in treating those who are enduring lengthy hospital stays.

When interacting with the delirious patient, communication should be concrete and brief. Use gentle touch to orient the patient's face to promote eye contact and face-to-face interaction. An amazingly effective method for soothing a delirious patient is to engage in deep abdominal breathing exercises along with the patient (Krupnik, 1993).

Perhaps most pragmatically, the patient's environment should be manipulated to promote soothing. Where possible, minimize irritating noise from air conditioning and oxygen administration. Take care to prevent startling noises and to use soothing conversational tones and comforting touch when interacting with the patient. As much as possible, fill the patient's environment with calming stimuli: soft illumination, quiet, the soothing presence of others, and so on. In addition, protect the patient from witnessing the suffering of other patients or traumatizing interventions with others.

Throughout the course of delirium, the patient should be reassured that his or her symptoms will pass and that self-control will soon be restored. This simple intervention is too often overlooked in administering typical clinical care to a delirious patient who seems to be out of touch with reality. It is important to remember that because delirium tends to be intermittent, most patients experience periods of vague awareness of their own behavior and react with feelings that this loss of self-control is unacceptable and worrisome. Offering reassurance during both lucid and delirious periods is tremendously important.

It is also wise to remember that delirium is traumatizing and patients need help in resolving this experience once the delirium has remitted. Mackenzie and Popkin (1980) offered the insight that people recovering from delirium are uniquely handicapped in their efforts to resolve the trauma of the experience because the cognitive impairment that characterized their condition prevents any accurate perception of the event once delirium passes. Patients retain fragmentary impressions and memories of what happened and how they behaved while delirious. These information fragments can be distressing, embarrassing, and inaccurate.

Fearing the meaning or the results of their behavior while delirious, many patients will only obliquely inquire as to what happened. It is a mistake to respond to such inquiries with scolding, humorous, sarcastic, evasive, or vague remarks. Doing so can reinforce the patient's suspicion, shame, or fear about what took place. On the other hand, it is not necessary to bombard the patient with embarrassing details of his or her bizarre behavior while delirious. Rather, give the patient the opportunity to discuss concerns privately. Describe specific events under question in a straightforward manner that assures the patient that delirium is a very common postsurgery occurrence and that its presence does not indicate any emotional illness.

Finally, patients who have been delirious should be forewarned that even though they will not recall all the details of their recent trauma, they might reexperience aspects of the trauma in flashbacks or dreams in the immediate future. In this sense, many postdelirium patients experience a variant of the posttraumatic stress disorder to be described later. This posttrauma syndrome can be especially bothersome because the patient may not be able to associate specific traumatizing stimuli with the overwhelming and intrusive negative affect that is experienced. Normalize that this syndrome might occur, and recommend that if these symptoms do not remit within

SUMMARY BOX

Treatments of Delirium

Preventive interventions
- Give presurgical counseling to patient and family
- Provide relaxation training

Secondary interventions
- Administer neuroleptic medications
- Help orient patient to reality cues
- Introduce yourself
- Repeat time and place
- Use visual cues, such as wall calendars
- Have family bring in familiar objects, home movies, or photographs of loved ones
- Employ simple, concrete, face-to-face communication
- Deep breathe with the patient
- Promote a soothing environment
- Reassure
- Protect patient

Postdelirium interventions
- Be sensitive to inquiries by patient regarding what happened
- Give specific information in a straightforward manner
- Avoid vague descriptions of the patient's behavior

4-6 weeks, further psychotherapeutic or psychiatric intervention should be sought. Advise the patient that supportive counseling during the immediate postdelirium period can be helpful, and offer to facilitate referral for such (Mackenzie & Popkin, 1980).

ORGANIC MENTAL DISORDERS

Survivors of cardiac arrest and COPD may be left with anoxic brain injury that manifests in disturbances of personality, judgment, and behavior. In fact, it has been purported that the vast majority of individuals who experience out-of-hospital cardiac arrest suffer serious neurological impairment (Earnest, Yarnell, Merrill, & Knapp, 1980; Reich, Regestein, Murawski, DeSilva, & Lown, 1983).

In clinical practice, the signs and symptoms of cerebral impairment in recovering cardiopulmonary patients are most often initially attributed to depression. However, Reich et al. (1983) presented six case studies demonstrating that cerebral dysfunction should be strongly suspected if the patient's clinical picture includes manifestations such as distractibility, excessive fatigue, diminished drive and mental acuity, diminishing self-confidence, emotional lability, passivity, poor judgment, and atypically inappropriate behaviors. Other patients may present with symptoms such as aphasia, rage attacks, or flat, humorless, or despairing affect.

As further pointed out by Reich and colleagues, a hallmark characteristic of cerebral dysfunction is its relentlessness: the syndrome is unresponsive to treatment or to interpersonal efforts to soothe and continues independent of the patient's cardiopulmonary status. Reactive depression associated with illness, on the other hand, tends to be episodic and lifts as the patient's physical status improves and is soothed by interpersonal comforting. These authors also caution that both depression and the effects of some anti-arrhythmic medications can cause organic dysfunction.

Treating such patients with a trial of antidepressants or psychotherapy may help clarify the extent to which depression is contributing to the overall syndrome. A full discussion of the signs and treatments of clinical depression will be presented later. More than anything, accurate diagnosis may require observing the patient over time. For example, the symptoms of cognitive impairment are likely to become magnified as the patient attempts to reenter the work environment or assume his or her typical family roles. Careful inquiry of the patient's family, formal neuropsychological testing, and neuroradiological assessment are recommended if such symptoms persist.

ALCOHOLISM AND SUBSTANCE ABUSE

Concerns about recognition and modification of alcohol and substance abuse in cardiopulmonary patient populations are based upon several facts: heavy alcohol use has adverse cardiovascular, pulmonary, and behavioral effects; the potential of sudden death is heightened by the use of drugs such as cocaine; and, in their efforts to soothe feelings of depression and anxiety, COPD patients often resort to use of alcohol and sedating drugs (Miller et al., 1990; Yellowlees, Alpers, Bowden, Bryant, & Ruffin, 1987).

Epidemiological data on this issue suggest that any health care provider will regularly come into contact with patients whose functioning is impaired by substance abuse, especially alcoholism. Thirteen percent of all adults and 21% of all males in the United States drink more than 60 alcoholic drinks per month (Kamerow, Pincus, & MacDonald, 1986). Fully 25% of hospitalized medical patients and 20% of patients seen in outpatient medical settings are alcohol dependent (Allen, Eckardt, & Wallen, 1988; Cleary et al., 1988).

Unfortunately, the vast majority of substance-abusing medical patients go undetected in the delivery of routine medical care (Rydon, Redman, Sanson-Fisher, & Reid, 1992). Matano and Bronstone (1994) offered useful clinical advice for assessing and intervening in this area.

Part and parcel of the substance abuse syndrome is a powerful ability to psychologically distort the truth about substance use or its effects in one's life. Thus, Matano and Bronstone recommend the routine use of brief, standardized questionnaires designed to assess substance dependence. Of the various instruments listed at the end of this chapter, special consideration should be given to use of the CAGE, which consists of only four items:

1. Cut down: Have you ever felt the need to cut down on your drinking?
2. Annoyed: Have you ever felt annoyed by someone criticizing your drinking?
3. Guilty: Have you ever felt bad or guilty about your drinking?
4. Eye-opener: Have you ever had a drink first thing in the morning to steady your nerves or get rid of a hangover?

Research has indicated that two or more affirmative responses on the CAGE indicates alcohol abuse or dependence with 85%-95% accuracy.

These questions can be worked into routine medical or psychosocial assessments. Here, as in many areas of assessment, it is best to broach the topic with broad statements that convey concern, not blame or shame, about the issue, followed by specific questioning. Care should be taken not to insult the patient's sensibilities by trying to trick him or her into discussing this topic. Examples of nonthreatening but direct ways to frame questioning regarding substance use are presented below:

"Mrs. Horwitz, I'm concerned about how stressful and depressing all of this has been for you. Many people in your situation simply don't know what to do to calm down, and they find themselves turning to alcohol to get relief from their troubles. Have you noticed yourself doing this? Has your drinking ever bothered you to the point that you felt the need to cut down? How has your family (or spouse, or friends) reacted? Have you ever felt annoyed by someone criticizing your drinking?"

"I can appreciate how complicated this gets. You do the best you can to cope, but then it sometimes backfires on you. Many people in your situation turn to alcohol to help calm themselves. Have you ever felt bad or guilty about your drinking?"

"It's hard to cope with feeling badly. Sometimes you just want to block out the pain. You mentioned that mornings are especially difficult times for you. Have you ever had a drink first thing in the morning to steady your nerves or to help you cope?"

If substance abuse is suspected, intervention that involves medical input from concerned health care providers is recommended. Matano and Bronstone recommend that such confrontation should include several elements: documentation of alcohol-related medical problems; notation of medical indicators of changes in tolerance or withdrawal symptoms; and reiteration of indicators of legal, occupational, familial, or social consequences of substance abuse. In addition, the patient's family should be coached and supported in their efforts to confront the patient about specific consequences of drinking, while conveying a spirit of care and support. The entire confrontation of the patient should be framed with compassion for the complexity of substance abuse and reassurance that help is available, but it should be made clear that you will not participate in denial of the truth that the patient has a substance abuse problem.

In this later regard, it is often helpful to emphasize to substance-abusing patients that successfully recovered addicts often admit that either by choice, due to naiveté, or through omission of caring confrontation of the issue, health care providers tend to inadvertently serve as enablers of their patients' ongoing substance abuse. Use of variations of the following case vignette from my own clinical experience can be helpful here.

In the midst of a busy day of office appointments, I walked past my waiting room and noticed a middle-aged man who looked vaguely familiar. When I returned to greet my next scheduled appointment, the man politely asked, "Excuse me, Dr. Sotile, may I have just a minute of your time? I know that you have an appointment, but this will only take a second."

We entered my office's coffee-break room, and the mystery became clear. "I know you probably don't recognize me. I put more miles on my face than anywhere else on my body in these past 10 years. But I'm James Breaux. I was in your stress management treatment program about 8 years ago. My family doctor, Dr. Smith, referred me to you because I was having stomach problems that nobody could figure out, and I got depressed over how bad my health was. You also counseled me and my wife for a while following that.

"Well, the reason I stopped by is this. Two years ago I bottomed out and faced the truth: I've been an alcoholic since I was 17 years old. I am seriously trying to put my life back together now, and as part of my AA program I'm trying to make amends with people and tell myself and them the truth. I came by to apologize to you: I didn't tell you the truth about what was happening with me back then. I even came to some of our sessions half lit up with vodka. I remember missing some of our appointments because I was hung over or drinking, and lying about that, telling you I was having another bout of stomach trouble. I'm sorry. I hope that you will forgive me for that.

"But I'd also like to tell you that, in all honesty, you and Dr. Smith were among my strongest enablers when I was drinking. You cooperated with me in calling my problems everything but what they really were: stress, depression, aggravation over my stomach problems, frustration with my wife, a midlife crisis, whatever.

"I know that I was responsible for my drinking and lying, not you. But I just wanted to tell the truth, for my sake and in hopes that you might be able to help other patients like me to get more ready to help themselves."

Presenting a variation of this vignette along with a compassionate statement of your intention to be helpful—not hurtful—to the patient and family can provide a very powerful intervention. Such confrontation should also include the offer to facilitate referral for specialized help. Here it is important to have readily available the names and phone numbers of inpatient substance abuse treatment programs, Alcoholics Anonymous or other self-help support programs, and specialists in substance abuse counseling.

PSYCHOSOMATIC INVALIDISM

The terms *psychosomatic, somatizing, cardiac neurosis,* and *cardiac invalidism* are sometimes used interchangeably to refer to patients who are unduly beset with symptoms of anxiety, somatization, dysphoria, and functional impairment that seem out of proportion to their actual cardiac condition. Some such patients show full-blown syndromes of hypochondriasis or panic disorder. A related condition is pseudoangina ("angina innocents"), which may or may not be accompanied by hyperventilation and/or documented CHD. Basically, these patients are overly sensitive to normal somatic symptoms; they overinterpret normal bodily sensations, often misattributing the physiological changes accompanying severe anxiety to a possible cardiac disorder (Bass & Wade, 1984; Costa, Fleg, McCrae, & Lakatta, 1982).

The causes of psychosomatic invalidism are difficult to pinpoint. In one form or another, at least partial invalidism is a common condition in recovering cardiopulmonary patients, and no universally occurring etiological factors are clearly implicated by the presence of this syndrome. However, higher rates of psychosomatic disorders are found in certain types of families. Specifically, patients who evidence this syndrome often come from "enmeshed" family systems. Enmeshment is signaled by emotionally close but constraining relationships that do not allow for individuality of reactions or open dealing with conflict (Meissner, 1973; Minuchin et al., 1979).

Waring (1983) proposed that psychosomatic patients tend to have marital relationships that can be characterized in eight specific ways:

1. Sparsity of verbally expressed affection

2. Low levels of expressed commitment to the marriage, a factor referred to as cohesion

3. Little overtly expressed conflict, argument, or criticism, resulting in a dearth of sharing of private thoughts, beliefs, and perspectives

4. Poor conflict resolution through open expression of thoughts, feelings, opinions, and so on

5. Limited sexual activity (a condition that is often acceptable to one or both spouses)

6. A collective tendency to normalize these patterns (i.e., the couple views themselves as no better or worse than other couples)

7. Isolation from friends and extended family

8. Interestingly, the couple's similarity and compatibility in background, values, and interests

Research has not yet clarified whether a cause-and-effect relationship exists between psychosomatic syndromes and such family dynamics or whether the relationship is purely correlational.

The literature regarding treatment of psychosomatic invalidism is rather sparse, is of generally poor quality, and focuses on prevention, not remelioration (Razin, 1982). Uncontrolled studies have reported success with treatment strategies such as systematic desensitization of anxiety, behavior therapy, biofeedback, and supportive psychotherapy and coaching regarding hyperventilation control. The importance of family interventions has also been emphasized in clinical case studies.

In my experience, patients suffering from psychosomatic invalidism are among the most difficult to treat in any brief therapy framework. The chronicity of their syndrome simply does not lend itself to quick cures. However, medical providers can help lessen their own and their patient's frustrations in several ways. First, focus on providing compassionate care for the patient and family, not on curing the invalidism. Avoid locking into the stated or unstated promise that you will be able to eliminate their distress. Instead, you should openly state your concern for the patient and his or her loved ones, and frame your role as providing consultation to them regarding ways they might better manage the process of living with their ailments. Teaching the patient fundamental coping skills such as relaxation techniques can provide at least moments of positive coping. However, the complex family patterns in which the patient's syndrome is embedded make it unlikely that simple interventions are going to provide lasting or dramatic change. Coaching the family to positively reinforce adaptive coping behaviors shown by the patient can be underscored with the simple advice to avoid allowing the patient to drift into a spectator's role within the family system (Sotile, 1992). In general, it is helpful to remember that treating patients suffering from psychosomatic invalidism requires patience and the ability to avoid becoming defensive in reacting to complaints from the patient or family. Go for small steps of relief, not for marked signs of progressive change.

DEPRESSION AND ANXIETY DISORDERS

Cardiopulmonary patients almost universally experience periods of anxiety and depression at some point during rehabilitation. Even in the absence of premorbid struggles with affective distress, the likelihood is that anxiety or depression will develop during hospitalization and rehabilitation.

THE SCOPE OF THE PROBLEM

Studies have reported that between 18% and 27% of hospitalized CHD patients suffer from major depressive disorders. In the months immediately following hospitalization, between 30% and 50% of recovering cardiopulmonary patients suffer clinically significant levels of anxiety or depression (Nickel, Brown, & Smith, 1990). Fortunately, these symptoms lift spontaneously within 6 to 9 months in most patients. However, between 5% and 15% of patients continue to show moderate to severe depression and anxiety symptoms. By some estimates, 70%-88% of discharged MI patients continue to feel either anxious or depressed for up to 3 years postevent (Stern, Pascale, & Ackerman, 1977). Growing attention is also being paid to the presence of anxiety disorders in patients with CHD (Taylor & Arnow, 1985).

Emotional struggle of some sort seems especially to be par for the course of living with COPD. The prevalence of high levels of anxiety in COPD patients has been unquestionably documented. This is quite understandable, given that "breathlessness itself is an anxiety provoking situation" (Rabinowitz & Florian, 1992, p. 73). According to some reports, COPD patients are not only anxious about their pulmonary functions; they seem to suffer a higher than average incidence of full-blown anxiety disorders and panic disorders when compared to the general population. In this later regard, definitive data are not available, but rough estimates suggest that as many as 34% of COPD patients suffer from anxiety disorders and that 24% suffer from the more severe form of anxiety, panic disorder, many with full-blown agoraphobic symptomatology (Yellowlees, 1987). The lifetime prevalence rate for panic disorder in COPD has been estimated to be as much as 5.3 times greater than in the general population (Karajgee, Rifkin, Doddi, & Kolli, 1990).

Other researchers have reported that the incidence of depression (but not anxiety) is significantly higher in COPD than in normal subjects of similar age. By some estimates, between 50% and 75% of patients with moderate or severe COPD are depressed (e.g., Emery, 1993). Yet it has also been estimated that only 16% of COPD patients suffer from full-blown clinical depression (Yellowlees, 1987).

THE CONSEQUENCES OF DEPRESSION AND ANXIETY

The physiological and behavioral consequences of unchecked anxiety or depression lend an even more pragmatic validity to focusing on the treatment of these conditions in caring for cardiopulmonary patients. In simple terms, highly anxious or depressed patients do not rehabilitate as well as non-distressed patients. For patients who have a chronic medical illness, depression and anxiety tend to compromise overall physical hardiness and to amplify the tendency to focus upon physical symptoms and decrease motivation for self-care. Cardiac patients with major depressive disorder are at greater risk of experiencing another major cardiac event than nondepressed, matched CHD patients. Both depression and anxiety have been shown to have a deleterious effect on the cardiovascular system and to decrease the likelihood of survival following MI (Dalack & Roose, 1990; Lowery, 1991). For these reasons, some researchers recommend that if a cardiac patient is found to be suffering from a major affective disorder, particularly major depression, entry into formal rehabilitation should be delayed until treatment for the affective problem is under reasonable control (e.g., Swenson & Abbey, 1993; Indexed Bibliography).

For COPD patients, too, the consequences of unchecked anxiety or depression can be formidable, if not lethal. Post and Collins (1981) proposed that anxiety is probably the single strongest predictor of not only psychological but also physical stress levels in COPD patients. With this population, self-ratings of depression have been correlated with self-ratings of breathlessness (Kellner, Samet, & Pathak, 1992). In fact, COPD patients with high depression scores on standardized testing tend to have a lower P_aCO_2 when the severity of airways obstruction is taken into consideration (Gordon, Michiels, Mahutte, & Light, 1985).

Despite these alarming data regarding the prevalence and consequences of affective distress in cardiopulmonary patients, estimates are that fewer than 10% of patients diagnosed with a major affective disturbance after MI receive psychiatric treatment (Schleifer et al., 1989). Swenson and Abbey (1993) reminded us that, although most recovering cardiopulmonary patients resist referral for psychiatric care, most will accept discussion and input regarding psychological issues delivered as part of their overall rehabilitation. This fact underscores the need for the general health care provider or rehabilitation specialist to develop at least a reasonable level of comfort in recognizing and responding to signs that a patient may be suffering affective distress.

WHAT CAUSES ANXIETY AND DEPRESSION IN RECOVERING CARDIOPULMONARY PATIENTS?

For the recovering cardiopulmonary patient, both depression and anxiety can occur secondary to psychosocial stresses, physical correlates of illness, or as by-products of treatment. Psychosocial stressors that can stir anxiety and depressive reactions for recovering patients include injury to self-esteem; feelings of powerlessness and vulnerability; helplessness in facing the unique adaptive challenges that come with illness; anticipated or actual losses of independence, financial security, or social networks; family discord; or concerns about loved ones (Clark, 1990; Sotile, Sotile, Sotile, & Ewen, 1993).

Depression and anxiety can also occur secondary to organic aspects of both cardiac and pulmonary illnesses. Depressionlike symptoms can come from physiologic factors such as electrolyte imbalances or hypoxia and from the physical effects of syndromes such as the weakness and fatigue caused by low cardiac output, anemia, or postviral syndrome (Clark, 1990; Malan, 1992; Silverstein, 1987; Smith & Leon, 1992).

As pointed out by Rabinowitz and Florian (1992), the cloudy picture of the prevalence of affective distress with COPD patients may be due to the difficulty in differentiating symptoms of affective syndromes such as depression from symptoms manifested by the illness itself. "These patients are often thin, have sleeping problems because of breathing difficulties, and are therefore often tired as a result of their illness. This compounding effect may lead to difficult diagnostic procedures" (Rabinowitz & Florian, 1992, p. 75).

Diagnosis of clinical depression in a COPD patient may also be complicated by the cognitive changes that occur with aging and that are often complicated by COPD and its sequelae. For example, blood gas changes that accompany COPD, such as hypoxia and hypercapnia, result in cognitive alterations and changes in neurophysiologic functioning associated with depression (Gift & McCrone, 1993). It is also possible that depression may be related to dyspnea level as well as to the actual level of oxygenation.

Such an intricate, circular relationship exists between the physiological consequences of chronically obstructed pulmonary functions and the physical and emotional correlates of anxiety that the diagnosis of anxiety disorders in COPD populations may also be complicated. These factors interplay to create the self-perpetuating nature of anxiety symptoms in COPD patients. It has been proposed that the feelings raised by dyspnea may trigger further attacks of dyspnea and thereby lead to a cyclic effect (Rabinowitz & Florian, 1992; Sandhu, 1986). Because COPD patients often come to perceive the locus of control for their breathing as being external to themselves, their feeling of lack of control may contribute to further episodes of dyspnea and result in further anxiety (Post & Collins, 1981; Rabinowitz & Florian, 1992).

Medications such as antihypertensives, sedatives, tranquilizers, corticosteroids, and some antiarrhythmics may have depressing side effects (Gift, Palut, & Jacox, 1986; Malan, 1992), whereas medicines such as theophylline and epinephrine can cause anxiety. Table 2.1, borrowed from Clark (1990), lists a number of commonly used medications that can cause depressive symptoms.

As shown in this table, the known depression-generating medications include a number of agents that are routinely given to cardiopulmonary patients. In fact, it is improbable that a recovering cardiopulmonary patient will get through hospitalization(s) and rehabilitation without being prescribed at least one medication that is known to cause depression.

Table 2.1   Medications That Can Cause Depressive Symptoms

Morphine	Propranolol	Methyldopa
Digoxin	Timolol	Nadolol
Guanethidine	Sedatives	Procainamide
Lidocaine	Clonidine	Reserpine
Nifedipine	Disopyramide	Thiazide diuretics
Prazosin	Hydralazine	Steroids

Note. From "Nursing Interventions for the Depressed Cardiovascular Patient," by S. Clark, 1990, *Journal of Cardiovascular Nursing, 5*(1), p. 57. Copyright 1990 by Aspen Publishers, Inc. Adapted with permission.

Depression that is contributed to by a patient's medical illness or treatment is often referred to as an organic mood syndrome (APA, 1987). Treatment of the underlying illness or changes in the medications causing depression as a side effect often lead to diminishment of depressive symptoms. However, it is important to note that such depressive disorders tend to be less responsive to typical antidepressant treatments (Popkin, Callies, & Mackenzie, 1985; Swenson & Abbey, 1993).

GUIDELINES FOR ASSESSING AFFECTIVE DISTRESS SYNDROMES

Given that the bulk of recovering cardiopulmonary patients experience at least transient periods of anxiety and depression, it is often difficult to discern who needs specialized psychosocial intervention. Several factors should be kept in mind in exploring this issue.

Keep Psychological Test Results in Perspective

It is prudent to exercise caution in interpreting results from the many simple interview strategies or self-report inventories typically used to assess affective distress in clinical and research settings. Cavenaugh, Clark, and Gibbons (1984) evaluated methods for assessing depression in patients with medical illness and postulated that cognitive and affective symptoms are more valid indicators of clinical depression in this population than the somatic or vegetative symptoms that are frequently charted in psychometric test instruments and clinical interviews designed to assess depression. For example, independent of physical symptoms (which may be rooted in the patient's medical condition), patients were more likely to have severe depression if they expressed that they had lost interest in people, felt like a failure, felt punished, or had suicidal thoughts.

In a similar vein, Gift and McCrone (1993) posed that depression inventories specifically designed for use with the elderly might be most appropriate for the COPD population. In this regard, the Geriatric Depression Scale (GDS) (Yesavage & Brink, 1983) holds particular promise. Developed specifically for use with healthy and medically ill older adults, the GDS contains no somatic items (such as decreased libido and early morning awakening) that may be indicators of both depression and the physical changes that are concomitant with aging or COPD.

Avoid False Positives: Don't Overreact

Both psychometric and clinical assessment strategies also fail to differentiate true affective disorder from other forms of emotional distress such as the normal grieving process that often accompanies illness (Knapp & Blackwell, 1985). In my experience, health care professionals not trained in mental health are often needlessly frightened by patient displays of strong emotions. They then either resort to erroneously diagnosing the patient or to referring for specialty care too soon, rather than offering simple and effective support and education regarding what the patient is experiencing. Labeling such patients as clinically depressed or as suffering from an anxiety disorder and therefore in need of specialized care is often premature, a fact supported by the frequently seen progression of psychologic response of the patient who participates in outpatient rehabilitation. Many patients enter outpatient rehabilitation evidencing symptoms of anxiety and/or depression; however, the increased sense of accomplishment, enhanced psychosocial support, and reassuring guidance that come with formal rehabilitation alleviate such symptoms for most patients within the first 3 months of entry.

Health care providers also may overreact to emotional displays by patients with excessive treatment. Evaluations of the medical treatment patterns delivered to asthma patients have found that independent of objectively determined measures of physical status, patients who evidence "panic-fear symptomatology" are typically kept longer in the hospital and sent home on higher dosages of medication, and that the prescribing of extra medications is not explainable by the patients' objectively determined physical status (Dahlem, Kinsman, & Fukuhara, 1982; Jones, Kinsman, Dirks, & Dahlem, 1979).

For both inpatients and outpatients, simply offering support or guidance regarding the normalcy of grieving or of depressive symptoms accompanying certain medications or physical conditions (e.g., low blood pressure, impaired oxygenation, or cardiac irregularity) can at once comfort the patient and serve as a diagnostic experience: if the patient does not improve with such intervention, then the need for a consultation from a mental health specialist is clearly indicated.

Learn to Differentiate Grief From Depression

Acute illness often stirs a relatively brief grief reaction. Living with a chronic illness almost always stirs episodic periods of grieving.

Kersten (1990a, 1990b) offered an insightful discussion of the damage to self-esteem that occurs for many COPD patients in reaction to the losses that come with their illness. These losses can include: loss of breath, loss of physical ability or appearance, loss of job, loss of a spouse, and loss of mobility and freedom—all of which can crumble the patient's former self-image. Until an equally valued new self-image is formulated, the patient will predictably mourn what has been lost. Now, beset with both grief and a floundering self-image, the patient is at significant risk of developing a depression-generating style of living. Reinforcing activities are restricted. Social isolation may become the norm. Discrediting definitions of oneself become cognitive habits. Selective perceptions of discounting or uncomfortable reactions from others fill one's frame of reference. Disappointments in the ways others respond to this illness and its sequelae may increase the burden placed on loved ones. As dependency and immobilization mount, so do the patient's intrapsychic and interpersonal tensions.

Although this scenario certainly underscores the need to include attending to personality and cognitive factors in designing psychosocial interventions (see the discussion of the Effective Emotional Management model in Part 2), it particularly highlights the importance of recognizing and comforting patients who are grieving.

For both cardiac and pulmonary patients who show affective distress, the importance of differentiating whether the patient is mourning losses associated with the illness or is suffering from clinical depression has been underscored (Clark, 1990; Sotile, 1992). As shown in Table 2.2, the symptoms of grief and clinical depression overlap in many ways.

One factor listed in Table 2.2 is especially crucial in differentiating grief from depression: Grief is time-limited; depression, for all practical purposes,

Table 2.2 Symptoms of Grief and Depression

Grief	Depression
Denial	Poor concentration
Shock	Loss of energy
Despair	Anhedonia
Confusion	Vegetative symptoms
Bargaining	Thoughts of death
Anger	Agitation/retardation
Acceptance	Preoccupation
Negative affects lift	Feelings of worthlessness
	Negative affects persist

is not. The emotional distress of grieving is at least momentarily relieved by supportive interaction with others. Clinical depression, on the other hand, is not alleviated by support or by the passage of time (Sotile, 1992). In addition, the despair that comes with clinical depression is often associated with feelings of worthlessness and suicidal thoughts, neither of which are common occurrences during normal grieving.

A final word about grief is in order. As mentioned above, if the patient's grief is being triggered solely by his or her illness and its accompanying losses, improvement should be forthcoming within several months. However, it is wise to remember that we often encounter patients who are at once facing their own illness and are mourning the death of a loved one. Clinical experience strongly suggests that few people are prepared for the fact that adjusting to the death of a loved one typically takes at least several years. The notion popularized by the work of Elizabeth Kubler-Ross (1969) that mourning occurs over a 6- to 12-month period actually promotes unrealistic expectations that simply serve to shame the aggrieved, in my opinion. More realistic—and infinitely more helpful—is the scheme depicted in Figure 2.1.

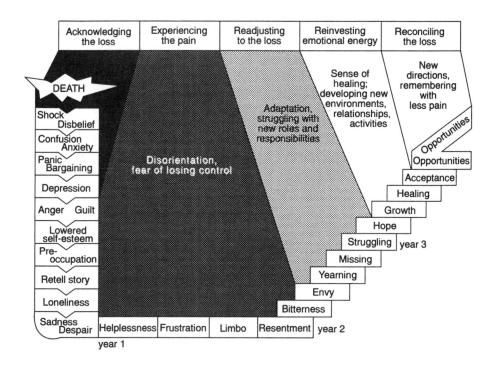

Figure 2.1   The stages of grief.
Jack LoCicero, "Stages of Grief" slide, Grief-Net Systems, Inc., P.O. Box 15723, Winston-Salem, NC 27113.

Developed by hospice grief counselor Jack LoCicero, of Winston-Salem, North Carolina, Figure 2.1 illustrates the fact that the stages of mourning unfold over several years, with each major section of the table representing roughly 1 year of the grieving experience. Elizabeth Kubler-Ross's stages of grief do, indeed, seem to occur during the initial months of mourning (the steps outlined in the left-hand margin of Figure 2.1). During this period and throughout approximately the next 6 months, the aggrieved person experiences a "year of firsts": anniversary reactions that are fraught with acute periods of grief, longing, and heartache. The second year of grief continues to be quite painful but not quite as reflexively emotional. Anniversary experiences are often accompanied by a combination of tearful and affectionate remembrances of the dead loved one. Clinical experience suggests that, for many, the frequency of acute periods of grief does not diminish significantly until the third or fourth year of mourning. By then, the survivor has created a new normal that incorporates loving memories of the lost loved one with resignation that, indeed, life does go on.

By recognizing the symptoms of ongoing grieving, a health care provider can compassionately normalize the patient's experience and offer needed support and education that might prevent misattributions that could otherwise cloud rehabilitation progress. The following case example demonstrates this point.

During a recent presentation to a community of recovering cardiac patients and their loved ones regarding psychosocial aspects of cardiopulmonary illness, I noticed an elderly man seated alone at the rear of the room. He seemed to be particularly interested in my comments regarding depression and to be bothered by comments about family relationships. The sources of both his interest and distress soon became obvious. During the question-and-answer period of the program, he spoke up:

"I have a question. I had bypass surgery 8 months ago, and I still am having trouble concentrating and getting on with my life. I can't remember things; my mind just drifts off. I don't feel much like doing things, either. Can bypass cause this? Also, I take medicine for high blood pressure. Does this medicine affect your mind? I think my doctors just messed me up. I'm seriously thinking about throwing that medicine away. I have to do something."

During further discussion of the possibility that stress or depression might interfere with cognitive functions and deplete energy levels, the patient offhandedly commented: "Well, I was stressed for a while—my wife died 19 months ago. But I should be over that by now. [trembly voice; with regained composure] It just feels like my surgery or this medicine has messed up my brain in some way or another."

Simply reassuring and educating this grieving gentleman seemed to provide him with immediate relief of at least one of his concerns: that his difficulties with concentration and memory did not necessarily signal any major problematic reactions to his medications or surgery. Perhaps even more important, compassionate conversation about the normalcy of his grief taking years to resolve and about the fact that—despite regular periods of despair—the second year of his grief was progressing with somewhat less emotional pain, proved to be helpful.

Use Unstructured Interviews for Diagnosis

The unstructured interview is currently the most frequently-used method of assessing affective disorder in cardiopulmonary patients (Kersten, 1990b). These interviews should target certain circumstances and syndromes that signal the need for further help in coping with anxiety or depression. For example, although experiencing moderately high levels of anxiety is certainly the norm during the initial phases of rehabilitation, extremely high levels of anxiety on the night before intervention have been found to predict more mood disturbance in CABG patients 6 months later (Shaw et al., 1986). This finding suggests that, at minimum, highly anxious patients should be given extra attention and follow-up to ensure that they have a realistic appraisal of their medical condition and of their capabilities.

Furthermore, Swenson and Abbey (1993) recommended that special attention be paid to any patient who:

- has a history of anxiety or depressive disorders;
- reports having thoughts about wanting to die, or has had past suicidal thoughts or has actually attempted suicide;
- has a history of unstable interpersonal relationships or social isolation;
- has sustained repeated major losses in recent years;
- has a pattern of alcohol use or abuse; and/or
- has either an individual or family history of psychiatric illness.

In outpatient settings, particular attention should be paid to those whose distress does not lift within a reasonable period after entry into rehabilitation or whose functioning is significantly compromised by any combination of the symptoms described below.

THE SYMPTOMS OF CLINICAL DEPRESSION

The U.S. Department of Health and Human Services recently published clinical practice guidelines for the office management of depressive disorders (U.S. Department of Health and Human Services, 1993). This publication encourages diagnosing as depressed any patient who evidences any combination of five or more of the symptoms listed in Table 2.3 for at least 2 weeks.

In addition to major depression, many cardiopulmonary patients may evidence an adjustment disorder with depressed mood (Swenson & Abbey, 1993). Here symptoms include anxious or depressed moods that are out of proportion to a normal reaction to the stressors at hand or altered behavior that may create difficulties in the patient's life. By definition, such adjustment struggles last less than 6 months, and when the acute stress abates, the patient resumes previous levels of functioning. In adjustment disorders, the patient's affective symptoms are less severe and less pervasive than those of a major depression. Swenson and Abbey (1993) also observed that many elderly depressed patients do not complain directly of depressed mood. Rather, they often present with complaints about somatic symptoms, particularly fatigue, insomnia, and anxiety-related symptoms such as lightheadedness, dyspnea, tachycardia, nausea, or chronic pain. Such patients also often evidence a lack of interest in everyday living, a condition that they may blame on their physical problems.

Finally, many recovering cardiopulmonary patients meet the diagnostic criteria for dysthymia. Here the patient is chronically depressed or irritable for most of the day, more days than not, for at least 2 years and exhibits two of the following symptoms: poor appetite or overeating; insomnia or hypersomnia; low energy or fatigue; low self-esteem; poor concentration or difficulty making decisions; and feelings of hopelessness (Gift & McCrone, 1993).

Table 2.3   Symptoms of Clinical Depression

Ongoing struggles to control mood or remain energized enough to cope with daily stressors

Preoccupation with fears, regrets, aches, pains, and thoughts of death

Loss of ability to experience pleasure

Disruption of appetites, resulting in changes in sleep, eating, and sexual drive

A recurring sense of being overwhelmed by current stressors

Agitation and frustration

Self-blame and pessimism

Irritation with others

Obsessive focus on insecurities about the future

Psychomotor retardation

Disrupted concentration and memory

Supportive interaction with others is ineffective in alleviating symptoms of depression

Persistent thoughts of suicide

SYMPTOMS OF ANXIETY DISORDER

Table 2.4 presents an integration of the descriptions offered by a variety of authors regarding how to flag a patient who is suffering from an anxiety disorder (APA, 1987).

In addition to the symptoms listed in Table 2.4, patients who suffer from anxiety disorders often report some combination of terrifying fears, including fears of dying, fainting, going crazy, having a heart attack, losing control, causing a scene, or not being able to get back to a safe environment such as home. Some patients also experience episodes of panic, with or without associated phobias. Phobias may develop when the circumstances in which the panic occurs get paired with the traumatic reactions. For example, many anxiety-disordered patients are diagnosed as suffering from social phobia or from claustrophobia, conditions that can result from avoiding stimuli that have, through conditioning and generalization, become associated with the dreaded episodes.

A special variant of anxiety disorder is obsessive-compulsive disorder. Here the patient's functioning is paralyzed by ruminative, intrusive thoughts and/or by the compulsion to engage in ritualized, patterned behaviors that provide momentary relief from free-floating anxieties. In practice, cardiopulmonary patients who evidence anxiety disorders most often manifest either panic or generalized anxiety (Swenson & Abbey, 1993). To my knowledge, no extensive information regarding the incidence of phobias or obsessive-compulsive disorders in cardiopulmonary populations is available. However, it appears to be the case that a fair number of recovering medical patients may experience a final form of anxiety disorder—posttraumatic stress disorder (PTSD).

SYMPTOMS OF POSTTRAUMATIC STRESS DISORDER

The anxiety being manifested by a given cardiopulmonary patient may be occurring secondary to the trauma of hospitalization and medical interventions. Such patients are said to be suffering from posttraumatic stress disorder. According to the official source of diagnostic guidelines for the

---

Table 2.4 Symptoms of Anxiety Disorder

Nervousness	Shortness of breath	Trembling and shaking
Agitation	Blurred vision	Feelings of paralysis
Weakness	Feeling unable to cope	Sweating
Numbness	Dizziness	Pressure in head or chest
Stomach churning	Heart palpitations	Feeling that things are not real

---

Table 2.5   Symptoms of Posttraumatic Stress Disorder

Recurrent, intrusive, distressing recollections of the trauma, including images, thoughts, or perceptions

Recurrent, distressing dreams of the trauma

Obsessive ruminations regarding details of the trauma

Recurrent tearfulness or anxiety

Sleep disturbances

Acting or feeling as if the traumatic event were recurring

Uncontrollable startle responses

Avoidance of stimuli associated with the trauma

General difficulty controlling mood, concentration, or irritability

---

American Psychiatric Association, the diagnosis of PTSD should be considered if, after exposure to a traumatic event, the event is persistently reexperienced in one (or more) of the ways outlined in Table 2.5 (APA, 1994).

Such symptoms signal an acute posttraumatic stress reaction if they occur during the initial 3 months after exposure to the traumatic event. The PTSD is considered chronic if symptoms persist for 3 months or more. Onset of symptoms of PTSD can also be delayed as much as 6 months after exposure to the traumatizing event.

SPECIALIZED INTERVENTIONS
WITH ANXIOUS OR DEPRESSED PATIENTS

Specialized consultation from a mental health professional should be considered for any patient who shows protracted struggles with anxiety or depression and who does not respond to brief crisis management interventions. Several factors should be considered here.

When Is Psychotropic Medication Warranted?

Although the benefits of cognitive/behavioral therapy in facilitating coping with anxiety and depression cannot be questioned, it is also true that, at its core, a protracted affective disorder is a medical condition. Like most medical conditions, appropriate therapy for anxiety and depressive disorders should combine pharmacologic and psychologic treatments. This recommendation has been supported by empirical investigations of the most effective ways to treat these conditions (e.g., Kahn, 1990). Extensive discussion of the many factors important to consider in prescribing or monitoring reactions to psychotropic medications is beyond the scope of this book; however, an overview of several factors that should be kept in mind regarding this issue is in order.

The overall safety and advisability of using antidepressant or anxiolytic therapy has been demonstrated, both with CHD patients and with those suffering from COPD. However, certain special considerations should be kept in mind in using psychotropic medicines with these populations.

Until the past decade, practitioners were hesitant to treat cardiopulmonary patients with the antidepressant medications then available due to fears of the ventricular arrhythmias and conduction blocks seen in overdoses and concerns about side effects such as respiratory complications, tachycardia, and hypotension. For example, patients taking tricyclic antidepressants may complain of anticholinergic side effects such as dry mouth, dizziness, blurred vision, and constipation, as well as fluid retention and antihistaminic effects such as daytime drowsiness. Further complications from certain of these drugs can include postural hypotension—a fact that should be underscored in treating elderly patients already at risk of injury from falling—and priapism. Also, for some elderly patients, tricyclic antidepressants can trigger central anticholinergic syndrome, a form of delirium characterized by confusion, disorientation, agitation, visual and auditory hallucinations, anxiety, and sometimes delusions (Swenson & Abbey, 1993). On the other hand, positive benefits of tricyclics in treating cardiopulmonary patients have also been noted (Gordon et al., 1985).

Several points should also be kept in mind regarding the effects of anti-anxiety medications. Benzodiazepines may have an adverse effect on memory and other cognitive functions in elderly patients (Wengel, Burke, Ranno, & Roccoforte, 1993). Other anxiolytic agents (e.g., Versed) actually cause amnesia for short-term memories. This fact should be especially noted when providing educational interventions to patients medicated with these agents; the patient's memory for the material presented may be lost in a medication-induced memory gap. In addition, benzodiazepines may cause such untoward side effects as respiratory depression. Thus, researchers have recommended that short-acting psychotropics (e.g., lorazepam, oxazepam, and alprazolam) may be better tolerated than long-acting benzodiazepines (Wengel et al., 1993; Wise, Schiavone, & Sitts, 1988). Although it is true that use of psychotropics such as benzodiazepines and antidepressants may help many patients with COPD, Thompson and Thompson (1984) pointed out that many psychotropic medications contain tartrazine, a dye that often provokes allergic bronchospastic attacks.

Swenson and Abbey (1993) offered helpful guidelines for choosing a psychotropic medication for a cardiopulmonary patient. Factors that should be taken into consideration include: the patient's past history of use and reactions to psychotropic medicines; the extent to which the patient is in need of sedation or activation; the anticholinergic side-effect profile of the medication; the overall cardiopulmonary status of the patient; and the patient's age. In reference to this last factor, it should be emphasized that elderly patients who have complex medical illness are most often best treated with one-third to one-half the usual initial dose of antidepressant medication.

Similar guidelines for prescribing psychotropic medicines are available for treating both cardiac patients at risk of sudden death (Vlay & Fricchione, 1985) and COPD patients (Gift & McCrone, 1993).

Gift and McCrone (1993) offered advice for prescribing psychotropic medicines for COPD patients that can also be applied to use of these medicines with many cardiac patients: "Because patients with COPD are elderly, the ideal antidepressant for use with this population would have a low side-effect profile, a short half-life, and no active metabolites. It would provoke few drug interactions and could be given once a day" (Gift & McCrone, 1993, p. 293). The newer generation of antidepressants such as fluoxetine (Prozac), sertraline (Zoloft), paroxetine (Paxil), and trazodone (Desyrel) seem to hold particular promise in this regard. Another antidepressant in this group is bupropion (Wellbutrin), but this medicine typically has to be taken three times a day. These medicines have been found to be effective in treating depression in CHD patients with no adverse side effects (Swenson & Abbey, 1993). Unfortunately, these medicines have not yet been definitively studied in specific COPD populations (Gift & McCrone, 1993).

Although a wide range of idiosyncratic reactions to psychotropic medications do occur, when used appropriately, these medicines are generally safe and effective in treating cardiopulmonary patients. In fact, some psychotropic medicines seem to have beneficial physiological effects on important target syndromes for cardiopulmonary patients other than anxiety and depression. For example, Borson, McDonald, Gayle, & Deffebach (1992) reported that, compared to controls, COPD patients treated with nortriptyline evidenced significant improvements in anxiety, respiratory symptoms, physical comfort, and day-to-day functioning, even though physiological measures of pulmonary insufficiency were unaffected by treatment. In addition, some researchers have reported that the atropinelike effects of tricyclics promote bronchodilation and improve airway obstruction (Wise et al., 1988); however, this finding has not been consistently replicated in further research, and, as noted above, some negative side effects of tricyclics have been reported in studies of COPD populations. Finally, a novel anxiolytic agent, buspirone (BuSpar), is now available. This medicine is free of many of the drawbacks of other anxiolytics in that it does not promote psychomotor impairment, interaction with alcohol, or addiction. In addition, it has been found to stimulate respiration and therefore can be quite effective in treating patients with lung disease, where other anxiolytics such as benzodiazepines might be contraindicated (Swenson & Abbey, 1993).

It should be reemphasized that effective use of psychotropic medication often requires psychiatric consultation. Referral for such consultation should be considered for any patient who evidences protracted syndromes suggesting the presence of an affective disorder.

ASSESSING SUICIDE RISK

A frequent symptom of clinical depression is suicidal ideation; however, the vast majority of clinically depressed people do not commit suicide. It is therefore important to develop strategies that can be used to assess which patients may be at serious risk of suicide and which are experiencing suicidal ideation as par for the course of their clinical depression.

Suicide has been studied in both COPD and cardiac populations. Sawyer (1983) indicated that the clinical course of COPD can lead to a progression toward despair and suicide for some patients. Feelings of hopelessness and discouragement may escalate in such patients as they come to recognize that recovery from COPD is not possible. Some patients are especially devastated by the disappointment that comes with realizing that COPD is irreversible and that rehabilitation can, at best, slow deterioration. Some patients then become susceptible to extremes of depression and develop suicidal ideation. Suicidal trends in patients with hypertension, asthma, and other cardiorespiratory illnesses have also been described (Dorbonne, 1966; Levitan, 1983). Specific characteristics of cardiopulmonary patients at high risk of suicide have been described (Clark, 1990; Farberow, McKelligott, Cohen, and Dorbonne, 1966). Thirteen factors should be especially considered in flagging patients at high risk of suicide:

- Excessive emotional distress in reaction to the illness
- Low tolerance for pain and discomfort
- High need to control the course of treatment
- Demanding behavior and a high need for attention and reassurance
- Alertness and good orientation
- Lack of active family support and general isolation and withdrawal
- Exhaustion
- Severe symptoms of depression
- Prior or present suicide threats
- Verbalized suicidal plan, complete with the means to carry it out
- Self-destructive behavior such as alcohol or drug abuse
- Hostile attitude
- Poor impulse control

No definitive guidelines exist for specifying the degree of suicide risk for a given patient. However, in an excellent, practical discussion of ways to assess suicide risk with cardiovascular patients, Clark (1990) noted that patients having vague, passing thoughts of death versus those with true suicidal planning can be differentiated with direct and compassionate questioning regarding lethality. Ask the patient:

- Are you thinking of hurting (or killing) yourself?
- How have you thought about doing it?

- When and where are you thinking of doing it?

- Do you already have the means to carry out your plan?

- Would you be willing to contact someone if you begin to feel that you will actually follow through with your plan so that you can get some help?

Any indication of serious intent or fear of suicide, or of severe depression, warrants immediate referral to a qualified mental health professional for further assessment and treatment. If need be, such patients should be hospitalized, either voluntarily or upon commitment proceedings implemented by the patient's family or by the concerned health care provider. Although such hospitalization is often resisted or resented by the patient, it is important to remember that a severely depressed individual may not be able to rationally problem solve. It is therefore neither fair nor reasonable to ask such a person to make complex decisions such as whether or not he or she needs treatment. Depressed people need compassion, help, guidance, and a caring system of support and active treatment to help them regain their functioning; depressed suicidal patients may need protection from themselves.

TREATING PATIENTS FOR DEPRESSION AND ANXIETY

As mentioned earlier, depressive and anxiety disorders are most often treated with a combination of psychotropic medication and psychological counseling. The counseling component of treatment often combines interventions from cognitive, behavioral, problem-solving, and psychodynamic schools of thought (Clark, 1990). The initial stages of treatment should focus on alleviation of affective distress (with the help of medication), retraining regarding cognitive habits that might be fueling such distress (see chapter 9), and orchestration of behavioral experiences that promote more adaptive functioning. In this latter regard, the specific targets of intervention vary in treating depressive and anxiety disorders.

The cognitive/behavioral approach to treating depression basically revolves around coaching, support, and contracting. The patient is encouraged to orchestrate daily living to foster three experiences, each to a moderate degree: some that foster a sense of accomplishment; some that allow a sense of having fulfilled important obligations; and some that are purely for pleasure (Beck, 1979). As behavioral changes occur, interventions should help the patient replace self-blaming or minimalizing cognitions with appropriately nurturing and soothing frames of reference. Works by Burns (1980) and Beck and colleagues (Beck, 1979; Beck, Rush, Shaw, & Emery, 1979) can be referred to for step-by-step descriptions of the actual course of cognitive/behavioral treatment of depression. An excellent, detailed description of a care plan that operationalizes the problem-solving component of treating depression in cardiovascular patients was published by Clark (1990).

Anxiety disorders, too, are most often treated with a combined psychological-biological approach. Often, some combination of anti-depressant, anxiolytic, and, in some cases, beta-blocker medications is used in treating anxiety disorders. The reader is referred to the previously mentioned works of Swenson and Abbey (1993) and Vlay and Fricchione (1985) for general guidelines in using these medicines with cardiopulmonary patients. A general discussion of psychiatric treatment of anxiety disorders is available in Sheehan (1984). Interestingly, antidepressants with sedating qualities—and not anxiolytics—are most often the medications of choice in treating anxiety disorders. This is due to the addiction potential of many anxiolytics and to the fact that the neurochemical causes of anxiety states are more directly treated and corrected by antidepressants than by any other class of medicines.

The psychological aspect of treating anxiety disorders combines support, guidance, and coaching in ways to overcome the residual emotional or behavioral consequences of anxiety or panic episodes or of the traumatic experiences that resulted in posttraumatic stress syndrome. Primary targets of such intervention are amelioration of anticipatory anxiety, reversal of any avoidant behavior that the patient may have developed, and restoration of the patient's confidence in his or her ability to return to normal functioning (Swenson & Abbey, 1993). A combination of relaxation training, cognitive retraining, behavioral rehearsal, and exposure to anxiety-provoking situations (either through imagery or in vivo), paired with relaxation, is used to promote systematic desensitization of the patient's anxiety. Extensive discussion of such strategies is available from Sheehan (1984) and Wilson (1987).

Finally, extended psychotherapy is also sometimes helpful and may be necessary in treating patients who are anxious or depressed. Suffering from anxiety or depression can shake one's self-confidence and magnify long-standing unresolved psychodynamic issues and stir new levels of concern and insecurity. When chronic illness is added to the list of stressors, serious examination of the meaning and direction of one's life often ensues. Such grave self-examination can correlate with depression and anxiety. This vul-nerability creates both pain and the opportunity to learn new ways of under-standing oneself and others who influence one's life. In the hands of a competent and compassionate psychotherapist, the depressed or anxious cardiopulmonary patient can be helped to benefit from the dual crises created by illness and affective distress.

PSYCHOLOGICAL AND PSYCHOSOCIAL ASSESSMENT TOOLS

Psychometrically based instruments for assessing a wide range of psycho-social concerns of medical patients are currently available. Some of these are relatively brief instruments that target a specific issue within a specific medical population; many are designed to provide an overview of general psychological or psychosocial functioning; some are designed to assess general quality of life; some address health-related quality of life (the patient's perceptions of the functional effects of an illness and its consequences); and some target specific health-related behaviors. Due to space limitations, the reader is referred to Rose and Robbins (1993) and Keefe and Blumenthal (1982) for more extensive discussions of this topic. In addition, Emery (1993) provided a thoughtful discussion of this topic with an emphasis on the importance of neuropsychological assessment in treating COPD patients. An extensive listing of available psychosocial assessment instruments follows.

GENERAL, SIMPLE PSYCHOLOGICAL SCREENING TOOLS

- Brief Symptom Inventory (Derogatis & Spencer, 1982)
- Profile of Mood States (POMS) (McNair, Lorr, & Droppleman, 1971)
- Beck Depression Inventory (Beck, 1978)
- Beck Depression Inventory—Short Form (Reynolds & Gould, 1981)
- Center for Epidemiological Studies—Depression Scale (CES-D) (Radloff, 1977)
- State Trait Anxiety Scale (Speilberger, Gorsuch, & Luschene, 1970)
- Denial Rating Scale (Hackett & Cassem, 1974)
- General Health Questionnaire (Goldberg & Blackwell, 1970; Vieweg & Hedlund, 1983)
- Kellner Symptom Questionnaire (Kellner, 1987)

MAJOR PERSONALITY AND NEUROPSYCHOLOGICAL ASSESSMENT INSTRUMENTS

Note. These instruments should only be used by licensed psychological examiners or licensed practicing psychologists who are trained in their administration and interpretation.

Personality Assessment Instruments

- Minnesota Multiphasic Personality Inventory (MMPI) (Dahlstrom, Walsh, & Dahlstrom, 1975)
- MMPI-2 (Hathaway & McKinley, 1989)
- MMPI-168—Short Form (Newmark, Cook, Clarke, & Faschingbauer, 1973)
- Hopkins Symptom Checklist—Revised, the SCL-90 (Derogatis, Brand, & Jenkins, 1983)
- NEO Personality Inventory (Costa & McCrae, 1985)

Neuropsychological Assessment Instruments

- Wechsler Adult Intelligence Scale—Revised (Wechsler, 1981)
- Mini Mental State Exam (Folstein, Folstein, & McHugh, 1975)
- Wechsler Memory Scale—Revised (Wechsler, 1987)
- Trailmaking Test (Reitan, 1958)
- Halstead-Reitan Aphasia Screening Test (Heimberger & Reitan, 1961)
- Aphasia Screening Test (Halstead & Wepman, 1959)

ALCOHOLISM SCREENING INSTRUMENTS

- Michigan Alcohol Screening Instrument (Selzer, 1971)
- The CAGE Questionnaire (Ewing, 1984)

MEASURES OF TYPE A BEHAVIOR PATTERN

- Type A Structured Interviews (Hecker, Chesney, Black, & Frautschi, 1988; Matthews, Glass, Rosenman, & Bortner, 1977; Rosenman, 1978)
- Jenkins Activity Survey (Jenkins, Rosenman, & Zyzanski, 1974)
- Framingham Type A Scale (Haynes, Feinleib, & Kannel, 1980)

MEASURES OF HOSTILITY

- Cook-Medley Hostility Scale (Barefoot, Dahlstrom, & Williams, 1983; Cook & Medley, 1954; Shekelle, Gale, Ostfeld, & Paul, 1983; Williams et al., 1980)
- Buss-Durkee Hostility Inventory (Buss & Durkee, 1957)
- Potential for Hostility (Dembroski & Costa, 1987)

SCALES THAT MEASURE ADJUSTMENT TO PHYSICAL HEALTH STATUS

- Psychosocial Adjustment to Illness Scale (Derogatis & Lopez, 1983)
- Cardiac Health Concerns Questionnaire (Stanton, Jenkins, Savageau, Harken, & Aucoin, 1984)
- Chronic Respiratory Disease Questionnaire (CRQ) (Guyatt, Berman, & Townsend, 1987)
- Transitional Dyspnea Index (TDI) (Guyatt et al., 1987)
- Pulmonary Functional Status Scale (PFSS) (Weaver & Narsavage, 1992)
- McGill Pain Questionnaire (Melzak, 1975)

- Millon Behavioral Health Inventory (Millon, Green, & Meagher, 1982)
- Medical Outcome Study (MOS) Questionnaire (Tarlov et al., 1989)
- Medical Outcomes Study—Short Form SF-36 (Mahler et al., 1992; Stewart, Hays, & Ware, 1988)
- Nottingham Health Profile (Hunt, McEwen, & McKenna, 1980)
- Sickness Impact Profile (DeBruin, DeWitte, Stevens, & Diederiks, 1992; Gibson et al., 1975)
- Quality of Well-Being Scale (Kaplan, Atkins, & Timms, 1984)
- Additive Activities Profile Test (ADAPT) (Daughton, Fix, Kass, Patil, & Bell, 1979)

FAMILY ASSESSMENT INVENTORIES

Marital/Family Assessment Instruments

- Family Environmental Scale (Moos & Moos, 1981)
- Family Adaptability and Cohesion Evaluation Scale (Olson, 1985; Olson, Bell, & Portner, 1978)
- Beavers-Timberlawn Family Evaluation Scale (Lewis, Beavers, Gossett, & Phillips, 1976)
- Family Assessment Method (van der Veen, Huebner, Jurgens, & Beja, 1964)
- Family Assessment Device (Epstein, Bishop, & Levin, 1983)
- Card Sort Procedure (Oliveri & Reiss, 1981)
- Dyadic Adjustment Scale (Spanier, 1976)
- Barbarin Family Process Scale (Barbarin & Gilbert, 1979)
- MATE (Schutz, 1976)
- Family Assessment Measure (Skinner, Steinhauer, & Santa-Barbara, 1983)
- Locke-Wallace Marital Adjustment Scale (Locke & Wallace, 1959)
- Family Apperception Test (Sotile, Julian, Henry, & Sotile, 1990)
- Revealed Differences Test (Olson & Ryder, 1975; Strodtbeck, 1951)

Health Behavior Family Assessment Scales

- Family Adjustment to Medical Stressors Scale (Koch, 1983)
- Health Behavior Scale (Miller & Wikoff, 1989)
- Marital Responsibility Scale (Kline & Warren, 1983)
- Marital Functioning Scale (Kline & Warren, 1983)

- Miller Social Intimacy Scale (Miller & Lefcourt, 1982)
- Family Adjustment to Crisis Scale (Dhooper, 1983)
- Perceived Beliefs of Others Scale (Miller, Johnson, Garrett, Wikoff, & McMahon, 1982)
- Compliance Questionnaire (Johnson, 1974)
- Spouse Support Questionnaire (Hilbert, 1985)
- Marital Conflict Scale (Waltz & Badura, 1988)
- Life Satisfaction Questionnaire (Myrtek, 1987)
- Adaptive Balance Profile (Heller, Frank, Kornfeld, Malm, & Bowman, 1974)
- Needs Assessment Questionnaire (Orzeck & Staniloff, 1987)
- Health and Daily Living Form (Moos, Finney, & Gamble, 1982)
- Partner Interaction Questionnaire (Mermelstein, Lichtenstein, & McIntyre, 1983)
- Spousal Coping Instrument (Nyamathi, Dracup, & Jacoby, 1988)

SOCIAL SUPPORT INSTRUMENTS

- Interpersonal Support Evaluation Schedule (Cohen, Mermelstein, Karmack, & Hoberman, 1985)
- Inventory Schedule for Social Interaction (Henderson, Byrne, Duncan-Jones, & Scott, 1980)
- Inventory of Socially Supportive Behaviors (Barrera, Sandler, & Ramsay, 1981)
- Perceived Social Support from Friends and Family (Procidano & Heller, 1983)
- Social Support Questionnaire (Sarason, Levine, Basham, & Sarason, 1983)
- Medical Outcomes Study—Short Form SF-36 (Stewart et al., 1988)

SUMMARY

The patients we serve belong to family teams, and—as individuals and as teams—they are stressed by the crises that face them at the time of our interventions. Their combined psychological and interpersonal reactions have much to do with the outcomes of our interventions and should be caringly considered in designing and delivering our clinical services. Here, as in any branch of medical care, effective treatment depends upon accurate assessment. The structure and focus of psychosocial assessment might differ in inpatient and outpatient settings and according to the illness being treated. Whether it is done through the use of formal psychosocial testing, structured clinical interviews, or simply through the use of clinical impressions and intuition, such assessment should, minimally, answer the following five questions (AACVPR, 1994):

Assessment Question 1: Is the patient's ability to positively adapt to his or her daily demands of living being disrupted by crisis that is caused by the illness or by entry into rehabilitation?

Assessment Question 2: Is the patient evidencing affective or cognitive impairment of his or her ability to cope with the adaptive demands of illness or of rehabilitation?

Assessment Question 3: Is the patient receiving adequate psychosocial support to aid his or her ability to cope with the stressors of medical intervention or rehabilitation?

Assessment Question 4: Does the patient evidence any behavioral or emotional patterns that warrant aggressive, immediate psychosocial intervention?

Assessment Question 5: What are the major concerns of the patient and of his or her family regarding anticipated psychosocial adjustment challenges in the immediate future?

Once gathered, assessment information needs to be presented to the patient and his or her loved ones. Guidelines for approaching such feedback sessions are presented in the following chapter.

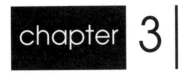

APPROACHING CARDIOPULMONARY PATIENTS FOR PSYCHOSOCIAL INTERVENTION

The goal of psychosocial interventions is to influence the patient's emotional experience and shape his or her behavior. Effective clinicians, whether they are aware of it or not, use a fundamental strategy to accomplish this goal: They establish rapport and then lead the patient in desired perceptual, behavioral, and emotional directions (Grinder & Bandler, 1981).

MATCHING, THEN LEADING

Within medicine, the systemization of this method of influencing others was first presented by the renowned medical hypnotist, Milton Erickson (Erickson, Rossi, & Rossi, 1976). The relevance of this strategy to general medical care was first underscored by Janis (1958), who called attention to the importance of matching "reassurance mechanisms" to the personality styles of surgery patients. In retrospect, Janis's advice foreshadowed the current recommendation to be careful in dealing with patients who are experiencing positive benefits from coping mechanisms such as denial or repression. For example, Johnson and Morse (1990) found that the goodness of fit between the health professional's and the heart patient's perceptions of the patient's progress can enhance, confirm, or devastate ongoing psychosocial adjustment. We should remember that too abruptly stripping patients or families of their ways of coping with crisis can hurt the effectiveness of our interventions.

WHO IS RESPONSIBLE FOR MATCHING?

Whether you are attempting to help a patient change in some needed way or simply providing support to a distressed patient or family member, it is incumbent upon you, the health care provider, to match frames of reference with the targeted individual, not the other way around (Dracup & Meleis, 1982). Respectful acknowledgment of the issues that are psychologically relevant to the individual is an essential first step in leading the distressed patient or loved one to a more helpful way of coping; one that promotes mastery of the adaptive tasks at hand and that prepares the individual for the next stage of psychosocial adjustment to rehabilitation challenges (Prochaska & DiClemente, 1984).

For example, the hard-driving Type A patient who is accustomed to coping with stress by ignoring pain and competitively striving to the point of exhaustion may be more distressed than soothed by recommendations to slow down and pace recovery efforts. Similarly, smoking cessation or nutritional interventions might disrupt the camaraderie experienced by an individual while indulging in such behaviors (Doherty & Harkaway, 1990). Finally, illness or entry into rehabilitation can even disrupt healthy developments that are going on for an individual or a family team (Rejeski, Morley, & Sotile, 1985; Sotile, 1992). For example, a college student's individuation from the family nest may be disrupted by her concern about the stresses faced by her parents when one of them enters rehabilitation. Both individual and family-level issues need to be considered in determining what needs to be matched when interacting with a given patient. The remainder of this section provides an overview of concepts that can help clarify what needs to be matched to establish and maintain rapport with patients and their loved ones.

REPRESSORS AND SENSITIZERS

It is clear that the style in which an intervention is delivered can have an iatrogenic interaction with the patient's coping style (Shaw et al., 1986). In this sense, the intervention itself can be seen as an important variable determining the patient's level of risk following treatment. This concept is particularly relevant for repressors and sensitizers.

Sensitizers are said to be more comfortable with high levels of information. These patients are best matched when they are given explicit details regarding upcoming medical procedures or rehabilitation tasks. Sensitizers thrive under treatment conditions that fill their senses with information. They prefer high degrees of exposure to stimuli relative to the stressor at hand, and they have negative outcomes when they are not given high enough levels of information.

Repressors, on the other hand, feel more comfortable with minimal amounts of information. These patients require minimal information in preparation for medical procedures and only simple principles or guidance during posthospitalization recovery; information overload simply serves to distress repressors (Shaw et al., 1986).

Research with heart patients has documented that matching the patient's coping style with the appropriate amount of information promotes recovery, both during hospitalization and upon discharge. Purposeful mismatching has led to negative outcomes, including: higher rates of heart monitor alarms and greater noncompliant behavior by recovering heart patients (Cromwell, Butterfield, Brayfield, & Curry, 1987); greater medical complications, sleep disturbances, depression, and general psychosocial distress for 6 months postintervention (Weinberger, Schwartz, & Davidson, 1979); and greater postintervention medical and psychosocial complications in coronary angioplasty patients (Shaw et al., 1986). Although no universally accepted method for assessing patient coping style is currently available, useful work has been done in this area and is discussed below.

THE STAGES OF CHANGE

One way of approaching the problem of matching our style of intervention to the patient's frame of reference has been developed by Prochaska and DiClemente (1992). They offered a conceptualization regarding the stages of change that occur as an individual attempts to modify behavioral patterns. These stages and their accompanying psychological frames of reference are as follows:

- Precontemplation: No intention of changing.
- Contemplation: Serious intention of changing.
- Preparation: Laying foundation for change.
- Action: Change in progress.
- Maintenance: Seeking to avoid backsliding.

Prochaska and DiClemente (1992) have proposed that the change process involves a cyclical pattern of movement through various stages and that each stage of change revolves around certain identifiable perspectives.

Precontemplation

During precontemplation, an individual finds ways to rationalize continuing in their old ways. Patients seem unmotivated and unresponsive to input during this stage. Such a person may demonstrate temporary change if pressured by loved ones or authority figures (e.g., employers or health care providers), only to quickly return to their old ways once the pressure is off. Despite the concerns of others, they may selectively perceive the positive effects of their current behaviors, intellectualize, rationalize, or discount the possibility or importance of changing.

To assess whether or not a patient is in precontemplation with reference to an area of change (e.g., smoking cessation), Prochaska et al. (1992) recommend asking whether he or she is seriously intending to change the problem behavior in the near future, typically operationalized as within the next 6 months. If not, he or she is classified as a precontemplator. It is emphasized that precontemplators may wish to change but lack any serious intention of changing.

Contemplation

The contemplation stage is one of consciousness raising. The individual becomes more introspective about health behavior choices, may verbalize a serious intention of changing in the near future, and is responsive to input and education. This is a stage in which the individual is aware that a problem exists and is seriously thinking about changing but has not yet made a commitment to take action. Prochaska et al. (1992) emphasize that people can remain stuck in contemplation for years, knowing where they want to go but not yet ready to commit to the journey that takes them there.

During contemplation, individuals actively weigh the pros and cons of the problem and the solution to the problem. Important here are perceptions of the amount of effort, energy, and loss associated with overcoming the problem. Serious consideration of changing the problem behavior is the central feature of the contemplation stage. Contemplators typically state that they are seriously considering changing the targeted behavior in the next 6 months.

Preparation

Next comes preparation, a stage characterized by the intention to take action in the next month but lack of success in taking such action in the past year. Typically, individuals in this stage report some small behavioral changes such as a slight reduction in the number of cigarettes smoked daily or a slight increase in the amount of exercise engaged in each week. However, these individuals have not yet reached a criterion for effective action; they are intending to take action in the very near future, but they have not yet accomplished a goal such as abstinence from smoking, alcohol, or drug use.

Action

Most patients in outpatient cardiopulmonary rehabilitation are in the action stage of changing some health behavior, even though a given patient may be at a different stage in the change process in various areas of importance to overall rehabilitation. Here the individual actively modifies behaviors, experiences, or the environment to overcome a targeted problem. In the Prochaska and DiClemente schemata, individuals are classified in the action stage if they have successfully altered a targeted behavior for a period of from 1 day to 6 months.

Maintenance

Once a change has been successfully implemented for approximately 6 months, the individual is usually in the maintenance stage for that particular health behavior. The work of the maintenance stage is to prevent relapse and consolidate the gains attained during action. Interventions that teach strategies for furthering self-efficacy and that safeguard relapse prevention are especially important at this stage of rehabilitation (Bandura, 1977a, 1977b; McKool, 1987; Prochaska, DiClemente, Velicer, Ginpil, & Norcross, 1985).

During maintenance, individuals benefit from help in seeing that the advantages of having made the change outweigh the costs of implementing the change, and from interventions that enhance self-confidence to maintain the change. Prochaska et al. (1992) emphasized that, although for some behaviors maintenance is a stage that lasts a lifetime, it is also imperative to remember (and to teach) that most people move through these various stages in a spiral, not a linear, pattern. Relapse occurs, and when it does, the individual regresses to an earlier stage. For example, many individuals relapse from maintenance to the contemplation or preparation stage, skipping the earlier stage(s) during the next attempt to change.

A major point of the work of Prochaska and DiClemente is that it is fruitless to mismatch intervention strategies and patients' naturally occurring progression through the stages of change. They emphasize that failing to frame interventions with respect for the patient's current concerns runs the risk of either underserving, misserving, or not serving the patient. In this regard, Prochaska et al. (1992) warn of two frequent mismatches: (a) attempting to get patients to modify behavior—through use of such strategies as reinforcement management, stimulus control, or counterconditioning—without first increasing their levels of awareness; and (b) trying to modify behaviors by simply increasing awareness through the use of strategies such as consciousness raising and self-reevaluation. In the authors' words: "Overt action without insight is likely to lead to temporary change" (Prochaska et al., 1992, p. 111). And, "Insight alone does not necessarily bring about behavior change" (Prochaska et al., 1992, p. 110).

Guidelines for matching interventions to specific stages of change are available (e.g., Prochaska et al., 1992) and will be presented later in this chapter.

PSYCHOLOGICAL REACTIONS DURING CORONARY CARE AND REHABILITATION: IS DENIAL ADAPTIVE OR MALADAPTIVE?

In addition to anxiety and depression, the trauma of medical crisis leads to high levels of denial for many recovering patients and for their loved ones. Twenty years of research of this factor has yielded inconclusive data as to whether denial is beneficial or detrimental to recovery following illness (Malan, 1992).

On the positive side, a number of studies have documented that denial can be associated with an improved medical outcome during an acute coronary crisis. It appears that denial lessens stress and therefore may help a patient avoid the catecholamine elevations and other physiological stress responses that may complicate cardiac functioning (Bertel, Buhler, Baitsch, Ritz, & Burkart, 1982; Smith & Leon, 1992).

Indeed, patients evidencing high levels of denial have been found to become medically stable twice as quickly as those who score low on measures of denial (Levenson, Kay, Monteperrante, & Herman, 1984). High deniers hospitalized for MI or CABG tend to complain of less angina and are less likely to require intravenous nitroglycerin to control angina during the CCU stay. They also spend fewer days in intensive care and evidence fewer signs of cardiac dysfunction during hospitalization (Levine et al., 1987). High levels of denial during initial hospitalization have been found to correlate with higher levels of survival of the cardiac event and also with earlier return to work, enhanced sexual behavior, and greater physical activity levels after hospitalization (Havik & Maeland, 1988).

On the negative side, many maladaptive correlates and consequences of denial have been noted. Although few researchers argue that brief use of denial can be adaptive, it appears that continued denial can interfere with both acute and long-range adjustment to CHD. High levels of denial can impair attention, concentration, and retention and therefore lessen the integration of information about the medical condition during hospitalization and rehabilitation (Shaw, Cohen, Doyle, & Palesky, 1985). Patients who evidence chronic posthospitalization denial have been found to show greater morbidity and mortality (Bartle & Bishop, 1974; Soloff, 1977). Signs of maladaptive use of denial can include:

- clinging to the erroneous belief that the medical condition is minor;
- attributing symptoms of illness to some minor health problem, such as stomach upset;
- refusing to believe that an illness event has or is occurring at all;
- denying and resisting the need for hospitalization;
- denial that the illness will have any impact on one's life;
- denial of any distressing emotions (such as anxiety or depression) that typically accompany acute illness (Malan, 1992; Marsden & Dracup, 1991; Smith & Leon, 1992).

Putting Denial in Context

One school of thought calls for initial support of denial, followed, as the crisis subsides, by confrontation with realistic views of illness and rehabilitation (Smith & Leon, 1992). Certainly, initial interventions should be respectful of the patient's evident level of denial (Hackett, Cassem, & Wishnie, 1968). But it is possible that for the sake of providing "support of denial," the emotional needs of recovering cardiac patients often go undertreated in acute care settings. There is some suggestion in the literature that as many as 20% of patients who do not show emotional upset in the hospital following MI present emotional problems 4 months after discharge (Havik & Maeland, 1990; Lloyd & Cawley, 1983). This reaction resembles a delayed crisis reaction that perhaps could be prevented by more attentive care to the emotions that are often left to fester during inattentive hospital care.

A number of writers (e.g., Doehrman, 1977; Malan, 1992) have provided convincing arguments in support of this concern. It appears that researchers of this issue often mislabel patients and therefore mismatch their clinical needs. For example, Thomas et al. (1983) documented that patients can both freely admit fears and deny the seriousness of their illness within a 20-min interview, a phenomenon that is not likely to be picked up in a simple paper-and-pencil psychological test or in a hurried clinical assessment of denial. Many patients who hide feelings about their illness during brief interviews or on paper-and-pencil tests are quite willing to discuss issues that are emotionally distressing if they are given longer term contact in a supportive environment (Doehrman, 1977).

FOUR THEORIES ON PSYCHOSOCIAL ADJUSTMENT

A number of theories regarding the patterns of psychosocial adjustment to cardiopulmonary illness and rehabilitation have been proposed, but none is universally accepted. Several efforts in this regard deserve consideration when assessing what psychological frames of reference need to be matched to effectively intervene with a cardiopulmonary patient.

Constellation of Factors for Risk

The first comes from Havik and Maeland's (1990) long-term (3- to 5-year) follow-up study of the emotional adjustment patterns of 283 MI patients. These investigators found that there is no constant or typical progression of psychological adjustment in recovering MI patients. Some patients evidence high levels of denial, only to be followed by high levels of distress after discharge. Others evidence pronounced distress from hospital throughout follow-up. Still others evidence low levels of emotional upset that gradually increase during long-range adjustment.

According to Havik and Maeland's data, a certain constellation of factors characterized patients who were at high risk of suffering prolonged, long-range adjustment struggles. The at-risk patients in this study tended to be those who:

- were younger in age (average age of 52 years versus 55 years for positive copers);
- were unemployed at the time of hospitalization;
- had a history of high frequency of previous hospitalizations for heart illness;

- had a history of previous angina pectoris;
- had received psychiatric treatment prior to hospitalization;
- had suffered pre-MI physical limitations in activity level; and
- had high pre-MI levels of marital conflict.

Patients who evidenced this constellation of factors tended to also evidence high levels of hopelessness, low levels of denial of the impact of illness, worse self-rated global health, and more negative expectations regarding the consequences of MI.

Four Stages of Recovery

In a second study, Johnson and Morse (1990) reported on extended clinical interviews of 14 MI patients conducted from 1 to 45 months following their first MI. Although the study sample here was quite small, the authors provide a useful hypothetical guide for further evaluations of the adjustment process of recovering cardiopulmonary patients. They highlighted four major phases in this adjustment process.

First, with the onset of symptoms, denial is used to reduce fear and anxiety. The second phase, coming to terms, begins 3 to 8 days after MI. Here the patient focuses on determining the cause of the illness. This phase often brings feelings of guilt, self-recrimination, and irritability with others for blaming or shaming them about having "caused" this illness. Future adjustment seems to be much affected by the patient's degrees of optimism or pessimism during this phase.

According to Johnson and Morse, patients begin to progress toward positive adjustment in the third phase, learning to live. This stage is characterized by lessening of uncertainty, solidification of new guidelines for living, and struggles with the role changes that have come with the illness. Positive copers at this stage are able to set small goals and derive a sense of achievement at each step of progress.

Finally, patients enter what Johnson and Morse call the living again phase: they accept their limitations, emphasize their residual capabilities, refocus their attention from worrying about health and illness to other aspects of life, and gradually attain a sense of mastery in their ability to attend to the tasks of their daily lives.

Psychological Progression in Rehabilitation

Cassem and Hackett (1971) developed a model of the psychological course of reacting to acute cardiac care that can also be used to categorize the reactions of many patients upon entry into outpatient rehabilitation. According to Cassem and Hackett, psychological reactions to acute care progress as follows:

- Anxiety predominates on post-MI days 1 and 2, then declines.

- Depression peaks on days 3-5, as the full impact of the MI is felt.

- Chronic character traits surface later (days 4-6).

The "typical" psychological progression of patients who enter outpatient rehabilitation is impossible to define, given the heterogeneity of patients enrolled in outpatient rehabilitation programs. For example, some patients enter rehabilitation immediately following diagnosis or hospitalization; some enter years later. Some have endured surgery; some have not. In addition, premorbid personality traits and the patient's general life circumstance shape coping patterns in obvious ways.

With this caveat in mind, I want to note that in my experience, patients often evidence a fairly predictable course of psychological adjustment following entry into outpatient rehabilitation.

Stage 1: Anxiety predominates the first 3 to 6 weeks of participation, then declines. During this time, the patient's premorbid personality-based coping tendencies predominate his or her clinical presentation. For example, the orderly may become compulsive; the grouchy may become hostile and cynical; the fearful may get paralyzed with anxiety; and so on. These personality-based coping reactions diminish as the patient gains familiarity with the rehabilitation procedures, social support from the rehabilitation team and from fellow patients, and, perhaps, the emotional benefit that comes with the regular exercise and structure offered in formal cardiopulmonary rehabilitation.

Stage 2: The patient's motivation is typically bolstered and anxieties further soothed as documentation of progress in physical rehabilitation accumulates throughout the initial 3 months of formal rehabilitation. For example, many patients evidence improvements in exercise capacity, blood lipid levels, pulmonary functioning, and so forth, culminating in marked improvements in these parameters upon their initial retesting 3 months after entry into rehabilitation.

Stage 3: Failure to continue at this same rate of improvement or, worse yet, regression in measured levels of physical rehabilitation upon a second reassessment (typically 6 months after entry into rehabilitation) often lead to a period of depression and/or renewed anxiety.

Stage 4: Next, characterological coping patterns surface, both for the patient and for the patient's concerned loved ones. Family teams often seem to get stuck in this last stage of coping; their stress-driven, personality-based coping patterns are not only exaggerated, they become seemingly concretized on both individual and family levels, often to the detriment of rehabilitation efforts. Family systems researchers have established that family-based coping paradigms solidify somewhere between 3 months and 1 year after onset of illness (Patterson, 1988, 1989).

Thus, a patient may enter outpatient care or a formal rehabilitation program having already solidified two factors that must be dealt with by the rehabilitation team—the individual and the family patterns of coping with the illness. For some patients (i.e., those who enter outpatient care or rehabilitation within weeks after being discharged from the hospital), these same factors—the individual and family-level coping patterns—may develop during the immediate course of treatment. This fact underscores the tremendous opportunity that health care providers working in outpatient and rehabilitation settings are given to help shape the adaptations of the patients being served.

Finally, it is wise to remember that the course of psychological adjustment is cyclical, not linear. Many patients experience setbacks in recovery, only to move forward again. Other patients become stuck in some earlier phase of adjustment. Johnson and Morse (1990) pointed out that this cyclical pattern may explain the discrepancies in research findings regarding the "typical" frequency and duration of such symptoms as anxiety and depression in recovering heart patients.

GUIDELINES FOR OFFERING FEEDBACK REGARDING PSYCHOSOCIAL FUNCTIONING

What should be done with the information that comes from psychosocial assessment? Several factors should be kept in mind in making this decision (AACUPR, 1994; Razin, 1982; Rejeski et al., 1985; Sotile, 1993).

KEEP THE RESULTS OF ASSESSMENT INFORMATION IN PERSPECTIVE

The perfect psychometric tool has yet to be invented. No clinician, no matter how experienced or perceptive, can override an individual's expertise in understanding him- or herself. We should be humble as we evaluate clinical impressions and formal psychometric assessment data: whether we understand it or not, the patient's behavior always makes some form of adaptive sense, at least to the patient. Patients tend to appreciate advice and guidance about their needed treatments. However, most people do not appreciate judgmental statements about themselves or their loved ones, especially if such statements are drawn from only a brief acquaintance with you or even briefer assessment procedures.

Always offer feedback from psychosocial assessment with a degree of questioning. It is useful to frame feedback with a statement such as the following:

"I appreciate your taking the time to speak with me and to respond to these questionnaires. I would like to give you feedback from this assessment. Before I do, though, let me emphasize that these psychological questionnaires are designed to generate questions, not answers. These are shortcut ways to develop guidelines for deciding what you and I might talk about. You are the expert on yourself and on your life. I am the expert on ways that folks can better cope with the unique challenges that come with rehabilitation. My hope is that you and I can put our heads together and design a program that will help you meet the challenges that come with your illness. Based on the information from this assessment, I have several observations about obvious strengths that you have, several specific areas of concern about you, and a number of questions."

REMEMBER THAT INTERACTION IS INTERVENTION

Actively offering feedback to the patient and his or her loved ones regarding their styles of coping is an obvious event of psychosocial intervention. However, it is also important to remember that feedback is often given by default; the patient may attend as much to what is not said as to what is said during interactions with a health care provider.

For example, despite being preoccupied with certain issues or questions, patients often remain silent about these concerns during consultation with health care providers. Unaware of the patient's concerns, the provider may fail to address those particular topics during consultation. The patient may then interpret the provider's silence on these issues as confirmation of their worst imagined fears—all without uttering a word regarding their concerns.

This silent scenario can unfold with reference to virtually any aspect of rehabilitation, but it is especially prevalent regarding two concerns: sexual adjustments and substance abuse. Despite the fact that anxieties about sexual functioning are pervasive both for recovering cardiac patients and their loved ones, these concerns often go unaddressed—both by patients and providers—during routine medical or rehabilitation care (Papadopoulos, 1978; Papadopoulos, Larrimore, Cardin, & Shelley, 1980). As will be discussed in chapter 11, the result can be unnecessary, paralyzing fears and anxieties about postillness sexual activity. In addition, clinical experiences such as the one highlighted in the preceding chapter's case study of a recovering alcoholic have led me to believe that both patients and their loved ones often quietly monitor whether or not health care providers inquire about the patient's use of alcohol, nicotine, and other drugs. Here silence from the professional tends to be interpreted as permission to continue ongoing patterns of substance use.

Based on these observations, I recommend that your feedback to patients contain both questions and statements. Don't just deliver messages of concern based upon your observations; take the time and effort to also inquire about patients' concerns and fears and those of their loved ones.

RESPECT THAT THE PATIENT IS COPING IN A MANNER THAT MAKES SENSE TO HIM OR HER

Be respectful of the fact that everyone copes in ways that make sense to him or her. Remember that the question is whether the patient's coping style is "adaptive or maladaptive," not whether the patient is "right or wrong." Although an individual patient's coping style may not match our model of preferable behavior, that coping style might be working adaptively for the patient. For example, advice to a feisty patient about the importance of controlling hostility should be delivered with respect for the fact that research has documented that, in some cases, open expressions of anger—particularly if such correspond with a healthy "fighting attitude" toward not giving in to the illness—can be rehabilitation-enhancing (e.g., Derogatis, Abeloff, & Melisaratos, 1979; Greer, Morris, & Pettingale, 1979). Furthermore, feedback regarding Type A behavior patterns (TYABP) should be offered with respect for the evidence that postinfarction patients who evidence TYABP may survive longer than their Type B counterparts and that TYABP sometimes enhances response to formal cardiac rehabilitation (Ragland & Brand, 1988).

Kendall et al. (1979) pointed out that too quickly jumping to the teaching of coping strategies conveys the metamessage to patients that their own methods are not as useful as those being presented. The effect may be to unintentionally increase the patient's distress and interfere with his or her subsequent adjustment.

Before offering advice about new ways of coping, validate the positive benefits of the patient's and the family's predominant coping styles. At minimum, the positive intentions underlying ongoing coping efforts should be acknowledged.

A patient may be so urgent to rehabilitate that he proudly proclaims, "I know that you told me to exercise four times a week, but I want to speed this recovery up! So, I've been exercising at least three times each day." Validating the positive intention underlying this patient's misguided coping strategy is important as an entree into giving him constructive feedback: "I admire your commitment. With that kind of an attitude, I am confident you will do well in your rehabilitation. But let me offer a suggestion and a bit of information about how the exercise component of rehabilitation really works best."

A COPD patient might respond to advice to "Take it easy; pace yourself" with the report, "I've been taking it slow and easy, just like you said. In fact, I haven't been out of my house since I last saw you. Mainly, I've been sitting around, taking it easy."

The positive intention underlying this extreme reaction might be framed as "an obvious willingness to follow our recommendations" or "a nice initial effort."

Try to find in your patients' responses at least the germ of an attitude that will enhance rehabilitation. Once this underlying positive intention is validated (matched), the patient is more likely to respond to feedback about ways to structure more truly adaptive coping efforts.

SPEAK TO ISSUES THAT MATTER TO THE PATIENT NOW

It is difficult to resist the temptation to educate, Educate, EDUCATE! recovering cardiopulmonary patients. However, it should be clear by now that, no matter how profound or diagnostic, the findings from psychosocial assessments will not likely be perceived as relevant to the patient unless they are offered in terminology that matches the patient's psychological frame of reference.

The psychological frames of reference outlined in the stages of change theory (see list on page 49) can help clarify which forms of advice and feedback are most likely to be helpful to a given patient regarding a given rehabilitation issue. For example, action-oriented therapies are most effective with individuals who are in the preparation or action stages of change. However, these same intervention strategies may be ineffectual or detrimental to individuals in precontemplation or contemplation stages, during which feedback that raises cognitive and emotional awareness of the importance of attending to a targeted problem area are most effective. Here interventions such as confrontations, interpretations, bibliotherapy, and other consciousness-raising techniques that increase information about self, about the problem, and about the effects of the problem on the patient's loved ones are recommended.

SET GOALS

Official guidelines for both pulmonary and cardiac rehabilitation have emphasized the importance of goal setting in providing care to recovering patients. A legion of researchers in this area (e.g., Mayou, 1990) have emphasized that careful attention must be given to the specifics of patients' lives—individually and socially—in designing goals and evaluating the effects of interventions.

Goal setting can be difficult, given the passive/aggressive approach to rehabilitation evidenced by some patients. A COPD patient who was coerced by his pulmonologist and spouse into seeing me for smoking cessation once introduced himself to me with the statement, "I don't know why I'm here or who you are, but I understand that you are supposed to do something to me. So do it, and let's get it over with."

As mentioned previously, other patients are motivated to change in some ways but not motivated enough to address all of the important issues of comprehensive cardiopulmonary care. Often, these are the patients who are only willing to focus on establishing one major health behavior change at a time. In clinical practice, such patients are often found to be contemplating change in other areas of concern; they hope that changing the targeted concern will lead to a foundation of success and self-efficacy upon which further changes can be implemented.

Still other patients seem motivated to change in whole-scale ways, reasoning that modifying multiple risk factors requires no more effort than focusing on single areas of change. This is the approach of various whole-scale, intensive programs targeted toward regression of illness (e.g., Ornish et al., 1990).

Goal setting with an individual patient needs to be done with respect for the patient's personal motivations. Accordingly, rehabilitation recommendations should, where appropriate, be couched in terms that tie advice and

---

Form 3.1   Personal Goals Statement

Name _____ **Date** _____

People often come to health care centers with specific needs/goals they would like to meet. For example, one person may be concerned with losing weight or stopping smoking, whereas another may want to learn more about proper nutrition or how to manage stress in his/her life.

In an attempt to more fully understand these personal needs, please list them in the space provided below. (If you do not have any specific areas of need, you should indicate by writing "None" on the first line.)

1. _____

2. _____

3. _____

4. _____

5. _____

6. _____

7. _____

8. _____

information to any targeted behavior change for which the patient is preparing to take action.

The way we structure our initial rehabilitation recommendations at the Wake Forest University Cardiac Rehabilitation Program is an example of how this concept can be used. Upon entry into the program, each patient is asked to list three to five rehabilitation goals that are personally important to him or her. The form used for this is reproduced in Form 3.1.

Following comprehensive, multidisciplinary evaluations of the patient, staff members meet and decide how to best frame our collective recommendations, given the implications of our assessment data and the patient's stated goals.

For example, if a sedentary patient who is also a smoker indicates that her primary goal in attending rehabilitation is developing a lifetime exercise program, she might be instructed in exercise motivation strategies and told that stopping smoking will enhance the positive (and positively reinforcing) results of exercising.

Even patients who initially fail to specify personally meaningful goals can often be helped using the concept underlying this technique. The following case vignette demonstrates how this can be done.

Mrs. Rosenthal was a 58-year-old CABG patient who returned her Personal Goals Statement blank. Our multidisciplinary assessment data indicated that she was highly depressed and quite physically deconditioned. In addition, she admitted to smoking approximately one pack of cigarettes per day. Rather than ignoring her unsigned Personal Goals Statement during her feedback session, I chose to broach this topic in a quizzical manner that was respectful of her right to determine to what extent she was open to discussing her issues and motivations.

WMS: "I was wondering about your Personal Goals Statement. [holding up the blank form] Can you fill me in on this?"

Mrs. R: "Oh, yeah. That thing. I don't know. I just didn't know what to write."

WMS: "Yeah. Sometimes it's hard to figure out exactly what is most important when life is complicated."

Mrs. R: "Oh, God, how true, how true."

WMS: "You've been going through a rough time, haven't you?"

Mrs. R: "The roughest."

WMS: "I'm sorry that all of this has happened to you, Mrs. Rosenthal. I know that you have been coping as well as you can."

Mrs. R: [tearfully] "Well, I have been trying. But I just am not getting any better. I miss the way I used to be."

WMS: "I know. This is a hard time for you. Can you say some more about what you miss about the way you used to be?"

Mrs. R: "I just miss having energy. I don't have energy to do things like I used to, and it's messing my life up—mine and my husband's."

WMS: "Your husband's, too?"

Mrs. R: "Well, you know what I mean: our 'relationship.' I don't have any energy to do anything—not in the morning, not at night; no time. No energy for us; no energy for me. I didn't even plant my tomatoes this year, and I've been making a vegetable garden for 20 years. No energy."

WMS: "So it sounds like one thing you might want to get out of this program is some energy, right?"

Mrs. R: "Well, yeah. I guess so. I didn't think of that. But that is what I want: my energy back."

WMS: "If you got your energy back, then you could start enjoying your personal life more—in a lot of ways, right?"

Mrs. R: "I hope so."

WMS: "Enjoying your hobbies; enjoying your husband."

Mrs. R: "Yeah. And my husband enjoying me enjoying him." [laughs]

WMS: "It's nice that you and your husband care about what is going on between you. Some couples don't even notice each other."

Mrs. R: "Oh, not us. We notice each other. I just don't have energy enough to do the things we used to enjoy doing, especially in the bedroom."

WMS: "This is important stuff, Mrs. Rosenthal. You having energy enough to do the things that please you—including planting your tomatoes and making love to your husband—is important. Helping you find that energy is something that we can do. Would you like some ideas about what it might take to get back to the point where you can enjoy more?"

Mrs. R: "Yes, sir, I would . . . but I'm still not filling out that little form you keep holding up." [smiles]

WMS: "That's alright. We don't need the form. We just need to agree on what's important here. Now let's talk about things that might be taking energy away from you, and things that you might consider doing—now or later—to help get that energy back."

With this 2-minute conversation as a backdrop, Mrs. Rosenthal and I were then able to talk about the various "energy drainers" that were also important aspects of her rehabilitation: her depression, her smoking, and her lack of physical conditioning. My advice and feedback was couched in terms of the energy-boosting and sex-enhancing benefits that can come from a combination of smoking cessation, regular exercise, brief counseling, and use of antidepressant medications. Mrs. Rosenthal was not willing to pursue counseling or to stop smoking during her initial stage of rehabilitation, but she was open to immediate referral for evaluation of the need for antidepressant medication and she committed herself to giving regular exercise a 3-month trial. In short, speaking to issues that mattered to her was crucial in at least planting the seeds of motivation to change in ways that were important to this nice woman's overall rehabilitation.

The goal-setting process can be formal or informal. Formal strategies often incorporate the signing of behavior change contracts committed to by the patient. Where appropriate, help the patient identify both a long-term goal regarding the target concern and a tangible, measurable step that can be taken immediately and that begins the change process. Remind the patient that change often requires heroic efforts, and that his or her efforts deserve rewarding. Encourage the patient to identify intrinsic and extrinsic rewards to be associated with successful completion of this first step toward his or her broader goal. Then help the patient to specify people who might provide support during this process, and encourage him or her to ask for their help.

ASK WHAT WILL HAPPEN NEXT FOR THE PATIENT AND FAMILY

A significant percentage of recovering cardiopulmonary patients and their families feel ill-prepared for the long-range course of rehabilitation (Razin, 1982; Stanton et al., 1984). Clinical experience suggests that this statement applies especially to cardiac populations; many cardiac patients are symptom-free and have an unrealistically short-term view of the rehabilitation process. On the other hand, their symptoms typically force COPD patients into awareness of the lifelong nature of rehabilitation.

With this concern in mind, it is important to help patients and their loved ones realistically anticipate the hurdles they will face during the next phase of rehabilitation or family life, whatever that next phase may be for a given patient. It is important to emphasize that "rehabilitation is not an event with a clear beginning, middle, and ending; rehabilitation is a process that begins with the onset of illness and lasts for the rest of your life" (Sotile, 1992, p. 9).

SPECIFIC COMPONENTS
OF EFFECTIVE PSYCHOSOCIAL INTERVENTIONS

Effective agents of psychosocial change employ a combination of treatment strategies to match and then lead their patients into more adaptive areas of functioning. The factors discussed in the remainder of this chapter have been gleaned from a broad research that has examined what might be done to help heart and lung patients adapt to both acute and long-range coping demands. Although some of these strategies (e.g., manipulation of the patient's environment by the provider) apply specifically to dealing with inpatients, most can be applied across treatment settings and regardless of the psychosocial issue of concern. In addition, these strategies can be helpful regardless of the structure or level of intervention (e.g., crisis intervention, psychoeducational presentation to a group, individualized counseling).

INTERVENTION STRATEGY 1: THINK CRISIS INTERVENTION

Bearing in mind that patients can experience hospitalization, routine medical care, or entry into rehabilitation as a crisis-generating stressor, it is useful to consider crisis intervention theory. In overview, crisis intervention theory proposes that patients and their loved ones are helped to cope with crisis when they are proactively offered a combination of reassurance, advice, challenge to cope cooperatively together, and follow-up—all delivered during a series of brief therapeutic contacts that address the stressed person's current concerns and that use that person's current support systems (Caplan, 1964; Pimm & Feist, 1984). When possible, such intervention should begin by helping patients anticipate what will be encountered once they enter the stressful situation that is upcoming, a technique referred to as anticipatory guidance. Several factors should be kept in mind when structuring crisis intervention.

Normalize the Patient's Reactions and Your Interventions

In crisis counseling, interventions are framed in terms that are palatable to the patient and that address the crisis at hand. Avoid terms that are esoteric, threatening, or vague, and any exploration of psychological material that is not directly relevant to the crisis at hand. Simply normalize the patient's experience and then deliver the psychosocial intervention (or the recommendation to seek specialized intervention) within frames such as those offered in the following examples.

Framing Example 1: "Busy people like you can never get enough help in managing the stress that comes with so many roles and obligations. I'd like to talk with you about how you might look at stress from some new perspectives."

Framing Example 2: "Families who care about each other almost always struggle in the ways you folks are struggling. Let me suggest that you spend a little time with [name a referral source], who is an expert on family stress management."

Framing Example 3: "One of our goals is to help you get through this [hospitalization, medical treatment, or rehabilitation] as smoothly as possible. If it's acceptable to you, I'd like to talk with you about a few tools that we have found very helpful for patients who were facing some of the same problems you are currently facing."

Your judicious use of self-disclosure can be quite effective in both normalizing the patient's struggles and modeling adaptive ways of coping. The patient's concerns can be normalized by pointing out similarities between his or her current experience and one of your own relevant past experiences. An alternative to this strategy is to discuss the patient's concerns in light of similar experiences you have noted with many other patients. A further excerpt from the case of Mrs. Rosenthal demonstrates this point:

Mrs. R: "I'm sorry, but I'm just not ready to do all of this. I'm not going to lie to you. I'll go see my doctor about depression medicine, and I will come here regularly for the next 3 months to exercise. But I'm not going to say that I'll stop smoking; at least not yet."

WMS: "I sure do like your honesty, Mrs. Rosenthal. And I certainly do understand and respect what you are saying. In fact, in the 17 years that I've been counseling medical patients, I've noticed that the most successful patients tend to start out their rehabilitation just like you are starting—feeling anxious and overwhelmed about all of the changes they think they should make . . ."

Mrs. R: "Lord, that's the truth!"

WMS: "They wonder if they have energy enough to change anything . . ."

Mrs. R: "That's me."

WMS: "But they are courageous enough to commit to starting someplace by changing at least something . . ."

Mrs. R: "Well, I don't know about 'courageous' . . ."

WMS: "Once they get that something done, they then go on from there with a little more confidence . . ."

Mrs. R: "I hope so."

WMS: "My own experiences and the research in this area clearly show that what you are doing is the way that many successful rehabilitation patients go about changing. They take one or two steps at a time, but they are willing to really commit to following through with those first steps."

Mrs. R: "Well, I don't know if it will help, but I will do what I said I'd do."

WMS: "Great. You've got the right attitude about this. You are dynamite, Mrs. Rosenthal."

Mrs. R: "No, I'm not. I'm just tired of being tired." [smiles]

Make the Intervention Relevant

Patients tend to be more adherent to rehabilitation recommendations if time is taken to explain how the proposed intervention relates to the goals of rehabilitation. In short, the goals of the treatment intervention (e.g., teaching the patient to physically relax, to better negotiate conflict with a loved one, or to stop smoking) need to be justified as being related to the patient's dual tasks of coping with the stressors at hand and progressing in long-range rehabilitation.

For example, a stress management intervention that revolves around teaching relaxation strategies for patients anticipating surgery should be framed as treatment that has been found to help recovery from surgery progress with fewer complications and with less pain. Or coaching a Type A patient in the differences between assertive and aggressive behaviors should be prefaced with information about the importance to health of curbing hostility and aggressive behaviors.

INTERVENTION STRATEGY 2: PROVIDE SUPPORT AND COUNSELING

There are many ways to provide patients with support and counseling. During the preoperative period, something as simple as roommate assignment can be important in promoting physical and emotional adjustments for cardiac patients facing surgery. Kulik and Mahler (1987) demonstrated that patients hospitalized for upcoming CABG benefited from room assignment with a postoperative CABG patient. Benefits included less anxiety and earlier ambulation and discharge.

You can also provide patients with direct, supportive counseling. This is done by soliciting the patient's concerns; reflecting back to the patient an awareness of his or her concerns; normalizing the patient's fears; and offering reassurance. Such supportive counseling prior to medical or surgical intervention is not only the compassionate, humane thing to do; it is also a wise way to practice your profession. Research has shown that medical care that incorporates brief supportive counseling leads to shorter stays in CCU and the hospital, less emotional distress, and fewer arrhythmias when compared to routine CCU care (Gruen, 1975; Schindler et al., 1989). In the general medical population, even a single supportive interview delivered on the evening before surgery has been found to lessen postoperative psychosis (Layne & Yudofsky, 1971). In addition, during both hospitalization and outpatient rehabilitation, supportive counseling of family members of patients has been shown not only to soothe the family but also to enhance the family's support of the recovering patient (Sotile, Sotile, Sotile, & Ewen, 1993).

Various forms of support are more or less effective at different stages of the recovery process. Knowing what kind of support to provide and when to provide it is crucial. For example, although CABG patients benefit preoperatively from informational discussion with a recovered CABG patient, they are most helped postoperatively by emotional support from family and friends, not by information (King, 1985).

There are no definitive guidelines for structuring supportive interventions. However, I offer the following brief overview of literature that has examined this issue as food for your own thoughts and experiences in this area.

Support Through the Stages of Recovery

Both patients and spouses tend to emphasize cognitive needs and deemphasize affective needs in the early convalescent phase of recovery (Orzeck & Staniloff, 1987). Immediately beyond the crisis of hospitalization, intimacy seems to be an important form of support for both patients and their loved ones. But in some ways, intimacy-type support also seems to reach a point of limited effectiveness. For example, Fontana, Kerns, Rosenberg, and Colonese (1989) found that during the first 6 months after hospitalization, intimacy was influential in ameliorating the effects of threats and distress and thereby lessening symptoms of dyspnea and angina, even though over the second half of the first year of recovery, threat overwhelmed the protective effects of intimacy. The authors concluded that the period immediately after hospitalization may not be the best time to get a patient to modify risk behaviors. Rather, this might be a time when the patient needs maximal emotional support, caring, and reassurance. In a thoughtful analysis, Antonucci and Johnson (1994) pointed out the need for understanding social support as an evolving, dynamic factor in the course of rehabilitation.

Some support relationships may be an asset at one point in the disease continuum but not another. Being warm and loving may shelter or insulate an individual with predisposing factors to cardiovascular disease, because it minimizes the impact of stress. It may also be very helpful post-cardiac event. On the other hand, such a network may be detrimental to the long-term rehabilitation of an individual if it encourages dependency. Similarly, multifaceted, extended networks may be more helpful when one is recovering from a cardiac event by connecting the patient with others who have experienced similar health crises or who can help facilitate life style changes. (p. 34)

Dhooper (1990) proposed a simple way of estimating the support needs of recovering cardiopulmonary patients. During crisis, people need emotional support. As rehabilitation progresses, so do the degrees of personal and relational changes, and coping with such transitions is aided by cognitive support for grasping the meaning of the changes experienced. Because long-term rehabilitation may lead to deficit state stresses (i.e., the person's life is defined by chronically excessive demands), material aid and direct action are needed to provide support that helps remedy the imbalance between needs and resources.

Finally, the family systems perspective on cardiopulmonary rehabilitation reminds us that, depending upon stage of life and family dynamics, different family members may at once need different forms of support and be asked to provide various forms of support to each other. For example, the spouse of a recovering MI patient may need information to enhance his or her sense of control of the rehabilitation process but may also be facing requests (or demands) to provide emotional support to the recovering patient and to other family members who have been frightened by the patient's illness.

The point is that here, too, interventions need to be individualized based on an appraisal of the specific needs of the targeted individuals. Failing to do so runs the risk of mismatching support efforts and the patient's or family members' needs. Studies of distressed individuals who retrospectively appraised the supportive efforts delivered by others have documented that if efforts to provide support mismatch the stressed individual's needs, these very efforts to be supportive prove to be stressful, not soothing to the already stressed individual.

For example, Lehman, Ellard, and Wortman (1986) found that bereaved persons were more stressed than soothed by certain forms of "supportive" input: patented reassurance; unsubstantiated remarks to the effect that "I know how you feel"; minimization of the crisis; forced cheerfulness; or provision of unwanted tangible support during this time of emotional need.

Support Throughout the Stages of Change

The forgoing observations underscore the importance of bearing in mind who the person in need of support is and what constitutes support for that person, given that person's current situation. Amick and Ockene (1994) discussed the varying roles of social support in modifying risk factors within the stages of change theory discussed above. Types of social support activities that facilitate movement from one stage to the next during the process of changing are as follows:

Support Through the Stages of Change
Precontemplation

- Encourage person to adopt a more socially acceptable, healthy lifestyle.

- Provide information to increase awareness of the impact of lifestyle behaviors on health.

Contemplation

- Encourage activities that increase awareness of the problem behavior, its impact on health and quality of life, how to change the behavior, and the benefits of changing.
- Give feedback to increase positive affect to avoid the effect of negative self-image.
- Direct attention to messages and symbols of greater social acceptance of a healthy lifestyle.
- Encourage efforts to resolve conflicts arising from greater awareness of the problem behavior by attempting to change the behavior.

Action

- Encourage focusing on past successes of changing the problem behavior or other troublesome behaviors to increase self-efficacy.
- Provide rewards for avoiding the targeted behavior and encourage self-rewards.
- Assist in activities that are not compatible with the problem behavior.
- Assist in removing objects in the person's environment that trigger the problem behavior.
- Encourage the person to express feelings regarding the behavior and the consequences of changing. Encourage the person to view his/her new behavior and changing self-image in a positive light.

Maintenance

- Remind the person of his/her prior condition before the problem behavior or encourage other activities that he/she might enjoy that are not compatible with the problem behavior.
- Remind the person to avoid cues that might trigger a relapse.
- Remind the person of current success in changing.

Relapse

- Help the person avoid getting distressed if relapse occurs.
- Remind the person of the reasons why he/she wanted to change in the first place.
- Avoid situations that might encourage the person to continue the problem behavior.
- Appeal to the person's sensitivity to his/her role as a model to others. Remind the person of the availability of special people who can be a resource.

Note. From "The Role of Social Support in the Modification of Risk Factors for Cardiovascular Disease," in *Social Support and Cardiovascular Disease* by T.L. Amick and J.K. Ockene, 1994, S.A. Shumaker and S.M. Czajkowski (Eds.) (p. 266). New York: Plenum Press. Copyright 1994 by Plenum Press. Adapted with permission.

Support during the early stages of change (precontemplation and contemplation) should emphasize cognitive processes, whereas more support for behavioral processes is most appropriate in the later stages of change (action and maintenance). Amick and Ockene (1994) pointed out that although little is known about how to influence precontemplators to make health behavior changes, it may be that coaching a person's support system in ways to exert influence during a health crisis will, because of the targeted individual's need for belonging, promote movement to the contemplation stage of change for a given health behavior. For example, a cardiopulmonary patient who is in precontemplation for smoking cessation might be motivated to move to the next stage of change if peer influence indicates that, now that this health problem has developed, the old behavior (i.e., smoking) is not as acceptable in his or her social network as it once was.

In the contemplation stage, network ties may be important as sources of information and consciousness raising, through both discussion and role modeling. This effect can be promotive of either positive or negative health behaviors, depending upon the norms regarding a given health behavior evidenced by the social network.

During the action stage, the interplay between the changer's behaviors and the reactions of supportive others is crucial in either promoting or sabotaging change attempts. As will be discussed in chapter 8, it is important at this stage to review the role that health behaviors may play in regulating relationship factors such as inclusion, control, or affection.

Finally, during the maintenance and relapse stages of change, social support can be offered in various direct and indirect ways: minimization of interpersonal and environmental stressors; conveying high expectations for success; and bolstering confidence to reimplement change during backslides.

Being an agent of support for recovering patients and their families is integral to providing effective cardiopulmonary care. Regardless of the stage of recovery or the stage of change, two facts about social support are important to bear in mind: (a) the mere perception that sufficient help is available from others if one needs to turn to another during a time of need is crucial in deriving benefits from social support (Wethington & Kessler, 1986); and (b) one's degree of satisfaction with the available support has much to do with well-being (Sarason et al., 1983). At minimum, you should regularly reassure patients and their loved ones of your concern and availability (within realistic limits) for offering various forms of support, and you should regularly inquire regarding their degree of satisfaction with the support that is available to them.

INTERVENTION STRATEGY 3:
INCREASE THE SENSE OF CONTROL

As will be discussed in chapter 4, patients cope better if they feel reasonably in control of their coping process. Three specific examples of how to increase the individual's sense of control are empowering the patient to be physically active and involved in his or her rehabilitation; coaching in the recall of effective coping strategies; and encouraging rehearsal.

Encourage Control Over Physical Factors

In both inpatient and outpatient settings, the enhanced sense of self-efficacy that comes with physical movement or exercise has been shown to benefit overall psychosocial adjustments for both COPD (Toshima, Kaplan, & Ries, 1992) and cardiac patients (Oldridge & Rogowski, 1990). Patients not yet able to exercise can be helped to develop a sense of control over the recovery process by instructing them in physical activities to perform after surgery that might improve flexibility and minimize postsurgical discomfort (Pimm & Feist, 1984).

In addition, manipulating environmental factors and allowing and encouraging the patient to be actively involved in the recovery process can have pronounced positive effects on the postoperative clinical course. For example, Cromwell et al. (1987) found that CCU patients who received a great deal of information about their condition and who were then placed in a stimulating environment or played an active role in their treatment were transferred from the CCU earlier and discharged from the hospital sooner than were patients who received similar educational interventions but who were placed in a dull recovery room environment in which they played a passive role. In the words of the authors: "It is unhelpful when patients are simply left to lie and worry" (Cromwell et al., 1987, p. 452).

In addition, research with gall bladder surgery patients (Ulrich, 1984) found that simply having a postsurgical room with a view of a parklike setting was associated with a shorter hospital stay (by nearly 1 day), less postsurgical narcotic use, and fewer postoperative complications.

Finally, research summarized by Ornstein and Sobel (1987) has documented that the effects of high versus low levels of environmental stimulation vary depending upon individual differences in psychological and physiological variables. A simple intervention in this regard is questioning the patient about what he or she finds most soothing and, where possible, matching the patient's preferences for stimulation level. Ideally, such individual differences should be considered in both the preparation and postsurgical periods of care.

Help the Patient and His or Her Loved Ones Access Already-Existing, Effective Coping Strengths and Strategies

Although the coping demands that come with illness are unique in the experiences of many patients, it is also true that adaptive coping seldom involves doing anything esoteric. Most of our patients have well-developed coping repertoires; they enter our treatment facilities with coping tools that have served them well throughout their lives and that can enhance their sense of control in managing the tasks of rehabilitation. However, given the uniqueness of the challenges that face them, patients and their loved ones often need to be reminded to use their already-existing, effective coping capabilities.

This can be done by simply asking the targeted individuals (patient and/or loved ones) about past times in which they faced the same or similar circumstances, and then helping them frame the past experience as one from which certain valuable lessons were learned. Where appropriate, point out that he or she was able to cope with such experiences as childbirth, a medical crisis of a loved one, or prior attempts to change some health behavior such as smoking. Emphasize that even if these experiences were stressful or traumatic, he or she did, in fact, survive and therefore accumulated a degree of coping experience with a variation of the stress currently being faced. In this way, confidence in the ability to cope with the current stressor can be bolstered.

Encourage Rehearsal

An effective way to enhance self-efficacy for coping is to rehearse adaptive coping strategies. This can be done both cognitively and behaviorally. Engaging the patient in discussion and education can provide cognitive rehearsal. Another simple form of cognitive rehearsal is systematic desensitization. Instruct the patient to imagine the anxiety-producing cues associated with the upcoming stressor and to then imagine using positive coping tools (such as relaxation) as the stressful situation unfolds in imagery. Research has shown that patient distress subsequent to a variety of medical procedures can be lessened through the use of various forms of psychological rehearsal, including the provision of detailed advice regarding ways to cope with an upcoming medical stressor and its consequences (Kendall et al., 1979).

Behavioral rehearsal, in which the patient is instructed to actually practice the coping skills that are being taught, is the logical next step. As discussed previously, even brief periods (e.g., 2 days) of such practice can be quite effective in enhancing coping responses to acute medical stressors.

In simple terms, the patient should be encouraged to replace maladaptive coping strategies with adaptive ones. The adaptive strategies may involve coping mechanisms that the patient already knows about and has been encouraged to access, or the patient may be helped to develop and use new coping tools such as those to be discussed in the following pages. This does not necessarily require lengthy counseling. In clinical practice, conversational interventions such as the following are often profoundly helpful.

"So, Mrs. Landry, I guess I won't be seeing you again until tomorrow, after your surgery. Remember, even though you will feel some pain when you wake up, as all of us women know, few things are as painful as what you have already gone through: it takes someone with stamina to give birth to four babies like you have! Just as when you delivered your babies years ago, recovering from this surgery will take a while. But remember to use your breathing techniques and the relaxation tape. Also, try to remember what you learned in the tape we showed you about the ways to move your body after surgery. More than anything, I want you to know that you won't be alone. We will be here taking care of you. Even though you won't be able to speak with us directly, we will be communicating with you regularly, and we will help you through this."

INTERVENTION STRATEGY 4: EDUCATE

Education has become a tenet of comprehensive medical care. Both research and clinical experience suggest that educating a patient about his/her disease and treatment is a crucial factor in promoting adherence to medical recommendations. Teaching health management techniques to both inpatients and outpatients has become an integral aspect of comprehensive cardiopulmonary rehabilitation, and has been shown to be a key element in promoting a wide range of risk factor changes such as smoking cessation, control of hypercholesterolemia, lowered blood pressures, and enhanced levels of physical exercise (Ott et al., 1983; Sivarajan Froelicher, 1989). Educating the patient and his or her loved ones regarding what is to come in the course of hospitalization or rehabilitation may also be one of the most effective methods of increasing a sense of control over the coping process (Mumford et al., 1982).

Exactly why does education work to promote more adaptive coping in recovering cardiopulmonary patients and their loved ones? The literature is filled with both controversies and practical guidelines about this question.

Education Is Not Always Enough

Blindly delivering patented educational information with no regard for the patient's current stage of receptivity may, in some instances, reduce patient anxieties and help alleviate depression (Miller et al., 1990). But many researchers have argued that education, in itself, does not promote lasting behavior change. For example, several investigations demonstrated that simply providing health education material on CHD risk factors does not promote change in coronary risk profiles over a 12-month period (Lovibond et al., 1985). It has also been stressed that, in addition to education, truly effective psychosocial interventions incorporate skill building for habit change (Carmody, Fey, Pierce, Connor, & Matarazzo, 1982).

This last recommendation was echoed in the AACVPR position paper regarding pulmonary rehabilitation: "In addition to knowledge, most patients require specific, individual strategies for changing behavior along with encouragement, practice, and positive feedback" (Ries, 1990, p. 83). Indeed, evaluations of the effect of education for patients with COPD have generally indicated that health education does not significantly impact any measure of health status in this population, including measures of symptom status, physical function, or overall psychosocial functioning (Howland, Nelson, Barlow, et al., 1986).

A few investigations have actually reported negative effects from educational interventions with recovering cardiopulmonary patients. For example, in a controlled investigation, Dracup et al. (1986) found that teaching cardiopulmonary resuscitation (CPR) training to family members of cardiac patients at risk of sudden death actually elevated the levels of anxiety and depression, both for the heart patients and their spouses, over a 6-month follow-up. The authors theorized that the health education intervention heightened tension, and they emphasized the importance of following educational interventions with support sessions that facilitate adaptive integration of the information presented. In an important subsequent study, these same researchers (Dracup, Taylor, Guzy, & Brecht, 1991) found that a single nursing discussion of psychological issues following CPR training eliminated what earlier (Dracup et al., 1986) had been found to be the distressful outcomes from the training.

Similar findings have been reported in a study that evaluated the effects of a community-based education program that combined didactic presentations, demonstrations of self-help skills, and group discussion regarding ways to deal with various psychosocial aspects of COPD (Ashikaga, Vacek, & Lewis, 1980). This intervention was compared to the effects of a control condition that involved providing only written material to subjects. In addition to noting that treatment enhanced subjects' knowledge of COPD following intervention, the authors also expressed concern that control subjects showed a false expectation of improvement. The authors emphasized the importance of providing counseling in the proper interpretation of educational material presented.

The Benefits of Education, When It Does Work

On the positive side, an educational intervention can serve as a desensitizing experience. As mentioned above, education can provide a successful, cognitive, "dry run" experience with the medical procedure to be faced (Kendall et al., 1979). Increased knowledge may also serve to lessen anxiety by diminishing the likelihood that the situation being faced will overload the individual's coping repertoire. The importance of how such education is framed is underscored concisely by Kersten's (1990a) discussion of how COPD patients can be motivated:

> To help the patient with COPD increase or sustain motivation, enthusiastic, dedicated, and caring staff members might implement the conceptual motivational model thoroughly described by Craig and Craig (1979) and Kersten (1989). In brief, according

> to this model, motivation is developed when a person sees a discrepancy between his or her present state and anticipated future state. This discrepancy or difference between the present and future is called a motivating gap. The goal of psychologic intervention is to help the patient develop a motivating gap so that the patient has a goal, sees alternatives, and can choose the action best for himself or herself. (p. 457)

In other words, one purpose of education is to create a motivating gap by helping the patient formulate alternatives to his or her current way of coping.

SUMMARY

For patients to be helped to cope better, their existing coping strategies and frames of reference must be understood. Recommendations must be framed in terms that match their goals, concerns, and idiosyncratic ways of approaching rehabilitation. Psychosocial interventions are most effective if they are presented with respect of the crises that illness and rehabilitation may cause and the support needs of patients and their loved ones. Successful interventions at once increase the targeted individuals' sense of control of the coping process and educate them regarding effective coping strategies. Effective Emotional Management is an integrative model for structuring practical psychosocial interventions with respect for these factors.

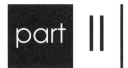

part II

THE EFFECTIVE EMOTIONAL
MANAGEMENT MODEL

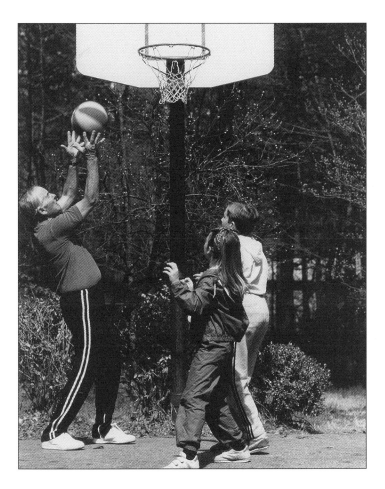

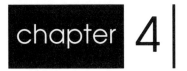

chapter 4 |

EFFECTIVE EMOTIONAL MANAGEMENT

A MODEL FOR STRUCTURING PRACTICAL PSYCHOSOCIAL INTERVENTIONS IN MEDICAL SETTINGS

In the pages that follow, my Effective Emotional Management (EEM) model for structuring practical psychosocial interventions in treating medical patients will be described. The EEM model was born of an attempt to answer a timely question: Based on existing research and clinical experience, what differentiates recovering cardiopulmonary patients who thrive from those who struggle with the tasks of living with their illnesses?

The importance of this topic has been recognized with the upsurge of attention being paid to the flip side of the stress research model that has dominated our thinking about emotions and illness since the 1950s: We are now turning attention away from redundant explorations of the undisputed fact that stress can have harmful effects on health to an emphasis on the importance of the link between positive emotions and health enhancement and stress hardiness. In truth, many people are able to thrive under high levels of objectively and subjectively measured stress. In fact, many cardiopulmonary patients and their loved ones report that the stresses of rehabilitation stir them to new levels of individual and family health and happiness.

THE ELEMENTS OF EEM

In my model, thriving individuals are described as being "effective emotional managers" because, as will be shown, in addition to managing stress per se, they also effectively manage their personality-based and family-level coping patterns. The defining characteristics of the EEM process are depicted in Figure 4.1.

As shown in Figure 4.1, the core of this model hinges on five factors:

1. Managing the physiological and psychological consequences of stress
2. Learning and using an effective method of relaxation
3. Controlling personality-based coping patterns
4. Managing marital and family issues
5. Controlling cognitive frames of reference

The EEM model borrows a key concept from the burgeoning research regarding stress hardiness and an overwhelmingly frequent observation in my own clinical experiences: nurturance benefits one's ability to make and maintain positive emotional, behavioral, and health changes (Pearlin & Johnson, 1977; Pearlin, Menaghan, Lieberman, & Mullan, 1981). Subsequent discussions of the cognitive element in stress hardiness (chapter 9) and of social support, well-being, and marriage and family life (chapter 8) will detail this observation. As will be shown, ample clinical and empirical data have suggested that patients who are best able to cope with the demands of daily living are those who maintain self-efficacious attitudes and live in environments and social networks that bolster them in many ways: their sense of worth is supported; the perception of their ability to cope with what faces them is enhanced; and cooperation with their efforts to change in healthy ways leads to greater flexibility in coping styles (Waltz, 1986).

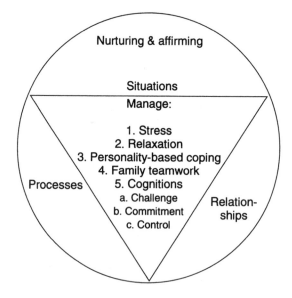

Figure 4.1 The Effective Emotional Management model.

In simple terms, the EEM model proposes that stress hardiness is enhanced when the "territory" within which an individual lives provides a reasonable "fit" between two broad factors: (a) the daily demands that come with living in that territory; and (b) the individual's inner needs, wants, and values. In the EEM model, this life territory is defined by three factors: the situations, processes, and relationships that fill the person's life.

Situations refers to the places in which the individual spends the time of his or her life: job, community, rehabilitation setting, church, clubs, and so on. Encompassed here are many of the factors typically referred to as "social support" within the health literature.

As the name implies, the relationship factor refers to the interpersonal relations that fill the individual's life. Included here are relationships with colleagues, acquaintances, family, intimate loved ones, friends, and health care providers.

Processes refers to the ways in which the individual cares for him- or herself, physically, psychologically, emotionally, and spiritually. Encompassed in the process factor are the typical "stress management" topics, such as exercise, thinking patterns, nutritional choices, and so on. Also, in EEM, patients are taught to pinpoint the steps in various of their coping processes. They are coached in ways to disrupt problematic coping progressions by making more adaptive cognitive, behavioral, physiological, or interpersonal choices. Here coping patterns are explained as being analogous to dominoes stacked on edge that are tipped by a stressor. The resultant coping process can be seen to unfold in fairly predictable steps, with each coping step serving to stir the next. Accordingly, stressors and attempted efforts to cope perpetuate certain ways of thinking, behaving, interacting with others, and so on until the last "domino" falls, creating the stress symptom.

In EEM, once such a sequence is identified, the patient is encouraged to substitute some adaptive coping strategy for at least one of the dominos in the progression. As will be shown in the pages that follow, this might involve a simple change in behavior (e.g., "At that point, when you notice the tension building, you might take 5 minutes to practice the relaxation technique that we discussed, rather than reaching for another cup of coffee."). Or a more complex psychosocial intervention might be necessary (e.g., "So, it seems clear that your anger outbursts signal a stirring of several factors: a sense of insecurity, thoughts of persecution—as though the other person is purposefully doing something to irritate you—and hyperphysiological reactions. At such times, I think it might be useful to do three things: (a) remember the information on personality-based coping patterns and their corresponding underlying needs; (b) use your 'coping with anger' self-statements sheet; and (c) practice the quick relaxation exercise we discussed.").

At its most fundamental level, the goal of EEM is to create and maintain situations, processes, and relationships that are fundamentally nurturing and affirming and to either weed out of one's life those that are toxic (i.e., those that yield a deep sense of distress and ill-being) or find ways to lessen the toxic effects of these factors. With a reasonably nurturing life territory in place, managing the core-level factors of the EEM model (physiological stress reactions; the ability to relax; personality-based coping patterns; family relationships; and cognitive habits) is facilitated.

EEM AND CARDIOPULMONARY CARE

Control of the sort promoted by EEM training can greatly facilitate making changes in any of the areas specifically important to cardiopulmonary rehabilitation. Figure 4.2 depicts the various aspects of psychosocial functioning that are important in cardiopulmonary care and that can be aided by attending to the key factors and processes of EEM.

Details regarding the individual components of comprehensive psychosocial adjustment to cardiopulmonary illness will fill the remaining chapters of this book. The information that follows should be considered against a unifying concept: An overriding goal of psychosocial intervention with recovering cardiopulmonary patients is to help patients and their loved ones realize that they are not alone and that they can learn to face the challenge of coping with rehabilitation successfully. In many ways, effective psychosocial

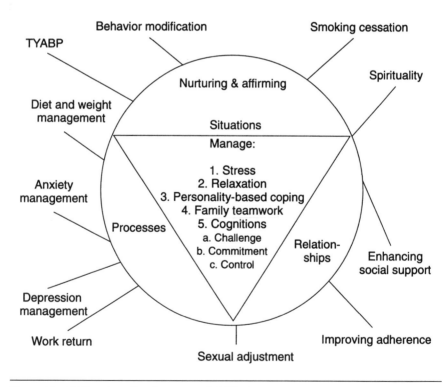

Figure 4.2   EEM and cardiopulmonary rehabilitation.

interventions provide nurturing "fencing" for patients and their significant others, while promoting a sense of control over the coping process they face. Support comes in many forms, in hospital, office-based, and formal rehabilitation settings.

Perhaps the most fundamental form of support is reflective listening: the patient's concerns are responded to with a compassionate statement that indicates awareness of the feelings or concerns being expressed. Formal support group programs make use of reflective listening coupled with practical advice that surfaces from patient discussions. Special efforts can also be made to provide supportive interventions directly to the patient and/or family (Gorkin, Follick, Wilkin, & Niaura, 1994). Staff support can take many forms, ranging from conveying information, to offering soothing touch, or to elaborate psychosocial interventions.

A readily available form of staff support—and a way to enhance coping control—is providing information and reassurance to concerned patients and family members. As mentioned previously, research has repeatedly documented that both cardiopulmonary patients and their family members clearly desire more information about the patients' recommended general activity level, sexual activity, and anticipated course of recovery than is typically given during the delivery of medical care (Bramwell, 1986; Papadopoulos et al., 1980; Thompson & Cordle, 1988). Both patients and family members have also repeatedly expressed a need for more reassurance from health care providers that the needs of their loved ones are being responded to (O'Malley & Menke, 1988; Sirles & Selleck, 1989).

THE IMPORTANCE OF EEM
IN CARDIOPULMONARY CARE

The importance of heath care providers conveying warmth, caring, and support has been emphasized in research spanning cardiac and pulmonary populations (Agle & Baum, 1977; Connors & Hilling, 1993). Some researchers have suggested that merely spending time with or attending to the needs of a patient will lead to enhanced compliance with rehabilitation recommendations due to the supportive factor that such attention provides (Atkins, Kaplan, Timms, Reinsch, & Loftback, 1984). In fact, it has even been shown that COPD patients given the minimal support provided from being included in a study but relegated to the delayed treatment control group improved on measures of psychological status during the 4-month delay until treatment began (Cockcroft, Sanders, & Berry, 1981). Even brief telephone follow-ups or caring inquiries regarding behavior change programs or behavior change diaries have been shown to provide significant support for both cardiac and pulmonary patients (Blake et al., 1990; Frasure-Smith & Prince, 1989; Gift et al., 1992).

Lynch, Thomas, Paskewitz, Katcher, and Weir (1977) showed that human contact from routine nursing care was associated with a significant reduction of premature ventricular contraction (PVC) rates, especially among patients with higher rates of PVCs (i.e., more than 3 ectopic beats/min). Weiss (1990) pointed out that a number of subsequent investigations (e.g., Longworth, 1982; Wakim, 1980) have documented that comforting touch (having the sole purpose of alleviating distress) is associated with reductions in physiological arousal and decreased anxiety. In her own empirical investigation of the effects of different forms of touching on 59 hospitalized CHD patients, Weiss found that both comforting touching (e.g., patting the patient's foot or hand while conversing, or holding the patient's hand while a medical procedure is being performed) and procedural touching (e.g., listening to the patient's chest with a stethoscope, checking the patient's blood pressure and pulse rate, checking the site of intravenous insertion, or adjusting the patient's oxygen mask) evoked heart rate deceleration in contrast to both baseline and conversational interactions with the patients. Specifically, diastolic blood pressure and state anxiety were lowered as a result of touching.

LEVELS OF PSYCHOSOCIAL INTERVENTION

Providing meaningful intervention within any level of the EEM model does not necessarily require that a busy professional find extensive time in an already overfilled work week. Psychosocial interventions can be addressed in a variety of ways and to varying degrees in hospital, office, and rehabilitation settings. Using the following continuum of care levels, any of the important areas of risk modification and psychosocial adjustment in cardiopulmonary rehabilitation can be effectively addressed, even if only briefly.

At Level I: General information regarding selected psychosocial issues is made available, either passively or in reaction to patient requests. Examples of Level I interventions include passively providing information regarding psychosocial issues through printed materials; or briefly mentioning relevant psychosocial issues during face-to-face delivery of some aspect of care (such as discharge planning).

At Level II: Detailed information is presented in a general psychoeducational format. Examples here might include: lectures; video- or audiotaped presentations regarding varying psychosocial issues; and presentation of general information regarding the availability of more specialized psychosocial interventions (e.g., lists of places to go for help in each of the areas of concern).

At Level III: Information and advice specific to a given patient's psychosocial needs are offered. Such intervention is based upon direct communication with the patient and his or her loved ones regarding their personal questions and concerns. Here the patient and, where possible and appropriate, the patient's spouse or significant other are seen briefly to (a) offer advice regarding the importance of the issue under consideration; (b) emphasize the importance of relationship cooperation in management of the issue; and (c) address any idiosyncratic concerns relevant to the issue (e.g., concerns regarding the effects of the patient's medication regimen on the psychosocial issue or concerns regarding family-level beliefs about rehabilitation recommendations).

At Level IV: In addition to providing tailored information, the health care worker proactively questions the patient and, where appropriate, the patient's significant others regarding their specific concerns, their reactions to the illness, their reactions to medical or rehabilitation advice, and their psychosocial adjustments. Here a counseling session is orchestrated, geared toward inquiring, identifying problems, and offering brief advice. Reactions to counseling are then monitored in follow-up sessions. If improvement in the targeted area of concern is not manifested within several sessions, referral is made for more specialized intervention.

At Level V: Systematic assessment, planned intervention, and extended follow-up are used. This level requires considerably more time commitment and more sophisticated counseling skill than prior levels and should only be attempted by health care providers who have received at least moderate training in the delivery of the intervention being provided. Here information is gleaned regarding the biopsychosocial factors that contribute to the difficulty being addressed, advice is offered regarding ways to modify behavior, and systematic follow-up is implemented to reassess and further tailor interventions. Such care can occur either in a multisession group format or in individual consultations delivered over several months. Referral for more specialized services is an option throughout treatment at this level. An example of a Level V intervention would be a six-session stress management class.

At Level VI: Interventions are delivered by mental health professionals who have received specialized training. How to select appropriate professionals for this level of intervention will be discussed in more detail in chapter 14.

SUMMARY

The Effective Emotional Management model encompasses several factors that are crucial in promoting positive psychosocial adaptation. These factors are understanding and controlling psychological and physiological stress reactions; learning to relax; controlling personality-based coping patterns; managing marital and family issues; and controlling cognitive frames of reference. Commonsense advice about the core components of this model can serve as the foundation for promoting both positive coping and enhanced adherence with medical recommendations. Details regarding ways to intervene in each of the foundation factors in EEM and for structuring positive, nurturing interventions fill the chapters in this section.

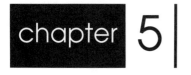

chapter 5

THE PHYSIOLOGY
AND PSYCHOLOGY OF STRESS

For obvious reasons, cardiopulmonary patients are concerned about the physiological consequences and correlates of their stress reactions. Mental stress response can trigger myocardial ischemia in CHD patients (Howell & Krantz, 1994; Rozanski et al., 1988) and impair pulmonary functioning in COPD patients (Dudley, Glaser, Jorgenson, & Logan, 1980). Many cardio-pulmonary patients assume that mismanaged stress either caused or will complicate their illness. My own anecdotal experience suggests that approximately 50% of patients who enter a formal cardiopulmonary program list the desire to learn to better manage stress as one of their prime motivations for entering rehabilitation.

Failing to provide information in this realm runs the risk of seriously mismatching concerns that are highly relevant to the patient and his or her loved ones. On the other hand, as will be seen, offering commonsense explanations of stress physiology and its emotional correlates can be a non-threatening way to match and then lead patients into needed areas of self-examination, such as their personality-based, stress-complicating coping patterns; their marital/family-based concerns; or their needs for changing exercise, diet, or other health behaviors—all in the name of quieting potentially dangerous stress reactions.

For these reasons, the first component of EEM with cardiopulmonary patients is explaining the physiology of the stress response and its various emotional concomitants. I recommend incorporating three commonsense explanations of physiological and emotional consequences and correlates of the stress response into EEM training.

EEM COMPONENT 1A:
EXPLAIN THE FLIGHT-OR-FIGHT SYNDROME

The flight-or-fight syndrome is the body's version of emergency response. It consists of a series of sympathetic activities marked by increases in circulating catecholamines and their consequences (Cannon, 1929). This reflexive "kicking into overdrive" in response to stress entails a series of physiological events that are inbred into every species of animal. The flight-or-fight response is triggered by any circumstance that is interpreted as being threatening, harmful, or demanding. Obviously, daily life is filled with such circumstances: threats to one's well-being; demands to change or adjust; or the perception that the circumstance being faced might override one's ability to cope comfortably. At such times, the adrenal medulla releases catecholamines and begins a series of alarm reactions that can have important consequences for cardiopulmonary patients: heart rate increases; more blood flows into the large body muscles as blood flow is shunted away from the liver and other internal organs; the peripheral vascular system constricts; and breathing patterns change from rhythmic to shallow.

Because more blood gets pumped into smaller spaces, this alarm reaction essentially creates a situation of momentarily elevated blood pressure. Although momentary elevation of blood pressure during stressful times does not typically create physical problems (Eliot & Breo, 1984), repeated activation of the fight-or-flight response and the concomitant failure to fully disengage this response with effective coping strategies has been said to be a major contributor to the etiology of essential hypertension and its sequelae (Farquhar, 1987).

In counseling cardiopulmonary patients, key points regarding the flight-or-fight syndrome can be conveyed in the following way:

"Fight or flight is your body's 'overdrive.' During fight or flight reactions, blood is forced away from your skin, liver, and digestive tract and redirected to your heart, lungs, and large muscles. This is your body's way of preparing you to literally fight or flee—you don't want blood near your skin, in case you get cut during the fight; and you need blood pumping through your large muscles to help you fight or run. Of course, the problem is that as we live civilized, responsible lives, we seldom fight or flee in reaction to stress. So we are often left with our bodies running in overdrive but going nowhere. This can be dangerous if it happens too much. Let me explain.

"Because blood is directed away from the liver during the fight or flight, this important organ becomes less efficient in performing one of its major roles: clearing the blood of cholesterol. In this way, repeated activation of the fight or flight response can lead to increased coronary artery clotting, a key factor in the development of atherosclerosis (or hardening of the arteries).

"Many folks hear this information and get frightened about two things: (1) 'If I don't learn to turn this thing off regularly, the fight or flight can lead to or complicate my heart illness'; and (2) 'It sounds like this big "overdrive" reaction could lead to my blowing a gasket—maybe a heart attack or sudden death.'

"In some cases, these fears are justified. You see, besides gradual long-term health complications such as hardening of your arteries, fight or flight also results in immediate changes in many physical functions: your blood pressure rises; your heart rate speeds up; your peripheral vascular system constricts; stress hormones flow causing clotting in your blood vessels; even your breathing can get fast and shallow. Little wonder, then, that over 60 years of research have demonstrated that the majority of acute cardiac events are triggered by the stresses of daily mental and physical activities rather than by atherosclerosis. In fact, the risk of having a heart attack is 5 to 9 times higher within 2 to 26 hours after a stressful event.

"Finally, let's talk about the emotions that come with fight or flight. The one most often experienced is anxiety, or a sense of urgency. If fight or flight occurs too often or lasts too long, you can develop a state of free-floating anxiety or alarm—all charged up, but not even aware anymore of what you are prepared to fight or run from. In getting through a regular day, most of us turn on the fight or flight 20 to 40 times. For all of these reasons it is very important to learn effective ways to turn the fight or flight off."

EEM COMPONENT 1B: EXPLAIN THE CONSERVATION/WITHDRAWAL RESPONSE

Many patients who are clearly in need of stress management interventions refuse to accept such because they do not identify themselves as being stressed. The reason for this is often that many people equate stress with anxiety. Explaining how conservation/withdrawal may follow prolonged activation of the flight-or-fight syndrome (Eliot & Breo, 1984), and how the emotions that accompany conservation/withdrawal are more numbing than anxiety-provoking, can help patients develop more open attitudes toward receiving needed psychosocial help. Modifications of the following script can be used to teach the specifics of this syndrome.

"Conservation/withdrawal can be explained as what happens if speeding up (that is, the flight-or-fight syndrome) does not work to calm your stress responses. To prevent a physiological burnout, your adrenal gland switches gears away from the part that is running the flight-or-fight reaction. Now the adrenal cortex secretes cortisol, which begins a series of events that automatically shuts down certain physiological reactions. This shutting down is the conservation/withdrawal response;

it prepares you for long-term survival by conserving your vital resources as you endure a highly stressful time. This tends to happen when you are stressed for prolonged periods but seem to have no control over a hostile environment.

"In many ways, conservation/withdrawal is the physiological opposite of the flight-or-fight response. The cortisol that comes form your adrenal gland moves throughout your body, slowing down your stress reactions: your blood pressure reactions slow; your body secretions of stress hormones decrease; your body tissues begin to retain chemicals such as sodium; clotting agents are released into your bloodstream; your production of sex hormones such as testosterone decreases; gastric acid production is increased; and your immune system's defenses are lowered.

"On the one hand, this reaction is protective: The shutting down that comes with conservation/withdrawal buffers you somewhat from the wear-and-tear effects of any major, unrelenting stressor, such as recurring health problems, financial worries, or relationship tensions. At first, this reaction may feel like a welcomed state of relief from the supercharged 'overdrive' of the flight-or-fight reaction.

"In many ways, it is accurate to think of conservation/withdrawal as your body's protection against a single, major source of stress. That's the good news.

"The bad news lies in the fact that none of us faces only one stressor at a time. We live in a stress epidemic, and each of us is constantly being bombarded by stresses that don't allow us to shut down for any length of time. When you are in conservation/withdrawal, you actually are in a state of increased vulnerability to toxic effects of the multiple stressors that fill your everyday life, and you are more vulnerable to many forms of stress.

"Plus, the 'relief' of conservation/withdrawal is not a restful relief. During conservation/withdrawal, you are in a constant state of vigilance, or watchfulness. In this sense, you become chronically aroused but do not react with emergency stress responses. Most patients I have known who were in conservation/withdrawal complained of emotional 'numbness.'

"Although it does not 'hurt,' this numbness is actually a rather dangerous state of affairs. This numbness can blunt the physical and emotional feedback that you need to make effective stress management adjustments in your daily life. Usually, these sorts of stress management adjustments happen automatically. If we get tired, we know that we need to rest; if we get bored or preoccupied, we notice it and do something to change our focus of attention.

> "But in conservation/withdrawal, we just stay numb, and this numbness
> can prevent us from making the adjustments necessary to interrupt the
> wear-and-tear effects that come with prolonged exposure to stressful
> circumstances. Unaware of feelings such as fatigue or boredom, we
> just keep on doing that which should be stopped. This numbness can
> even blunt awareness of body signals such as fear, hunger, or other
> bodily cues. The blunted concentration and attention that comes with
> this state can even increase the likelihood of your having accidents."

The interesting literature on vital exhaustion, the prevalence of exhaustion
during the prodromal stages of acute MI, and the major problem of delay
in seeking help by MI patients may relate to this conservation/withdrawal
stress phenomenon. Conservation/withdrawal numbness may be a mechanism underlying the observation that MI patients often spend months prior
to heart attack ignoring symptoms of their developing heart illness, such as
chest tightness, shortness of breath, and even crushing chest pain, apparently
plowing through life in a state of inertia and helplessness and quasi-
depression (Falger, Schouten, & Appels, 1988). Clinical experience also suggests that the emotional bluntedness shown by many COPD patients may
be related to the numbness associated with conservation/withdrawal.

EEM COMPONENT 1C:
EXPLAIN THE GENERAL ADAPTATION SYNDROME

A third way of explaining physical and emotional stress reactions is offered
in Hans Selye's General Adaptation Syndrome (Selye, 1974, 1976). This set of
concepts is especially effective in helping many recovering cardiopulmonary
patients understand coping struggles such as stress-related depression,
momentary cognitive impairment, and physiological and emotional exhaustion. In addition, it provides stress management motivation for engaging in
important physical rehabilitation changes such as exercising regularly and
controlling dietary choices.

One of the oldest and most original theories of stress response, Selye's
model offers a complex and detailed explanation of the physical changes
that occur as the body progresses from alarm to adaptation to exhaustion
when facing unrelenting stress. This complex series of reactions is mediated
by pituitary and adrenal cortical activation. For purposes of EEM, this theory
can be explained in the simple terms of the following analogy.

 "Your ability to cope with stress can be thought of as depending on
the availability of a precious fuel, called adaptation energy. Only a
limited amount of adaptation energy is available at any point in time,
and this energy is divided across a number of 'fuel tanks.' Each of

these tanks serves a specific purpose, depending upon your activities or stressors at the moment. Both positive and negative aspects of life can drain adaptation energy, because coping with both requires changing, and any change requires adaptation or adjustment. Here is a drawing that shows how this works. [Show Figure 5.1.]

"The General Adaptation Syndrome can be explained in this way: Whenever you need to adapt or cope, you draw adaptation energy from the appropriate fuel tank. There are two ways that you burn off fuel from the corresponding adaptation energy channel: if you are actually dealing with a stressor related to the theme of that channel; or if you are thinking about that stressor. In this way, you might burn adaptation energy from multiple channels at once. For example, while cooking dinner one evening, you may also be thinking of problems at work. The result: You immediately lose coping energy from the 'chores' and 'work' fuel tanks. This drawing shows what I mean here. [Show Figure 5.2.]

"Stress complications occur when energy is drawn from a given channel for too long a time. When this happens, the stress response progresses from alarm to adaptation to exhaustion. The alarm stage is similar to the fight-or-flight response. If it is not turned off (by coping successfully with whatever caused it, or simply by stopping your dealing with the stressor), you enter the adaptation phase. During alarm, you experience the same physical reactions that occur in the fight-or-flight response: a set of 'kicking your body into overdrive' responses. If you then enter the adaptation phase and stay in it for too long, you begin to suffer certain obvious physical consequences. For example, during this phase, some people might suffer from headaches, indigestion, insomnia, constipation, hives, muscle spasms, chest pain, or

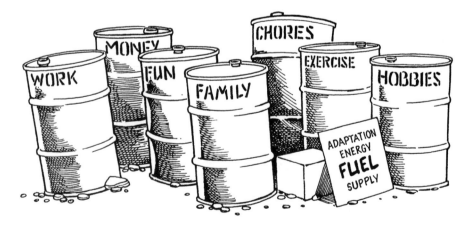

Figure 5.1   Adaptation energy.

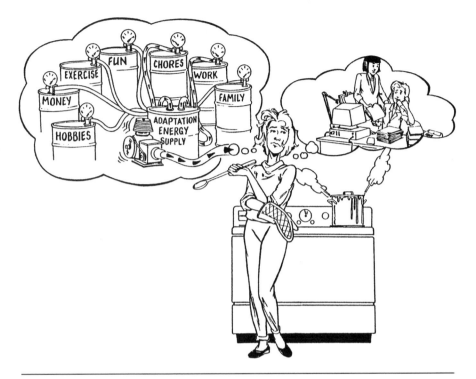

Figure 5.2   Energy drains from multiple channels.

breathing difficulty—to name but a few possibilities. These symptoms come and go, depending on the stress situation at hand and on whether or not the changes you make during the adaptation stage of the stress response are successful in alleviating the stressful situation. If not, you enter the dangerous exhaustion stage of stress.

"When you enter the exhaustion stage of the General Adaptation Syndrome, you get a new bath of stress hormones. These accelerate wear and tear on your physical system. Although certain physical reactions (such as those explained in the previous discussion of the flight-or-fight syndrome) occur in everyone when stressed, your specific version of wear and tear when you begin to suffer stress exhaustion will depend upon your particular physical makeup. Everyone reacts to stress in some unique ways; everyone has some physical systems that are especially stress-hardy and others that are more vulnerable to the effects of stress. Anyone with a major physical illness has the advantage of knowing definitively what, at minimum, is one of their most vulnerable physical systems (for example, your cardiovascular or pulmonary system). But your major illness is not all that you are about. Other of your physical systems also react to stress, and this

might explain why you sometimes struggle with _____ **[fill in information regarding the patient's specific coping struggles or somatic
symptoms]**. In general, it is important to accept that unchecked
exhaustion-stage stress responses can lead to new illnesses or to
complications in your already-existing illness.

"You know that you have moved from alarm to adaptation to exhaustion by noticing certain physical and psychological 'red flags' that
the General Adaptation Syndrome is progressing. Physical signals of
advancing stress might be fatigue, aching, or flare-up of your body
parts or physical systems that are most involved in responding to the
stress at hand or that are your 'weak links.' For example, anyone who
works for too long at a chore such as paying bills or trying to balance
their checkbook might start to get eyestrain and a neck ache from
leaning over and focusing on the figures at hand. These symptoms
come from wear and tear on the specific body parts that are being
used to face the stressor. For you, though, given that one of your
most reactive stress systems seems to be your _____ **[fill in blank
with information about the patient]**, it is likely that working too
long at a chore like this will also lead to the 'red flag' of your _____
**[symptoms related to the patient's most reactive physical stress
system, such as neck pain, stomach pain, chest pain, or breathing
difficulty]** flaring up.

"This General Adaptation Syndrome also leads to certain emotional
signals that a stress response is progressing too far. You might notice
a growing sense of restlessness or aggravation as it becomes hard
to find satisfaction in the things you deal with each day. You might
also find that you are becoming generally irritable and losing your
ability to be flexible when coping with your daily stressors. These
symptoms mean that you are getting dangerously low on adaptation
energy fuel—the stuff that has to be there for you to cope effectively.
In other words, these physical and emotional symptoms signal that
you are about to run out of coping gas.

"One more set of signals that you are entering the 'running on empty'
zone of adaptation energy comes from your thinking patterns. As a
backdrop to understanding what happens here, it is important to know
just a couple of facts about how your brain works to control your
thinking and your emotions. Basically, your brain is like a massive
electrical circuitry that is made up of a bunch of nerve endings that
don't join each other. In doing its 'stuff' that controls your thinking
and your emotions, your brain depends upon the exchange of certain
'juices' (called neurochemicals) between the nerve endings. Prolonged
stress can interfere with your brain's ability to exchange these precious
juices. If these neurochemicals aren't flowing correctly, your thinking
and emotional systems signal trouble. Your thinking might change in

many ways: you may have trouble concentrating; your ability for abstract reasoning might get blunted; and your memory may begin to fail you.

"If your neurochemical exchanges get too far out of balance, you might experience a full-fledged bout of clinical depression—the sort of depression that usually requires the help of antidepressant medicines to fix. A more temporary condition could be termed stress-related depression: you lose your passion and zest for living; your coping becomes more rigid than flexible; your mood is not exactly one of depression, but your emotions seem to be blunted and you settle into a general feeling of 'just getting by' in your day-to-day life.

"The beauty of the general adaptation syndrome is that sensibly responding to these warning signals can protect you from many of the harmful effects of stress and can lead to a replenishment of your stress-managing energies. By simply switching channels—changing your activity and your focus—you allow the exhausted channel to refill its drained supply of coping energy. In simple terms: Damage from stress can be prevented simply by changing your activity and your focus when you notice the signals of advancing stress. In this way,

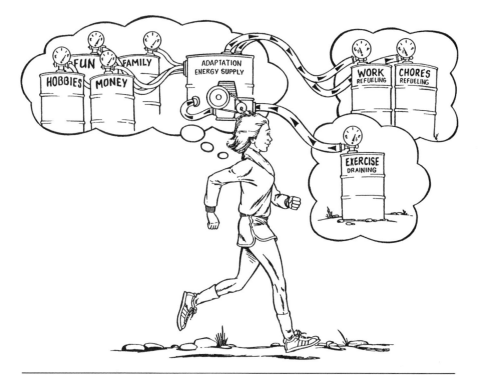

Figure 5.3   Diversifying to refuel coping energy.

energy-exhausting drain from the overused channel is stopped, and as drain from a more full adaptation energy 'tank' is started, the relatively drained tank is refueled. This drawing shows this process. [Show Figure 5.3.]

"Think of it this way: Your stress system is run by 'magical' fuel tanks that automatically refill if you simply stop using them periodically by switching to a different activity. This is only one of the many reasons for making time in your daily and weekly life to exercise regularly, spend time with your loved ones, practice your relaxation procedures, and so on."

SUMMARY OF THE MANY FLAVORS OF STRESS

In summary, stress can be explained as affecting the patient's physical functioning in various ways that can lead to different emotional symptoms:

- The fight-or-flight syndrome can cause feelings of anxiety, alarm, and/or anger.
- The conservation/withdrawal response can result in feelings of numbness.
- The General Adaptation Syndrome can lead to stress-related depression.
- Persistent neurochemical depletion or "jamming" can lead to clinical depression or anxiety disorder symptomatology.

Explaining these facts about stress sets the stage for making further rehabilitation-enhancing recommendations to recovering cardiopulmonary patients. The first of these in the EEM model is the recommendation to learn and to regularly use a guaranteed calmer of stress reactions—the relaxation response.

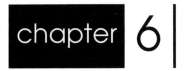

chapter 6

RELAXATION

The second component of EEM is relaxation training. What follows is a brief discussion of the physiological benefits of relaxation training, an overview of various relaxation methods that have been used in treating cardiopulmonary patients, and specific guidelines for teaching patients this important skill. This chapter closes with a discussion of the benefits of physical exercise as an aid to relaxation and stress management.

THE BENEFITS OF RELAXATION

In normal subjects, relaxation techniques have been found to lead to a number of physical changes that can be crucial in cardiopulmonary patients, including reduced anxiety, heart rate, respiratory rate, and muscle tension (Paul, 1969). The research-documented benefits of providing brief relaxation training to patients anticipating surgery have already been mentioned. These have included fewer incidences of postsurgical delirium, diminished medical complications, and shorter lengths of hospital stay. In addition, several investigations have reported positive effects from providing relaxation training specifically to recovering cardiopulmonary patients (Gift et al., 1992). A representative sample of these studies is summarized in Table 6.1.

Table 6.1 is not a comprehensive summary of studies in this area; its purpose is simply to show the diversity that exists in the various uses of relaxation interventions. As can be seen from Table 6.1, "relaxation training" is used to refer to a variety of interventions that can benefit patients in ways that go far beyond simply helping them feel more comfortable. Positive effects have been demonstrated from various forms of relaxation training (e.g., yoga, progressive muscular relaxation, autohypnosis) provided in various treatment settings (e.g., taped relaxation instructions, in vivo instructions, inpatient and outpatient settings) to various cardiopulmonary populations (e.g., asthmatics, recovering MI patients, and patients suffering from COPD).

An observation from this literature deserves special mention. Joint participation in relaxation training by a couple, one of whom is a heart patient, has been demonstrated to be effective in helping the cardiac patient to

**Table 6.1   Reported Benefits of Relaxation Training
With Cardiac and Pulmonary Patients**

Study	Population	Relaxation intervention	Results
Tandon (1978)	COPD outpatients	Yoga	Better work rate, exercise tolerance, and self-control of breathlessness
Acosta (1987)	COPD outpatients	Hypnotically induced relaxation	Lessened fear of breathing off ventilator
Alexander, Miklich, & Riff (1972)	Asthmatics	Progressive relaxation	Peak expiratory flow; decreased anxiety
Renfroe (1988)	COPD outpatients	Progressive relaxation	Decreased anxiety and decreased dyspnea
Acosta-Austan (1991)	COPD outpatients	Progressive relaxation and hypnotic suggestion	Pulmonary functions and patient confidence
van Dixhoorn, Duivenvoorden, Staal, Pool, & Verghag (1987)	MI patients	Relaxation plus exercise	Significantly improved S-T segment changes
Munro, Creamer, Haggerty, & Cooper (1988)	MI patients	Relaxation training	Significant reductions in Sickness Impact Profile
Aiken & Hendricks (1971)	Open heart surgery patients	15 sessions, taped relaxation training	Overall psychological adjustment

cope (Wadden, 1983). Interestingly, I am not aware of any study that has investigated the effects of relaxation training on the spouse of a cardiopulmonary patient. This notion deserves research attention.

RELAXATION TRAINING STRATEGIES

Many options for teaching relaxation exist, and there is no convincing evidence that one form of relaxation therapy is more effective than others in treating cardiopulmonary patients (Egbert et al., 1964). In practice, combinations of a number of relaxation training strategies are most often applied. Following are instructions for coaching patients in the use of several popular and effective methods of relaxation.

RELAXATION TRAINING STRATEGY NO. 1: TEACH DIAPHRAGMATIC BREATHING

To slow respiratory rate and increase tidal volume, pulmonary patients are routinely taught a form of breathing that is also a potent method for quickly inducing a relaxation response: diaphragmatic breathing (Barach, 1955). In the simple terms of Ries (1990), "This technique involves teaching the patient to coordinate abdominal wall expansion with inspiration and to slow expiration through pursed lips" (p. 85).

Diaphragmatic breathing can be taught in this way:

Have the patient place his or her hands on the chest and abdominal regions. Instruct the patient to inhale as much air as possible into the abdominal, not the chest, region. If done correctly, the hand placed on the abdomen will move outward, whereas the hand placed on the chest will remain relatively still. Next, instruct the patient to exhale twice as much air as was inhaled, signaled by movement of the lower hand inward toward the abdomen. With pulmonary patients, in addition to emphasizing the 2:1 exhalation/inhalation ratio, incorporate instructions for using pursed-lip breathing.

This technique is easily paired with other forms of relaxation, such as progressive muscular relaxation or meditation. The effectiveness of pairing various relaxation strategies with diaphragmatic breathing has been demonstrated in research with COPD populations spanning decades (e.g., Ambrosino et al., 1981; Becklake, McGregor, Goldman, & Braudo, 1954).

RELAXATION TRAINING STRATEGY NO. 2: ENCOURAGE THE RECALL OF NATURALLY OCCURRING OR PREVIOUSLY LEARNED RELAXATION STRATEGIES

Most people have experienced relaxation many times in their lives, even though they may not have identified the circumstance with the term *relaxing*. Helping a patient identify naturally occurring or previously learned relaxation strategies can greatly expedite relaxation training. Inquire, "When, during the course of your typical day or week, do you feel most relaxed, contented, or at peace?" Process the patient's response by helping him or her to elaborate the sights, smells, sounds, and bodily sensations experienced during such a time. The following excerpts from a case study demonstrate how this might be done.

WMS: "So, the most relaxing time for you is each morning, early in the morning, before anyone else in your home arises?"

Patient (Pt.): "Yes."

WMS: "Can you tell me what it is exactly that you find so relaxing about that time?"

Pt.: "I don't know; I just like it. It's peaceful."

WMS: "Peaceful?"

Pt.: "Yeah. You know, nice and quiet. Nobody running around, turning on the TV or anything."

WMS: "So one thing you like is the silence. That's relaxing?"

Pt.: "Yeah. There's too damn much noise in the world."

WMS: "During these relaxing, quiet times, where do you usually sit?"

Pt.: "Well, I'm usually in my kitchen, reading the newspaper, eating my cereal, and waiting for my coffee to brew."

WMS: "Do you usually sit in a certain chair?"

Pt.: "Yes. We all have our 'designated chairs' in my family."

WMS: "So you are in that quiet house, sitting in your favorite chair in your kitchen, eating your cereal. If you will, I'd like for you to breathe deeply and slowly, and practice filling your mind with the sensations of that time.

"Recall how it sounds. All silent and soothing. Maybe you hear little sounds that remind you of the peacefulness of this time: the refrigerator turning on, then off; the air conditioner or furnace running; the coffee dripping in its pot.

"As you hear it brewing, you might even recall how good the brewing coffee smells. With each breath, you relax and smell that coffee. You might even be able to taste it, waiting for it to brew.

"Recall how it feels to sit in that chair. Notice the weight of gravity pulling on you as your bottom pushes on the seat of the chair. Notice the feel of the back of the chair on your back.

"Notice, too, what you can see in this memory. The colors of the plates against the color of the kitchen table, the way the light comes into the kitchen, even the colors of the curtains on the window.

"Filling your head with these sounds, sights, and tastes, you might notice different body sensations: relaxed, peaceful, content, quiet."

This simple relaxation induction is borrowed from the school of neuro-linguistic programming and its related concepts regarding training in self-hypnosis (Grinder & Bandler, 1981). The concept here is simple: an "altered state" (for our purposes, this simply means relaxation) will occur reflexively if the patient's attention can be overloaded with material that comes from the suggestion to concentrate on two or three entries from each of three or more of the senses (e.g., "recall two images, two sounds, two bodily sensations, two tastes, and two smells from that special time").

An alternative is to have the patient simply recall a prior experience in which he or she systematically induced a relaxation response. Again, bear in mind that the patient may not have labeled such an experience as being relaxing. For example, few people would argue that any woman who success-fully employed Lamaze methods for childbirth is able to "alter her state." Reminding the patient of his or her already learned (but, perhaps, seldom used) tool for relaxing is an expeditious way to get the patient to reexperience and systemize a relaxation experience.

RELAXATION TRAINING STRATEGY NO. 3: TEACH PROGRESSIVE MUSCULAR RELAXATION

Here, while periodically employing abdominal breathing, the patient is in-structed to progressively tense, then relax alternating muscle groups. Suggestions for feeling and imaging the body relaxing are incorporated between instructions to tense, then relax the next body part.

 As in any relaxation dialog, it is important to avoid using terms that require the mind to attempt to process a negative. For example, in-structing a patient, "Don't worry about your tension, your problems, or the image of a white elephant" simply implants the suggestion to the patient to conjure up images of his or her tensions, problems, or white elephants.

It is better to tell the patient what to think: "Notice your body relaxing, with one part being especially relaxed and warm. That part begins to spread its comforting relaxation to all parts of your body."

The reader is referred to Benson (1975) for further discussion of progressive muscle relaxation training.

RELAXATION TRAINING STRATEGY NO. 4: USE HEALING IMAGERY

No definitive data exist showing that imagery creates cellular changes of the sort that control or reverse cardiopulmonary illness. However, few people would argue that recovering patients do tend to fill their minds with negative, fearful images related to their disease. Clinical experience suggests that heart patients tend to visualize cholesterol clogging their arteries following a meal, smokers tend to imagine their lungs growing blacker following smoking a cigarette, and so on. Relaxation is an opportunity for patients to replace distressing imagery with imagery that, at minimum, enhances a sense of well-being, even if it does not create changes in the illness progression.

This can be accomplished in two ways. First, once relaxed, instruct the patient to visualize a given body part (e.g., heart muscle, coronary arteries, lungs, air passages). Next, instruct the patient in some version of the following:

"Now keep that part of your body on one screen in your mind's eye. On another screen, I want you to notice what part of your body is most relaxed; most warm, heavy, comfortable.

"Now notice the two screens merging, coming together, as you move relaxation from screen No. 2 into that body part on screen No. 1. You might see and feel yourself healing." (Here offer specific suggestions for healing, such as: "See and feel your artery walls getting flexible and strong; your lungs clearing, gradually being warmed and softened to a healthy, pink color"; and so on.) Comprehensive guidelines for using imagery are available from Achterberg (1985) and Naparstek (1995).

In addition, it is helpful to encourage patients to use visual rehearsal techniques during the state of relaxation. This is a form of cognitive rehearsal that can help bolster the patient's confidence about functioning in certain anxiety-provoking situations. Such suggestions can take many forms. An example follows.

"Relax and breathe comfortably. Notice how easy it is to breathe while you relax. Now imagine taking the memory of *this* relaxation with you as you: walk toward your car—relax in *this* way; drive home, seeing traffic ahead—relax in *this* way; arrive home and greet your family—take *this* relaxation with you."

This method simply pairs an intonated word ("this" in the above example) with the state of relaxation, then bridges new stimulus-response connections by pairing the intonated word and its associated relaxation with imagery of upcoming events in the patient's life. This technique is borrowed from the seminal work in medical hypnosis by Milton Erickson, M.D., that was referred to earlier.

RELAXATION TRAINING STRATEGY NO. 5: BIOFEEDBACK

Finally, no discussion of relaxation training with cardiopulmonary patients would be complete without mention of the utility of providing biofeedback-assisted training in relaxation and psychophysiological monitoring. This technique has been used successfully in treating both cardiac and pulmonary patients (Parker, 1988; Sexton, 1987; Tiep, 1993). Of course, specialized training is required to learn the use of biofeedback techniques. Readers interested in a critical discussion of the use of biofeedback as a behavioral medicine intervention with cardiopulmonary populations are referred to Tiep (1993) and Patel, Marmot, & Terry (1981).

EXERCISE AS A RELAXATION AND STRESS MANAGEMENT TOOL

In clinical practice, stress management training seldom fails to emphasize the importance of regular physical exercise, a fact that is reflected in the inclusion of exercise as a component of EEM. The reported benefits of stress management interventions that emphasize physical exercise have included reduced exaggerated cardiovascular reactivity and enhanced control of arrhythmias and enhanced overall psychosocial functioning, both in healthy populations and in those suffering from cardiopulmonary illness (Feuerstein & Cohen, 1985; Gatchel, Gaffney, & Smith, 1986; Gayle, Spitler, Karper, Jaeger, & Rice, 1988). A key question in this line of inquiry concerns the benefits of exercise on cardiovascular responsivity and on overall stress management capacity and emotional well-being.

Many studies have suggested that physically fit individuals evidence less exaggerated cardiovascular reactivity to psychosocial stressors than do the physically unfit (e.g., Blumenthal et al., 1988). Specifically, when stressed, the physically fit have been shown to evidence:

- smaller increases in systolic blood pressure (Light, Obrist, James, & Stogatz, 1987);

- smaller increases in diastolic blood pressure (Hull, Young, & Ziegler, 1984);

- less increase in heart rate (Holmes & Rothe, 1985); and

- a faster heart rate recovery (Sinyor, Schwartz, Peronnet, Brisson, & Seraganian, 1983).

In this vein of research, responsivity is typically assessed by measuring cardiovascular and neurohumoral responses to standard laboratory challenges. These challenges include both mental tasks (e.g., viewing stressful films, performing mental arithmetic) and physical tasks (e.g., cold pressor test, exercise treadmill testing) (Emery, Pinder, & Blumenthal, 1989). Controversy hinges around the fact that less convincing research exists to suggest that physical conditioning effects stress responses during daily living.

It also is unclear whether or not regular physical exercise, in itself, leads to lasting psychosocial benefits. Extensive exploration of this debate is beyond the scope of the current discussion. For critical evaluations of this literature, the interested reader is referred to thought-provoking articles by Hughes (1984) and Emery et al. (1989). But in a nutshell, this debate involves two pockets of research. On the one hand, a number of researchers have suggested that in nonmedical populations, regular physical exercise has psychological benefits that include reduced anxiety, decreased muscular tension and depression, increased stress management, and a generally enhanced feeling of well-being (e.g., Ewart, 1989; Ross & Hayes, 1988). This research has also noted that regular exercise can reduce the cardiovascular impact of emotional stressors (e.g., Lake, Suarez, Schneiderman, & Tocci, 1985).

On the other hand, it has been argued that the enhanced well-being that often comes with regular participation in exercise programs is not necessarily due to increased levels of physical fitness. A number of studies (e.g., Blumenthal, Williams, Needels, & Wallace, 1982) have shown that changes in emotional functioning that were associated with participation in aerobic exercise classes were independent of actual changes in fitness. This finding seems to hold for healthy, cardiac, and pulmonary populations (Agle, Baum, Chester, & Wendt, 1973; Emery, 1993).

Although exercise is clearly not a panacea for promoting well-being in recovering cardiopulmonary patients (Emery, 1993), clinical experience strongly supports the efficacy of incorporating the recommendation to engage in even mild exercise as part of overall EEM training. Independent of the actual physical consequences of such exercise, this recommendation is based upon several observations:

- Exercise can provide a tangible way of "switching channels" to prevent stress-related exhaustion.

- When facing uncontrollable stressors, exercising is a way of creating an arena of control over some tangible factor, and the effects of this taking of control seem to generalize to enhance self-efficacy for coping in general.

- Regular exercise can be used as a positive coping tool when facing the difficult parts of managing virtually any of the areas of risk factor or psychosocial concern in treating recovering heart or lung patients (e.g., management of smoking, eating, depression).

I believe that this recommendation is especially relevant in treating COPD patients. Research has consistently indicated that, independent of changes in lung function, COPD patients evidence enhanced psychosocial functioning following even minimal participation in rehabilitation interventions that incorporate an exercise component. Research-documented benefits of such interventions have included: greater independence and self-esteem; improved activities of daily living; lessened fear related to dyspnea; and an enhanced sense of self-importance (Agle & Baum, 1977).

SUMMARY

Regardless of how they do it, it is important that patients regularly experience relaxation. Emphasizing this recommendation is a simple but important aspect of overall cardiopulmonary care. At minimum, you might encourage the patient to take brief relaxation breaks throughout the day. Taking many mini-breaks to calm one's stressed physiology and psychology is not only an effective way to abort the wear and tear of stress; it is also a way of reorienting oneself to awareness of the physical, cognitive, behavioral, and interpersonal chains of responses and counterresponses that are ongoing and that create the quality of one's life in the moment. Key components of the process of becoming an Effective Emotional Manager are (a) taking time to force into consciousness an awareness of one's own coping process; and (b) doing something, however small, that at least momentarily and adaptively disrupts what might otherwise be a problem pattern of coping. Learning to relax instead of tensing and remembering to use brief periods of relaxation throughout the course of daily living are examples of such adaptive pattern disruption.

Another arena in which EEM focuses on pattern disruption has to do with personality-based coping tendencies. We now turn to a discussion of this crucial aspect of the model.

chapter 7

PERSONALITY-BASED COPING PATTERNS

Researchers who investigate cardiopulmonary patients have been quite interested in the effects personality factors have on the developmental course of these illnesses. Convincing research has documented that coping styles can moderate the stress-health relationship during both pre- and postmorbid periods (Denollet, 1993; Krantz & Hedges, 1987). For example, literally thousands of research studies have examined whether TYABP leads to the development of CHD and how TYABP might affect the course of rehabilitation (Matthews, 1988). However, a valid understanding of how coping styles may have both functional and health consequences for recovering cardiopulmonary patients can only come from going beyond the mere investigation of Type A patients. In teaching cardiopulmonary patients to cope more effectively, it is important to bear in mind that the interplay between their own and their loved ones' personality-based coping styles may have important physiological, behavioral, emotional, and interpersonal consequences.

Accordingly, EEM emphasizes, at minimum, a commonsense appraisal of the personality-based coping styles of recovering patients and, where possible and appropriate, of their loved ones. Formal psychological assessment (see chapter 2) can yield information important in designing interventions that meet personality-based needs of individual patients. In EEM, the intent of assessing personality-based coping is threefold: (a) to facilitate matching delivery of information to the patient's psychological frame of reference; (b) to facilitate education regarding potential coping pitfalls that come with the patient's particular personality style; and (c) to educate regarding the possible interplay between the individual coping styles of various family members and the rehabilitation implications of such interaction. This last topic will be fully explored in chapter 8 in the discussion of families as teams. Here I will provide a brief overview of a commonsense way to assess personality-based coping tendencies, an extended discussion of the practical implications of research regarding TYABP, and keys for structuring interventions given the implications of these two sets of information.

UNDERSTANDING PERSONALITY-BASED COPING PATTERNS

Tables 7.1 and 7.2, taken from *Heart Illness and Intimacy: How Caring Relationships Aid Recovery* (Sotile, 1992), outline frequent ways in which individuals attempt to cope with fears and insecurities and the coping pitfalls that can come from blind adherence to each of these coping patterns.

The information in these tables can illuminate the circular patterns of interaction often manifested by families and individuals as they struggle with cardiopulmonary illness. For both individuals and families, coping problems most often result from rigid adherence to overlearned coping styles. For example, one family member might tend to react to stress by striving to try harder than anyone to attain perfection in adhering to rehabilitation recommendations. By referring to Tables 7.1 and 7.2, you can see that this individual is likely to approach rehabilitation with a sense of urgency and obsessiveness over the details of the process. Such a person would also be at risk for suffering guilt, anxiety, and obsessive preoccupation about the fact that rehabilitation never goes perfectly. These feelings may lead to aloofness, exhaustion, stress, depression, and joylessness.

Alternatively, another family member might tend to assume a "Pleasing others" coping pattern when stressed. Such a person is likely to adopt a caretaking quest and ignore his or her own needs in deference to encouraging, reassuring, and attempting to communicate and be affectionate with distressed loved ones. Such a person might also be at risk for exhaustion in the caretaking role, followed by withdrawal into depression or despair.

Table 7.1   Coping Patterns and Pitfalls

Driver	Underlying hope	Coping pitfalls
Being strong	To be nurtured	Numbness, loneliness, anger
Being perfect	To feel good enough	Guilt, anxiety, obsessive preoccupation, aloofness
Trying hard	To feel deserving of rest and enjoyment	Exhaustion, stress, depression, joylessness
Pleasing others	To feel understood and appreciated	Exhaustion, withdrawal, guilt
Hurrying	To feel finished	Frazzled and chaotic feelings
Being careful	To feel safe	Free-floating fear and obsessive worrying

Note. Sotile, Wayne M., *Heart Illness and Intimacy: How Caring Relationships Aid Recovery.* The Johns Hopkins University Press, Baltimore/London, 1992.

Table 7.2 Coping Patterns and Reactions to Illness

Driver	Maladaptive reaction to illness
Being strong	Quiet about one's own fears and needs; seeming denial of all concerns; eventual depression from perception that others do not care; focus on physical symptoms as indirect way to get soothed
Being perfect	Obsessiveness about details of health; all-or-nothing thinking; ignoring the spirit of the rehabilitation process; never soothed that adherence to details of rehabilitation is sufficient
Trying hard	Sense of urgency that interferes with pacing; attitude of "wait until" rehabilitation is completed before enjoying life
Pleasing others	Lack of self-expression; failure to soothe own needs; guilt over illness that interferes with needed relief from performing "well enough"; fear; discomfort telling medical personnel anything that might disappoint them
Hurrying	Frustration, irritability, and impatience with slowness of own or others' progress in recovering or adapting; demoralized; resort to "quick cures"
Being careful	Fear-based withdrawal from life; spectatoring; obsessive monitoring of own or others' reactions; depression

Note. Sotile, Wayne M., *Heart Illness and Intimacy: How Caring Relationships Aid Recovery.* The Johns Hopkins University Press, Baltimore/London, 1992.

This withdrawal leads to guilt, which results in a redoubling of caretaking behaviors, and the vicious circle starts all over again.

Tension can escalate as these two family members react to external and intrafamily stresses with further exaggerations of their respective personality-based coping strategies, all in misguided efforts to fulfill the "Underlying hopes" specified in Table 7.1. The more agitated and anxious the first person becomes over his or her failure to rehabilitate perfectly, the more stressed the caretaker might feel due to disconnection from the preoccupied partner. The caretaker might then push for more interaction. But these demands for communication and affection might simply serve to agitate the perfectionistic partner who is driven to "wait until" rehabilitation is "completed" before daring to enjoy life and its relationships.

Effective emotional management has much to do with the capacity to recognize and abort such stress-generating patterns of personality-based interactions. This means learning to identify and, in adaptive ways, soothe the hopes that underlie reflexive coping patterns. Your effectiveness in advising cardiopulmonary patients and their loved ones can be significantly enhanced if you match your input to the patient's personality-based coping style and its corresponding underlying hope. For example, using the guidelines offered in Table 7.1, the perfectionistic, driven person from the above example might be most effectively soothed (and therefore maximally open to further input) by feedback that is framed like this:

> "I know that you are willing to work harder than anyone to get rehabilitated. Your attention to the details of this process is amazing. From my many years of working with literally hundreds of patients who have faced this illness, I know that you are doing excellently. You should feel better than 'good enough' about your efforts. In fact, I think you deserve a little rest from your quest. The best way to make rehabilitation a lifetime affair is to pace yourself. Let me elaborate on what I mean by this."

In a similar vein, the underlying hopes and the coping styles of the caretaker from the above example might be matched in the following manner as a prelude to leading the individual into more adaptive perspectives on his or her role in rehabilitation:

> "I have noticed how concerned you are about your loved ones and about the reactions and feelings of everyone else. I admire your compassion and your perceptiveness. These are gifts that many people don't possess. I have found in working with many patients that giving support and encouragement to others—especially to loved ones—is an important aspect of rehabilitation. I have also found that it is important to remember that the better care you take of yourself—physically and emotionally—the better will you be able to continue taking care of the people you love. In this vein, I would like to offer you a little advice about how to balance your desire to caretake with my advice that you, too, be nurtured and taken care of."

An amplifier of any coping pattern is TYABP. As will be shown in the remainder of this chapter, learning to match and manage this high-powered coping style ranks among the most universal challenges faced by cardiopulmonary rehabilitation specialists on both professional and personal levels.

TYPE A BEHAVIOR PATTERN (TYABP) DEFINED

Type A behavior pattern is generally defined as "an action-emotion complex that can be observed in any person who is aggressively involved in a chronic, incessant struggle to achieve more and more in less and less time" (Friedman & Rosenman, 1974, p. 68). Essentially, TYABP is a style of reacting to certain situations; it is neither a personality trait nor a universal pattern of coping (Jenkins, 1971). In the research literature, the relative absence of TYABP in reacting to stressful circumstances is said to signal Type B behavior pattern.

TYABP is considered an independent risk factor for CHD, supposedly because many Type A individuals show greater sympathetic nervous system reactivity than Type B people under frustrating or competitive circumstances (Matthews, 1982; Razin, 1982). However, both the definition and assessment of TYABP have been under fire in recent years, primarily due to a number of well-controlled investigations that have questioned whether or not TYABP really relates to development of CHD, the prognosis of CHD, or to rehabilitation responses (Case, Heller, Case, Moss, & the Multicenter Post-Infarction Research Group, 1985; Haaga, 1987; Ragland & Brand, 1988).

In addition, a wealth of research has examined the question of whether TYABP represents a unidimensional or a multidimensional set of coping characteristics. The prevailing notion is that TYABP exists on a continuum ranging from some individuals exhibiting singular Type A coping characteristics to some who evidence multiple Type A characteristics in their coping style (Haynes & Matthews, 1988; Helgeson, 1989). The many characteristics of TYABP that have been presented in the literature were systematized by Sotile (1992), and a summary of this information is presented as follows:

SUMMARY BOX

Summary of Type A Response Styles

The Type A is driven by:
Conscientiousness and an inflexible sense of responsibility.
Perfectionism.
The need to prove self-worth through performing well.
Cravings for recognition and power.
Competition and challenges.
High needs for working long, hard hours.
The desire to be seen as a leader.
A vague mistrust of the motives or competency of others.

Type A behaviors include:
Tense, energetic movements.
Constant movement. Difficulty being still. May fidget, tap feet, drum knuckles, or shake leg or foot while attempting to sit still. Explosively emphasizing points during conversation with finger and hand motions.
Frequent use of profanity.
Forceful expressions of opinions, often using such words as "stupid," "idiotic," and "ridiculous" in response to opinions differing from one's own.

(continued)

Summary of Type A Response Styles *(continued)*

Flashing grimacelike smiles.

A clipped speaking pattern, the result of constantly tensing jaw muscles.

Irregular breathing pattern, often leading to expiratory sighs in the midst of conversations.

Constantly rushing and fighting against time—also known as "hurry sickness."

Overly aggressive and competitive reactions, even when the situation does not warrant such.

Doing several things at once.

The Type A's style and focus of thinking:

Tends to think on several levels at once.

Anticipates what is coming next and reacts in advance (Examples: interrupts conversations with answers to unfinished questions; prepares for departure from car or airplane well before the vehicle stops).

Hypervigilant: scans surroundings, noticing what might go wrong or what is irritating at the moment.

Constantly checks the time, noting time crunch, punctuality (own or other's), and efficiency (or lack thereof).

Preoccupation with all of the above results in poor observational abilities—especially of own behavior or of own impact on others.

Factors that affect interpersonal relationships for Type As:

Self-focused. Preoccupied with own stresses, anxieties, or tasks. Poor listener: interrupts, breaks rapport with distracted behavior, gives advice rather than empathy.

Easily bored by another's conversation.

Easily angered, and has difficulty not showing it (glaring, curt comments, honking horn while driving).

Makes critical, blaming, or shaming comments when someone makes a mistake.

Defensive in reaction to feedback, especially feedback regarding obvious hostility.

Shows overt bravado and confidence regarding own opinions, abilities, and power.

Often frustrated when working with others.

Very controlling: dictates, gives unsolicited advice.

Visibly uncomfortable with physical intimacy or with verbal expressions of tender feelings.

Note. Sotile, Wayne M., *Heart Illness and Intimacy: How Caring Relationships Aid Recovery*. The Johns Hopkins University Press, Baltimore/London, 1992.

It has been predicted that more than 70% of individuals living in urban populations and only a slightly smaller percentage of residents of rural populations evidence at least one characteristic of TYABP (Thoresen & Low, 1990; Ulmer, 1990). Indeed, it seems only logical that the stress epidemic in which we are living would inevitably result in various of the coping habits outlined in the Summary Box on pages 113-114, even in children and adolescents (Thoresen & Pattillo, 1988). After all, such coping styles are adaptive in many of the situations faced in daily life. It has been argued (Sotile, 1992) that, regardless of whether or not TYABP causes cardiopulmonary illness, unchecked TYABP will complicate both the treatment system and the personal adjustment.

What is to be done about this evidently universal phenomenon? Fortunately, numerous treatment outcome studies have assessed whether or not TYABP is modifiable (Haaga, 1987). An overview of this literature can provide guidelines for better understanding and helping any patient who evidences TYABP.

PERSPECTIVES ON TYABP

The various perspectives on TYABP that have been elucidated in the literature point to the complexity of understanding this coping pattern. For example, the mechanistic interaction model poses that TYABP is most likely to be fueled by the internal struggle for control that comes when one faces situations that represent opportunities or demands for achievement but that lack explicit standards of achievement (Glass, 1977; Matthews, 1982; Matthews & Siegel, 1983).

In the biologic interactional model (Krantz & Durel, 1983), TYABP is seen to reflect constitutional factors such as the predisposition for exaggerated sympathetic reactivity in responding to stressors. Here Type A reactivity is not seen as a reaction to conscious mediation. For example, Type As have been shown to evidence elevated blood pressure during but not prior to surgery (Krantz, Arabian, Davia, & Parker, 1982).

The biopsychosocial interactional model (Smith & Anderson, 1986) proposes that Type As do not simply respond to stressful situations; they also create additional challenges and demands in their environment through their TYABP. This perspective will be elaborated shortly, when the interpersonal aspects of TYABP are discussed.

HOSTILITY AND TYABP

In their efforts to link TYABP with the etiology or progression of CHD, contemporary researchers have offered a clear emphasis on the hostility component of this syndrome. Krantz and Manuck (1984) and Williams (1989) emphasized that such factors as competitiveness and time urgency (the factors that have traditionally been the focus of stress management interventions with Type As) are of less etiological importance in CHD than are hostility and anger and a predisposition to respond to frustration with reactions of irritation and contempt. This notion has been supported by a wealth of other researchers (e.g., Hecker et al., 1988; MacDougall, Dembroski, Dimsdale, & Hackett, 1985; Matthews et al., 1977).

HOSTILITY DEFINED

Similar to what has occurred in research on TYABP, the construct of hostility has been found to encompass various distinct factors. Smith (1992) proposed that the following differentiation is important in understanding research on hostility, because the different scales used in this research primarily measure one or another—but not all—of these factors. According to Smith, distinct components of what often is referred to as "high hostility" can include:

- Anger—an unpleasant emotion ranging in intensity from irritation to rage;
- Aggression—overt behavior, typically defined as attacking, destructive, or hurtful actions; and/or
- Hostility—the emotion of anger felt toward others that perpetuates a tendency to distrust others and to wish to inflict harm on them.

Smith pointed out that hostility is an emotion that is fueled by a set of negative attitudes, beliefs, and appraisals through which others are viewed as frequent and likely sources of mistreatment, frustration, and provocation (Smith, 1992). As a result, highly hostile individuals develop cynical skepticism regarding the trustworthiness of others (Williams, 1989).

HOW DOES HOSTILITY HURT?

Why is hostility so dangerous to one's health? Research has suggested a number of answers to this question (Smith, 1992) that can play important roles in motivating highly hostile patients to take seriously your recommendations that they learn to disrupt their hostile and aggressive reactions.

I have noticed in treating hundreds of highly hostile patients that they tend to dismiss the recommendation that they learn to manage their hostility. This dismissal is often due to the attitude that hostility should be curbed for the sake of others, not for oneself. By their very nature (i.e., they evidence high levels of hostility and cynicism), such people are not likely to be motivated by notions that have to do with enhancing the well-being of others. As one of my patients put it: "You are just wanting me to learn to be nice to fools who are aggravating me. I'm not so sure that biting my tongue off is worth it just to be nice to someone who (a) I probably don't care about and/or (b) just did something to piss me off."

This gentleman would never be motivated by the notion that he should become a fount of patience in dealing with others. But he was highly motivated by his fear of experiencing another MI or having to undergo a third CABG operation.

The Psychophysiological Reactivity Model

It may be that heightened cardiovascular and neuroendocrine reactivity leads to illness in highly hostile subjects (Williams, Barefoot, & Shekelle, 1985). Hostility increases cortisol, elevates lipid levels in plasma, and heightens overall physiological reactivity. Plus, the neuroendocrine responses triggered by frequent bursts of anger may impair immune functions, thereby increasing vulnerability to other diseases.

The Psychosocial Vulnerability Model

Perhaps highly hostile individuals live in more taxing interpersonal environments, the stresses of which accumulate and promote illness. As mentioned above, it has been proposed that the Type A style of reacting may create these taxing environments (Houston & Kelly, 1989; Smith & Anderson, 1986; Sotile, 1992). A specific variation of this pattern has been observed with COPD patients. The loss of resources and the symptoms of COPD can lead to increased angry behavior by the COPD patient, which, in turn, leads to increased anger in members of their support systems (Lane & Hobfoll, 1992). Whether they begin as highly hostile individuals or not, it is possible that the chronic stress that comes with living with COPD or with a loved one who has COPD may deplete both personal and social resources, making the individuals in the relationship system increasingly vulnerable to further stressful experiences. As will be discussed shortly, a wealth of clinical and research experience suggests that this notion applies not only to highly hostile individuals but to any individual who evidences any exaggerated Type A coping pattern.

The Transactional Model

Here the psychophysiological and psychosocial models are extended and integrated. Highly hostile people are seen as creating prolonged episodes of cardiovascular and neuroendocrine reactivity through their own thoughts and actions (Smith & Pope, 1990; Suls & Sanders, 1989). Indeed, research is affirming that such patterns elevate the risk of illness for highly hostile people. For example, highly hostile subjects have been found to experience pronounced physiological reactivity during conflictual marital interaction, the same forms of physiological reactivity that are thought to link stress and the development of CHD (Smith & Brown, 1991; Smith & Sanders, 1986).

The Health Behavior Model

Perhaps highly hostile people are at greater risk of disease simply due to their poor health habits (Leiker & Hailey, 1988). Research has shown that such people do tend to consume more caffeine, nicotine, alcohol, and calories and to more frequently engage in high-risk behaviors such as driving while intoxicated. They also engage in fewer positive health behaviors such as exercise, dental hygiene, or getting adequate sleep (Smith, 1992).

The Constitutional Vulnerability Model

It has also been proposed that people differ in their genetically determined autonomic lability. Highly hostile people may be more vulnerable to the development of illness simply due to some underlying constitutional or structural weakness (Krantz & Durel, 1983; Matthews, Rosenman, Dembroski, Harris, & MacDougall, 1984; Suls & Sanders, 1989).

TYABP AND MARRIAGE AND FAMILY LIFE

Whether or not any particular aspect of TYABP affects one's health, it is certain that unchecked TYABP will damage an important arena of well-being—relationships with others (Sotile, 1992). TYABP both affects and is affected by the inner workings of important relationships in the individual's life. The marital and family dynamics of recovering cardiopulmonary patients who evidence TYABP have received relatively scant research attention (Sotile, Sotile, Ewen, & Sotile, 1993). Instead, attention has tended to focus either on the solo experiences of individual patients or of their loved ones, not on their interactive dynamics.

This individualistic research of TYABP does have its merits. A wealth of laboratory research and clinical experience can be integrated into at least educated speculation regarding a systemic perspective of TYABP. In overview, this research has suggested that in interpersonal situations, Type As tend to:

- struggle to avoid loss of control (Glass, 1977);

- become distressed in reaction to stressors that are ambiguous regarding causes and effects (Helgeson, 1989; Suls, Gastorf, & Witenburg, 1979);

- react with irritation and contempt as frustrations grow (Krantz & Manuck, 1984; Williams, 1989);

- experience increased physiological reactivity when their dominance is challenged (VanEgeren, 1979; VanEgeren, Abelson, & Sniderman, 1983);

- generate conflict by selectively perceiving negatives and engaging in challenging behaviors (Smith & Anderson, 1986);

- show competitive and aggressive behavior when in small groups, and especially in reacting to other Type As (Blaney, Brown, & Blaney, 1986);

- become interpersonally reactant and then withdraw from contact once stressed (Blaney et al., 1986); and

- evidence poor ability to accurately observe their relationship styles and the effects their own behaviors have on others (Condon, 1988).

Because of such predispositions, the Type A is especially likely to find the intensity and complexity of ongoing family relationships stressful and is likely to react to such stress in ways that disrupt family harmony. This hypothesis is supported by research which has found that, regardless of whether it is evidenced by husband or wife, TYABP is rated as having a negative effect on the quality of daily family life (e.g., Becker & Byrne, 1984; Smith & Sanders, 1986; Sotile, 1992).

One area of family life that is clearly affected in negative ways by unchecked TYABP is parenting. Research has documented the negative effects of high levels of parental hostility on children (Trieber, Mabe, Riley, McDuffie, Strong, & Levy, 1990) and that Type As tend to: perceive children as stressors; lack effective parenting skills; project their own insecurities onto their children; and react to children's behavior more often with criticism than with nurturing comments (Price, 1982; Sotile, 1992).

Clearly, these and many other Type A characteristics create a negative impact on marriage and family living. In a landmark research project, Levenson and Gottman (1983, 1985) found that exaggerated sympathetic reactivity of the sorts that Type As have typically shown in laboratory studies accounted for over 80% of variance in marital satisfaction changes in 30 married couples, 19 of whom were followed for 3 years.

A summary of the implications of this research and of other extensive clinical descriptions of marriage and family life for Type As (e.g., Sotile, 1992) suggested a number of obvious ways that unchecked TYABP might disrupt marital/family harmony. Table 7.3 presents an overview of these patterns.

Similar to the other personality-based coping patterns discussed above, interaction within families that revolve around TYABP can become circular in nature. As the effects indicated in Table 7.3 accumulate, family patterns become more tense and tension-producing for all parties concerned. This tension becomes a variation of what Friedman and Rosenman (1974) identified as the hallmark factor that leads to Type A coping patterns: "an environmental challenge . . . serves as the fuse for this (Type A) explosion" (p. 10).

Furthermore, family life is typically a high-stakes arena in which the Type A individual lacks competency regarding needed adaptive skills. For the many reasons outlined above, Type As have difficulty establishing and maintaining intimate, empathic, nonjudgmental, relaxed, loving contact with others. In essence, I am proposing that unchecked TYABP can lead to the creation of family patterns that result in the Type A constantly feeling on the "outside" of his/her own family, struggling to gain acceptance but encountering criticism, frustration, or rejection.

This family process replicates the pain that is said to be at the core of the Type A's psychodynamic makeup. And what is the nature of this psychological pain? Research regarding the family experiences of Type As is mainly

Table 7.3   The Relationship Effects of TYABP

Type A factor	Relationship effects
Time urgency	Impairs connection with loved ones
Polyphasia	Yields poor communication; poor empathy
Impatience	Increases stress on others
Perfectionism	Increases criticism of loved ones and lowers levels of positively reinforcing interactions with loved ones
Irritation/hostility	Increases alienation and wounding of loved ones and leads to avoidance of attempts at intimacy by loved ones
Controlling	Loved ones cease to self-disclose and begin to avoid the Type A
Competitive	Loved ones avoid to escape being "put down" in Type A's efforts to bolster own shaky self-esteem

theoretical. However, most theorists and clinicians who have studied Type As agree that they tend to be people who harbor pain from having failed to receive adequate unconditional positive regard in their first family experiences. Excellent discussions of this literature (Matthews & Woodall, 1988; Price, 1982) have suggested that Type As tend to come from families characterized by

- unpredictable parental reactions,
- conditional parental approval,
- attention paid to outcomes,
- parental projections that lead to criticism,
- parents modeling tension and performance anxiety,
- vague performance criteria,
- parents' use of more physical discipline, and
- family patterns indicative of low levels of cohesiveness, support, and openness.

Interestingly, it appears that many Type As tend to parent as they were parented. Here, as in their marital interactions, Type As are at risk of responding to relationship stresses in ways that simply serve to further, rather than soothe, their stresses.

WHAT CAN BE DONE TO CHANGE TYABP?

Over 10,000 articles have been published in the professional literature regarding various aspects of TYABP. A wealth of treatment strategies have been shown to be at least partially successful in altering TYABP in both healthy and CHD patient populations. Various cognitive, behavioral rehearsal, physiological, and interactional strategies (e.g., assertion training, communication training) have been shown to be effective in treating different components of overall TYABP (e.g., Blumenthal & Wei, 1993; Haaga, 1987; Price, 1988).

Positive effects on TYABP have been noted from interventions that ranged from the use of simple, automated, brief educational treatment strategies (Oldenburg, Perkins, & Andrews, 1985) to those that involved extensive behavioral group therapy delivered over a 3-1/2-year period (Friedman et al., 1986). Extensive discussion of self-help strategies gleaned from this broad area of research have been published elsewhere (Sotile, 1992). Research and clinical experience have suggested that, in combination, the following factors can powerfully promote change in TYABP.

TREATING TYABP: GENERAL CONSIDERATIONS

There is no clear consensus in the literature regarding the most important focus of treatment with Type As. However, it is generally agreed that successful treatment programs include at least some versions of the following strategies (Razin, 1982):

- Encouragement to develop philosophies that promote self-reflection and compassion for others
- Self-monitoring through inventory-taking
- Guided practices or drills in self-observation
- Coaching regarding ways to develop behaviors that disrupt TYABP
- Advice regarding time management
- Discussion of work styles and the work environment

Treatment success seems to hinge on helping Type As to change either their expectations or the reinforcement values of TYABP. Rejeski (1983) cautioned that TYABP is a powerfully successful and familiar style of coping and that motivating an individual to change this coping pattern requires teaching the Type A that needs can be fulfilled by non-Type A behaviors and that such changes will eliminate considerable frustration from his or her life (i.e., the reinforcement value of non-Type A behavior can override the value of TYABP).

As mentioned above, cognitive, behavioral, and combination approaches have each been shown to successfully modify TYABP. Specific interventions that have been shown to be effective in changing components of TYABP include:

- retraining irrational beliefs that drive TYABP;
- reframing Type B behaviors as opportunities to prove oneself as an effective environmental and emotional engineer;
- aerobic exercise;
- coaching regarding the use of progressive muscle relaxation and self-monitoring in high-stress situations;
- anxiety management training;
- stress management training; and
- anger management training.

These various strategies and techniques can be combined in many ways to provide effective interventions with Type A patients. The remainder of this section is divided into two parts. First, specific strategies that should be kept in mind when treating Type As will be outlined, along with examples of brief interventions. Next, fairly detailed descriptions of more intensive and extensive treatment programs will be presented.

SPECIFIC TREATMENT STRATEGIES

Eight guidelines can help structure your treatment of Type A patients in any setting (Sotile, 1991). Both your comfortableness and effectiveness in treating Type As will be enhanced if you manage to

- be clear and specific,
- help soothe the Type A's shame or self-criticism,
- play to the Type A's need for control,
- use active interventions,
- educate the couple and coach effective interpersonal skills,
- teach tracking of sequences, and
- manage yourself.

1. Be Clear and Specific

Intervention with Type As should be respectful of their time-urgent, high-performing penchant and their need for structure. Accordingly, present rehabilitation information in a concise, data-based format that at once conveys respect for the patient's needs and your authority and expertise in serving as a consultant regarding the problems facing the patient. From the outset of your relationship, clearly specify treatment goals and the antici- pated course of the intervention, including the expected results. Where pos- sible, justify your intervention by briefly mentioning research that has documented the intervention's importance and effectiveness. Type As ap- preciate such orderliness and are likely to perceive any meandering, un- structured psychosocial intervention as being a waste of their precious time.

2. Help Soothe Shame or Self-Criticism

In many ways, TYABP is about perceived power; admitting the need for help can be an anxiety-provoking circumstance for such people. Such dis- comfort can take many forms. When forced to acknowledge their lack of control, Type As experience a variant of depression that has been termed "vital exhaustion" (Falger et al., 1988), a state characterized by overwhelming self-blame and discouragement, fear that all of life's obstacles will never be overcome, paralyzing levels of distress, and atypical passivity in responding to the challenges at hand. During such times, the Type A cardiopulmonary patient is especially likely to passively resist complying with medical recom- mendations (Rhodewalt & Fairfield, 1990).

Type As also tend to blame and shame themselves when they are faced with negative outcomes. When they most need the soothing that can only come from self-nurturing or from accepting nurturing from others, their excessively high standards and their tendency to selectively perceive nega- tive feedback propel them into a barrage of self-criticism that promotes momentary states of helplessness and depression (Cooney & Zeichner, 1985; O'Keefe & Smith, 1988; Wortman & Brehm, 1975).

By helping the patient develop new perspectives on the illness, on TYABP, and/or on the need for accepting help in learning to modify TYABP, you can help soothe these painful emotions and calm their accompanying alarm- ist frames of reference. You can calm the fear and shame that come with the notion that TYABP may have caused the illness with a brief summary of cutting-edge research that has refuted this perspective. Questions regard- ing the pathology of TYABP can be soothed with a summary of research which has shown that, in general, TYABP does not necessarily correlate with subjectively rated signs of stress or with objectively measured degrees of neuroticism or other forms of psychopathology (Rosenman, 1990). On the contrary, for some people, high scores on measures of TYABP tend to corre- late with personality traits such as extroversion, self-confidence, and a height- ened sense of mastery and vigor in coping with stress. Type A behavior has also been found to correlate with positive life experiences such as success in school, career distinction, and high occupational status (Bryant & Yarnold, 1990; Swan, Carmelli, & Rosenman, 1990).

Shame and distress over various components of TYABP (e.g., irritability, difficulty relaxing) can be soothed with a brief explanation of the physiology of Type A reactivity (Williams, 1989) and with input regarding the various ways that socialization and the stress epidemic of modern times promotes

TYABP (Sotile, 1991). Emphasize that the goal is to learn to avoid the extremes of TYABP; very few of us are able to completely avoid developing Type A tendencies, but each of us can learn to control these tendencies. The need for receiving help in learning to alter TYABP can be framed in positive terms such as:

"High-powered people often need specialized coaching to further hone their already powerful skills. Think of my input as a set of guidelines for organizing what you already know and systematizing what you do so that you can cope more effectively. I would also like to give you a short course on new information about TYABP (or anger management). I think you might find this information both interesting and helpful."

Finally, the Type A's distress can be soothed by ample use of cognitive frames that compliment. Seeking counseling can be labeled as "an indication that you are broad-minded enough to take an honest look in the mirror." The need for learning new anger control strategies can be framed as: "It is wise to learn to conserve your energy, saving those coping 'bazookas' for times when you will really need them." The need for making amends with other people can be framed in terms of: "Illness and crisis lead wise people to take a new look at what life is all about. People important to you probably need for you to be strong and wise enough to be the one to start building bridges of connection with them. Now, more than ever, they are afraid and in need of your help in connecting with you."

3. Play to the Type A's Need for Control

As mentioned above, Type As also tend to experience depression and a sense of helplessness when faced with crises over which they have no control. In the course of rehabilitation, many Type As attempt to satisfy their need for control by taking charge of the course of treatment. This dynamic can, and often does, result in nonadherent behavior: the Type A decides to take charge of some major aspect of treatment by ignoring or exaggerating his or her response to medical recommendations. More often, this dynamic is manifested in the Type A taking charge of smaller aspects of treatment: The format of treatment may be questioned ("Why is this a 3-month program? It seems that 2 months could do the trick just as well?"); attendance patterns may be altered in minor ways ("I'll have to leave 10 minutes early today; I have another commitment."); or modification of typical modes of delivering care may be requested or simply implemented ("I am not willing to fill out all of these forms. This is not why I came here." Or: "I didn't use the forms you gave me to keep a food diary. I made up my own form.")

Successful interventions with Type As match, rather than collide with, this frame of reference. When it does not really matter in promoting the safety and rehabilitation of the patient, such control maneuvers should be responded to by either ignoring, acknowledging, or—if appropriate— complimenting them ("You know, you have a good point there. I will take that into consideration in designing future programs."). In some instances, it may be appropriate to redesign procedural aspects of your care in response to patient feedback ("So, it sounds like the group would prefer for us to start 15 minutes earlier next week. If that's your vote, it's okay by me.").

4. Use Active Interventions

Remember that Type As tend to be action-oriented people who like to quantify their experiences. This penchant should be used to the advantage of treatment. Provide them with treatment interventions that require implementation of homework, charting of experiences, and documentation of progress. Have Type A outpatients journal their medication-taking, exercise, or dietary behaviors. Or use this same concept as a foundation for interventions that promote control of Type A tendencies by reframing desired goals and having the patient chart progress in reaching these goals. The following case example demonstrates various of these techniques.

I once treated a competitive, hot-reacting Type A heart patient who repeatedly experienced anger outbursts while driving the 50-mile commute to and from his place of employment. He explained the fuel for his anger in this way: "I have this little competition with myself: I try to break my record every time I drive this 50 miles. My best time to date is 36 minutes. I can't match that every day, though. Those fools driving in from Statesville always clog up the highway, going nowhere slowly."

An effective intervention with this patient consisted of several parts. First, I explained to him the dangers of unchecked hostility and that hurry sickness is a primary source of fuel for episodes of irritability and anger. I also had the patient (who was quite concerned about his hypertension) wear a 24-hr ambulatory blood pressure monitor to provide documentation of the physiological costs of his style of driving. Next, I had him calculate a reasonable pace of driving the 50-mile commute during rush hour traffic, using the frame of reference: "If one of your two teenage daughters was making the trip, how much time would you advise her to allow for making the commute, in order to be safe?" (His estimate was somewhere between 60 and 65 min.)

Finally, geared with this collective information, I suggested a new competition: The patient would begin charting his effectiveness in making the commute in as close to 60 minutes as possible. The new game became to make sure he was driving slowly enough to not arrive too early, according to these new rules.

In true Type A fashion, the patient modified the plan in several ways. To help remind himself to slow down, he decided to play soothing music while driving, and he taped pictures of his two daughters on the dashboard of his car—"To remind myself that the real competition is to stay alive long enough to see my babies' babies." He also calculated the amount of money he would save in fuel costs over the course of the upcoming year if he consistently made the commute driving 55 mph rather than his typical pattern of alternating between speeds of 65 mph and spurts of 70 to 90 mph. Each month, he multiplied the amount of money saved by two, divided the total in half, and placed equal amounts in savings accounts for his daughters.

This intervention demonstrates several points. It at once matched the patient's competitive strivings and his penchant for charting his experiences. It also promoted a pattern disruption in what typically was a stress- and anger-generating part of his daily life. The intervention recommendation ("slow down") was justified with data, both from research and from the patient's own experiences (his 24-hr blood pressure readings). Finally, the patient exercised needed (and, I thought, quite creative) control over the process by modifying and adding to the intervention's motivation strategies (use of his children's pictures as reminders of why he was driving more slowly and institution of immediate rewards for driving more slowly— "earning" money to give to his children). Also noteworthy is the lack of psychodynamic exploration in the intervention. Again, this was in response to the patient's frame of reference, expressed during our initial session: "I'm not interested in getting my head shrunk; I just want to get my heart healthy."

Examples of Active Interventions
In a similar vein, active interventions can be designed to facilitate changes in various aspects of TYABP. Patients can be encouraged to exert 20 minutes of effort each day trying on new behaviors such as:

- "Practice relaxation methods, and chart your subjective levels of attaining relaxation responses."

- "Monitor the actual number of hours spent working or thinking about work each day."

- "Visit a museum or art gallery and write a letter to a friend about the experience" (a strategy recommended by Friedman & Ulmer, 1984).

- "Experiment with a new interpersonal behavior such as remembering and commenting on the last conversation you had with an acquaintance or loved one."

- "Keep a pleasure log—a journal of how much pleasure or displeasure is associated with daily activities that are charted each hour, on the hour, throughout the day" (a strategy recommended by Roskies, 1987).

Further guidelines for active interventions geared toward altering Type A behaviors can be found in Friedman and Ulmer (1984), Roskies (1987), Sotile (1992), and Williams and Williams (1993).

5. Educate the Couple and Coach Effective Interpersonal Skills

Behind most Type A cardiopulmonary patients is a spouse or loved one, waiting to see what you will do about the patient's TYABP. As the Type A patient enters your care, it is important to at least briefly address relationship concerns that may have developed in reaction to the TYABP. At minimum, this should involve acknowledging to the loved one your awareness of the patient's Type A tendencies, debunking shame-generating mythologies regarding TYABP (see No. 1 above) but compassionately underscoring your advice that certain aspects of TYABP should be modified. Clarifying such issues with concerned loved ones can at once create allies in the treatment process and lessen tensions within the patient's household.

When possible, it is important to coach the Type A individual in effective interpersonal behaviors. As mentioned earlier, Type As tend to be over-powering and insensitive to the effects their behaviors have on others; however, clinical experience suggests that Type A patients can be motivated to learn more effective ways of managing themselves while interacting with others, especially if recommendations are framed in terms of "strategies for taking more effective charge of generating the outcomes you want when interacting with others." In this vein, the patient can be encouraged to experiment with and chart the results of a variety of new behaviors such as:

- "Increase the show of affection between you and one of your children or grandchildren by having the child teach you his or her homework without you giving any advice. Just listen and admire what the child knows."

- "Develop checklists to remind yourself of important interpersonal behaviors to work into your daily or weekly life. You might include on your list behaviors such as the following:

    Play a game with a family member and lose.

    Comment to a loved one, 'I was bragging about you today,' and explain why.

    Apologize twice each day.

    Smile.

    Have three conversations without giving advice.

    Instead: listen, reflect, empathize, admire.

    Express a self-doubt to at least two people each day."

In addition, it is important not to confuse the Type A's high-powered interpersonal style with effectiveness in managing conflict. Virtually every effective program for treating TYABP contains training in the ability to differentiate assertive from aggressive behaviors. The reader is referred to Alberti and Emmons (1982) for a guide to assertive training. In addition, those who want help in overcoming the awkwardness that accompanies attempts to change long-standing relationship patterns that revolve around TYABP are referred to Sotile (1992).

6. Use the EEM Model to Teach Tracking of Sequences

Clinical experience suggests that Type As respond readily to interventions that are framed using the terminology of the EEM model. In fact, this model was in large part developed out of my clinical experiences in treating Type A individuals and couples. Especially palatable to the Type A is the tenet of EEM that promotes awareness of the "domino coping progressions" that result in Type A symptomatology: the physiological/cognitive/behavioral/relationship processes that typically result in certain outcomes that are bothering the patient. This conceptualization provides an alternative to the "I can't help it" or "I can't change" mentality that many Type As evidence. The point is to acknowledge and normalize that, indeed, some aspects of Type A reactivity may be unchangeable (e.g., hyperphysiologic reactivity during certain types of stressful situations). However, what is always change-able—if the individual is willing to accept the challenge to learn new steps in their typically reactant progression of coping "dominoes"—is the next step of the process. Within this frame of reference, the patient can be helped to devise interventions that disrupt blaming, controlling, or catastrophizing cognitive or behavioral reactions during stressful times.

7. Manage Yourself

Finally, a word must be said about a crucial aspect of the treatment process as it affects TYABP: the health care provider's management of his or her own personal Type A tendencies. In my experience, health care providers often recoil at TYABP shown by patients due to their personal struggles with similar issues.

Remember that researchers have estimated that somewhere between 50% and 70% of men and women living in urban settings and only a slightly smaller percentage of residents of rural communities evidence at least one marked characteristic of TYABP. This coping pattern seems to be especially prevalent in people ages 30 to 55 and employed in white-collar occupations (Kelly & Houston, 1985; Thoresen & Low, 1990).

Given the prevalence of this coping pattern, clinicians working in any health care setting are faced with two probabilities: (a) you will treat a large numbers of Type A individuals; and (b) in the process of your own life, you, too, are likely to develop at least some markedly Type A coping styles. Effective providers of care to Type As are able to attain the delicate balance of showing strength but avoiding competition and power struggles with the patient. This can generally be done by some combination of the following.

- Compliment the patient freely, emphasizing the positive intention underlying his or her coping style.
- Judiciously use self-disclosure to relax the patient's embarrassment about seeking help from another (a particular problem for male Type As).
- Be respectful and caring in reacting to the patient's efforts to exert control (e.g., "I noticed that you missed our last scheduled appointment. I know that you are busy, and appointments sometime fall through the cracks of a busy schedule. But I'd appreciate you calling and keeping me posted; I was worried about you.").
- Finally, steadfastly avoid making statements that fuel blame, shame, or unwise competitive reactions.

Avoid statements such as:

"If you don't slow down, you're going to kill yourself. Your competitiveness is what got you sick in the first place."

"One reason you aren't showing progress is that you aren't taking your rehabilitation seriously."

"That's pretty good progress, but I've seen better."

"Come on! If I can manage to force myself to exercise and quit smoking, you can do the same."

Instead, use statements such as:

"I know that your life speeds you up, but it's important to learn how to pace yourself."

"I know that you aren't showing the kind of progress you'd like, but remember that this takes a while. You are making some good efforts in spurts, but we need to take a another look at your overall approach to your rehabilitation."

"Everybody I work with goes through rehab at their own pace. Your pace is fine for you."

"I really can appreciate that it's hard to make changes such as stopping smoking or getting into an exercise routine. I've struggled with those myself."

I do not mean to imply that you need to treat Type A patients in a coddling way or that they should be considered exempt from the need for limit setting or confrontation. Management of any therapeutic relationship requires a combination of respect for the patient and a healthy degree of self-respect and willingness to set limits in responding to the patient's needs or style of coping. Indeed, I have found that, as a group, Type A patients tend to respond adaptively to limit setting when the limits are set with respect and concern.

My point is to underscore the two key words at the end of the preceding sentence: respect and concern. As health care providers treating Type A patients, we are vulnerable to violating a credo that should govern our behavior while delivering health care: To be avoided at all costs when treating any patient are inappropriate expressions of one's own psychodynamics, competitive strivings, or struggles with issues of control or hostility— regardless of how much the patient may be struggling in these same ways.

EXTENSIVE TREATMENT PROGRAMS

A number of extensive treatment programs have been designed for the treatment of TYABP. The following discussions provide overviews of several such approaches. The interested reader is referred to the many citations listed in this section for extended details on how to structure such interventions. For others, a perusal of this section may prove helpful in underscoring basic concepts to keep in mind in determining who might be appropriate for referral to an extensive treatment program and in highlighting the overall features of such programs. In addition, the research findings that are summarized in the following can be very effective in motivating and reassuring Type A patients that changing this behavior pattern is possible and is a worthwhile investment of time and energy.

Anger Management Training

Extensive treatment programs for TYABP always incorporate cognitive/ behavioral approaches to anger control. In addition to sharing the physiological facts regarding the dangers of unchecked anger, you can motivate patients to change their angry behaviors with a simple fact: Research has shown that the expressive aspects of hostility, such as aggression or antagonism, may be more closely related to risk of CHD than subjective experiences such as angry feelings and thoughts (Siegman, 1989). This means that simply learning to control aggressive behaviors can lessen the risk of developing CHD.

Furthermore, contrary to the notion that "expressing anger helps relieve internal agitation," angry behavior simply leads to further aggression, not to calming (Green & Quanty, 1977). This information can be used to reassure and to motivate the Type A who fears that he or she simply cannot control anger reactions. Confronting such a person with the advisability of managing behaviors, even when feeling angry, creates leverage for promoting needed behavioral changes. Of course, as such behavioral changes accumulate, anger may be experienced less frequently, a notion that will be discussed further below.

From the outset of treatment, it is important to convey that you understand the positive, adaptive aspects of anger. Anger can serve to: energize a person to assertively confront a provocative or unjust situation; demonstrate potency; terminate feelings of vulnerability; and/or enhance one's sense of personal control (Novaco, 1976a).

The patient's personal underlying beliefs about anger should be elicited, examined, and made conscious. For example, many Type As believe that their anger is necessary to ward off injustice or to remain motivated or powerful. Women tend to have particularly complex beliefs about anger, probably due to socialization. Biaggio (1987) called attention to research which has shown that women experience more anxiety and guilt in conjunction with anger or aggression than do men (e.g., Frodi, Macaulay, & Thome, 1977). Prohibitions against the direct expression of anger—due either to socialization or, as is the case for many COPD and CHD patients, to fears of the physiological consequences of emotional arousal—can lead to unconscious suppression of anger. This can result in a blunting of any direct expression of anger and a fueling of a hostile attitude or of passive-aggressive behavior.

It is also important to help patients learn to differentiate between anger reactions that are justified and those that are not and between provocations that can be remedied and those that cannot (Biaggio, 1987). When anger is justified, the individual must learn to pause and examine potentially productive versus unproductive coping strategies. If the situation cannot be modified, the patient should be coached to employ cognitive coping strategies such as reinterpretation, relabeling, or distraction.

The literature on the treatment of anger examines various methods for helping people learn to cope constructively with provocation and anger arousal. Various treatment strategies that have been reported include:

- Coaching in assertive behavior directed toward removal of the provoking stimulus (Biaggio, 1987).
- Social skills training that combines cognitive training, skill acquisition, rehearsal, and imaginal and role-played practice for dealing with high-stress situations without showing aggressive behavior (Moon & Eisler, 1983; Novaco, 1975, 1976b). Here, for example, through didactic presentations and role-play, the individual is coached to increase the frequency of eye contact, decrease inappropriate requests, and increase appropriate facial mannerisms and affect during potentially stressful situations (Moon & Eisler, 1983).

- Cognitive training to control anger-provoking self-statements that occur in response to anger-provoking situations (Novaco, 1975).

- Cognitive self-instruction paired with relaxation training (Novaco, 1975).

- Coaching to disrupt anger and aggressive behavior by inducing an incompatible emotional or behavioral response such as empathy (Baron, 1979), humor (Mueller & Donnerstein, 1977), or relaxation (Hazaleus & Deffenbacher, 1986; Roskies et al., 1978).

- Coaching in effective expression of anger. For example, the following are characteristics of adaptive expressions of anger that might be taught, modeled, and role-played in an anger management class:

  1. Focuses on the problem at hand

  2. Involves a clear and genuine expression of personal feelings

  3. Avoids expression of opinions that belittle others

  4. Focuses on the speaker's internal reactions, rather than on the listener's actions

  5. Avoids any judgment about the listener's character

  6. Inflicts no harm; does not attempt to coerce the listener

  7. Suggests constructive remedies to the bothersome situation

  8. Conveys a spirit of intention to get beyond the tension at hand

  9. Results in both parties maintaining self-esteem

Clinical observation suggests that once highly hostile patients begin accumulating experience in acting differently (i.e., under more control) during stressful, anger-generating times, both their emotional experiences and their cognitions are likely to shift to more calming directions. This observation is supported by empirical research related to the aforementioned theory that the reinforcement value of non-Type A behavior must override the value of Type A behavior if lasting modifications in TYABP are to occur (Rejeski, 1983). Biaggio (1987) showed that during interpersonal conflict, calm assertion is much more likely to elicit understanding than highly emotional displays of anger. It is therefore likely that, if an individual can be convinced to experiment with restraining impulsive, angry expression and to instead practice calm assertion of feelings, "the new behavior is likely to be reinforced and, with repeated success, to be strengthened" (Biaggio, 1987, p. 668). This notion was leant further support in a comparison of three behavioral treatment strategies with an attention control group in the reduction of anger by Moon and Eisler (1983). These researchers found that social skills training not only decreased aggressive responding and increased assertive behaviors, but also led to improvement on a measure of the cognitive factor of perceived anger across various situations.

Many helpful self-help guidelines for controlling anger and hostility have been published. Two that deserve special mention are *When Anger Hurts* (McKay, Rogers, & McKay, 1989) and *Anger Kills* (Williams & Williams, 1993).

Anxiety and Stress Management Training

Suinn (1974, 1975) proposed that TYABP is a maladaptive means of coping with anxiety experienced when the Type A is not active. In the Cardiac Stress Management Training program (Suinn, 1975), a five-session treatment is used to help the patient learn to recognize tension cues and to use relaxation to promote alternative responses. This treatment basically hinges on a form of systematic desensitization: Deep muscle relaxation is taught; the patient's anxiety responses are aroused via imagery; and, with the aid of coaching to recognize the physiologic cues of anxiety, the patient is helped to evoke the relaxation response in the presence of these cues and imagery. Suinn also included a visual-motor behavioral rehearsal component that employed stressful imagery paired with practicing anti-Type A behaviors.

Suinn's technique has been modified to target treatment of anxiety (Suinn, 1977; Suinn & Bloom, 1978) and anger in noncardiac, Type A populations (Hazaleus & Deffenbacher, 1986). In the latter technique, instead of anxiety cues and scenes, anger-arousing cues and scenes are used. The reader is referred to the writings of Suinn for further specifics regarding these treatment strategies.

Training in Interpersonal Skills

It is recommended that any treatment of TYABP also incorporate at least minimal education and training regarding the interpersonal effects of TYABP and ways to manage interpersonal tensions (Sotile, 1992; Sotile, Sotile, Ewen, & Sotile, 1993). It is naive to limit one's understanding of TYABP and hostility to the implications of laboratory research. As pointed out by Biaggio (1987) in his review of research regarding the management of anger, laboratory settings contain social inhibitions and proscriptions regarding anger expression and involve less intense personal anger provocation than occurs in real life. Averill (1992) analyzed self-report data regarding anger expression and found that 88% of recent incidents of anger involved another person as the target of anger: 53% were either loved ones or someone known well, 26% were acquaintances, 8% were people known well but disliked, and only 12% were strangers.

Extensive discussion of ways to coach Type As to be more interpersonally effective is available in *Heart Illness and Intimacy: How Caring Relationships Aid Recovery* (Sotile, 1992).

Extensive, Combination Programs for Treating TYABP

The multiple strategies listed above have been coupled with group supportive interventions to create especially powerful programs for modifying TYABP. Such programs have been shown to be effective in treating both recovering MI patients (Friedman et al., 1986) and healthy Type As (Roskies et al., 1986). Perhaps the most noteworthy study in the professional literature on TYABP involved The Recurrent Coronary Prevention Project (RCPP), a randomized 4-1/2-year clinical trial that employed over 800 post-MI Type A patients (Friedman et al., 1986). The RCPP intervention was structured around a cognitive social learning approach. It used group support; cognitive/behavioral interventions geared to help patients recognize and counter TYABP and Type A lifestyles; encouragement to alter environmental cues that typically elicited TYABP; and relaxation training. A total of 44 treatment sessions were offered over a 3-1/2-year period, but the subjects actually attended an average of 29 sessions.

At 3-year follow-up, the treatment group had significantly greater reductions in indications of TYABP than controls and evidenced a 50% reduction in recurrent MIs compared to controls. These results were maintained at 4-1/2-year follow-up. It was also found that, for subjects who had singular, mild MIs, intervention reduced death rates during the 4-1/2-year follow-up by nearly 50%. This reduced mortality finding did not hold for those subjects who entered the program having already suffered either multiple MIs or a severe initial MI.

It is noteworthy that, although this treatment program was delivered over a lengthy period of time, the actual interventions used were quite simple. These involved such assignments as:

- purposely driving in the slow lane of traffic;
- once each day, sitting and doing absolutely nothing for 15 min;
- attending cultural events and writing a letter to a friend telling about the event;
- smiling more often;
- admitting personal vulnerabilities to friends and loved ones.

The method underlying these seemingly simple interventions was quite ingenious, given that a prerequisite for each was countering some major aspect of TYABP. For example, driving slowly forces a reprogramming of hurry sickness. Doing nothing counters polyphasia. Attending a cultural event counters work addiction, writing a letter about it requires attending to what is happening (countering polyphasia), and writing a friend about the experience facilitates social support. Smiling and self-disclosing provide rehearsal of effective interpersonal behaviors. Detailed descriptions of these and interventions used in the RCPP are available in *Treating Type A Behavior and Your Heart* (Friedman & Ulmer, 1984).

The strategies used in the RCPP have also been used successfully in treating healthy Type As (Gill et al., 1985). However, the most noteworthy study of a specific treatment program with healthy Type As was the Montreal Type A Intervention Project of Ethel Roskies and colleagues (Roskies et al.,

1986). This study compared the effects of 20 cognitive-behavioral stress management group sessions delivered over a 10-week period to those of aerobic exercise and weight training. Subjects were 107 healthy, male executives, 33 in the aerobic exercise group and 37 each in the other two treatment groups. Following treatment, the stress management group showed significantly greater changes in behavioral indices of TYABP than did the other two groups.

A major value of the Montreal Type A Intervention Project lies in the excellent description of the treatment protocol used in the study (Roskies, 1987). Treatment hinged on teaching the concept that TYABP had admittedly been proven (in research and in the group participants' personal experiences) to be effective in promoting such desirable outcomes as work accomplishment. However, it was also emphasized that most Type As fall into the pattern of overresponding to the inevitable hassles and challenges of daily living with automatic, stereotyped, all-or-nothing Type A reactivity. The result? Most Type As fail to use their coping energies efficiently. Participants were challenged to learn to recognize and minimize the "coping costs" of TYABP by learning to respond to stressors in new ways. This required learning to use a number of coping strategies with flexibility.

Indeed, Roskies and colleagues structured their program around the teaching of several coping strategies such as muscular relaxation, communication skills, cognitive relabeling, stress inoculation, and problem solving. Participants were also coached to differentiate "good" and "bad" stress perceptions and responses and were helped to devise and implement coping experiments in dealing with each form of stress. Group sessions were used to provide didactic interventions as well as feedback and social support. In addition, 19 graded homework assignments designed to promote application of the concepts covered in the group sessions were employed. Treatment focused on teaching participants to:

- increase their awareness of the situations that triggered dysfunctional chains of physiological, behavioral, and cognitive stress responses;

- learn new coping responses;

- more accurately assess the effects of various coping strategies on their mental and physical well-being; and

- expand their practice of the new coping strategies into a variety of situations until these new patterns became habitual.

Roskies and colleagues structured their intervention into seven modules. The first three were devoted to basic skill building, enhancement of self-monitoring, and the beginnings of experimentation with modulating physical, behavioral, and cognitive stress responses. Modules four and five taught participants to combine and apply the strategies taught in prior sessions and to troubleshoot regarding upcoming stressors. This phase of treatment also emphasized learning to regain control when suddenly confronted with unpredictable and initially uncontrollable stress emergencies.

Interestingly, module six focused on using self-management skills to integrate pleasures into one's daily and weekly life. Here the goal was to teach each individual to attain needed rest and recuperation. Roskies noted that many Type As drift into the trap of confusing "aversion relief" (i.e., accomplishment of pressing, anxiety-provoking tasks) with pure pleasure. Participants were coached to develop and heighten their awareness of what they found pleasurable and to dare to create time in their busy lives for such activities. The final module focused on relapse prevention, emphasizing the importance of not responding to slips with all-or-nothing thinking and of anticipating and aborting reversions to old habits.

Detailed descriptions of the many exercises used in the Montreal Type A Intervention program can be found in *Stress Management for the Healthy Type A* and its companion workshop leader's handbook (Roskies, 1987).

CONCLUDING THOUGHTS REGARDING TYABP

A growing legion of contemporary researchers are questioning the necessity of adding to what they consider an already exhaustive and somewhat circular body of published data regarding TYABP. In my opinion, this objection is shortsighted. Regardless of whether or not TYABP is associated with physical illness, many crucial questions remain to be answered regarding this coping style. Given the prevalence of TYABP in contemporary times and the problematic behavioral consequences of unchecked TYABP, attempting to find answers to these questions seems warranted.

I am not alone in my call for continued research into TYABP.

1. Houston-Miller et al. (1990) urged future researchers to determine: standardized measures of hostility and/or TYABP; long-term effects of interventions that change TYABP and hostility; whether behavioral approaches to modification of TYABP can reduce hostility in patients with established illness; and the long-term effects of these interventions.

2. Razin (1982) made the important point that further research into the effects and treatment implications of TYABP evidenced within medical care facilities is needed. Specifically, the effects of TYABP on patient responses to CCU stays or to the challenges of outpatient rehabilitation are underresearched. Razin astutely observed that certain aspects of TYABP, such as annoyance, suppression of awareness of psychological and physical symptoms, competitiveness felt toward other patients, agitation with the confinement of the CCU, or actual or perceived enforcing of a frustrating pace in outpatient rehabilitation settings, might differentially stress Type As compared to Type Bs. Such frustrations might even trigger cardiovascular hyperreactivity and thereby complicate the clinical condition evidenced by a Type

A. These possibilities raise an as-yet unanswered question: Should Type As be treated differently than Type Bs?

Finally, I again emphasize a relatively virginal territory of much-needed research in this area: the interplay between TYABP and interpersonal dynamics, particularly as these apply to the workings of intimate relationships in the Type A's life. These and other questions regarding TYABP remain to be answered by future researchers.

SUMMARY

A key component of EEM is the recognition and management of personality-based coping patterns. During stressful times, we all are compelled to cope in certain ways that, if magnified by the syndrome of TYABP, can become problematic. Through a combination of education, coaching, and support, patients can benefit from, rather than suffer the consequences of, their most habitual coping tendencies.

Regardless of the patient's personality-based coping tendencies, one thing is certain: his or her stress reactions will interplay with those of loved ones. The stresses of rehabilitation create special challenges and opportunities for recovering patients and their families. Learning to manage family relationships is the next component of EEM.

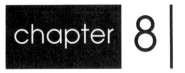

chapter 8

MARITAL AND FAMILY ISSUES

Traditionally, psychological assessment and intervention in cardiopulmonary rehabilitation have focused on the examination and treatment of the individual patient. The burgeoning field of family systems medicine reminds us that families function as teams and that rehabilitation efforts should, at minimum, consider the interactional processes within the family; how the challenges and stresses of illness and rehabilitation impact the family; and how family-level reactions to these challenges and stresses affect the course of rehabilitation for a given cardiopulmonary patient.

Over 1,000 articles pertaining to the family are published each year in the medical literature. Unfortunately, less than 5% are reports concerning research on the family and health, and less than 5% of these are empirical studies (Campbell, 1986). Furthermore, the most often cited of these studies within cardiology are social epidemiological investigations that use a disease model which is targeted on the examination of a disorder (i.e., heart illness) that is seen as existing entirely within the patient. Accordingly, a unidirectional (linear) causality relationship between such variables as family demographics (e.g., marital status) and illness variables (e.g., death or presence of heart illness) is assumed.

Because social epidemiological research employs quantitative methods to investigate discrete relationships between specified variables, highly valid results are possible (e.g., the effect of bereavement on mortality)—results that contain important implications for the relationship between family functioning and health outcomes (Campbell, 1986). Noteworthy examples of such studies with a focus on heart disease include: the Alameda County study (Berkman & Syme, 1979); the Framingham study (Haynes, Eaker, & Feinleb, 1983); and recent studies regarding the importance of social support—especially of the presence of a confidant—in preventing mortality in recovering male MI patients (Case et al., 1992; Williams et al., 1992).

From a clinical management standpoint, the problem with such epidemiological research is that it provides no direct examination of the richness of family systems operations in the wake of illness. Such studies provide important input to answer the question of whether or not family factors play a role in the etiology or course of heart illness. But these studies—just as with traditional psychological assessment that focuses on examination and treatment of the individual medical patient—ignore a factor that is crucial to better understanding who responds how to various aspects of cardiopulmonary illness and rehabilitation: the complexities of human relationships and families. For example, the Framingham study employed a 300-question psychosocial interview and 20 separate scales but included only two questions involving the family (marital dissatisfaction and disagreement) (Campbell, 1986).

The comments of family systems medicine pioneers William Doherty and Thomas Campbell (1988) regarding the historically narrow range of research and practice in health psychology also applies to many of our efforts heretofore in cardiopulmonary rehabilitation: It appears that we have been developing more of a biopsychological model than a true biopsychosocial model of rehabilitation.

In delivering clinical care, a number of questions are more important than whether family factors affect the development of illness. These include:

- How might family factors affect the process of rehabilitation?

- How might illness and medical interventions affect the family's functioning?

- Finally, what signals that family-level consultation might benefit overall psychosocial adjustment for the recovering cardiopulmonary patient and his or her loved ones (Hill et al., 1992; Sotile, 1992)?

When these questions are considered, perspectives on the delivery of medical and rehabilitation care shifts from a linear to a family systems framework.

FAMILY SYSTEMS THEORY

The family systems approach to medical care and rehabilitation is rooted in general systems theory (von Bertalanaffy, 1968). This school of thought includes a diverse group of family theorists and practitioners who share the view that families function as highly integrated teams composed of interdependent parts, organized within a discernible structure and bound together by a system of shared values and beliefs. A family systems perspective on rehabilitation is distinguished by:

- seeing patients as parts of larger wholes;

- seeing behavior as being determined by interaction and as serving a purpose for family systems;

- understanding circular cause-and-effect patterns in family relationships;

- seeing rehabilitation (or illness behavior) as one of the most consistent "forces" around which family relationships revolve; and

- pinpointing attempted family solutions that are actually serving to perpetuate anticipated family problems.

Family teams are said to be governed by rules and interaction patterns that are driven by habit. Often, the rules that are most salient in determining the behavior of individual family members go unarticulated (Barbarin & Tirado, 1984). For example, based on the roles that have historically been assigned and assumed within a family team, different family members, when stressed, will be compelled to lock into the roles of peacemaker, rational problem solver, emotional symptom bearer for the family team, and so on (Satir, 1964; Sotile, 1992).

From the family systems perspective, cardiopulmonary illness and rehabilitation of one family member is seen as a potential stressor for all members of the family team, and interplay between individuals within the family results in emotional and behavioral consequences at both the individual and family levels (Sotile, Sotile, Ewen, & Sotile, 1993). Accordingly, in the family systems model, the focus of assessment and intervention is the system of interactions among: reactions by individual family members; the reactions and attitudes of the family as a team; the adaptive tasks of rehabilitation; and the health care provider's style of relating to the family (Harkaway & Madsen, 1989; Stein & Pontious, 1985).

DO MARITAL AND FAMILY FACTORS REALLY MATTER IN CARDIOPULMONARY REHABILITATION?

William Doherty has proposed that health behaviors such as smoking, dietary choices, or alcohol use can be viewed as a form of interpersonal communication that regulates inclusion, control, and affection processes in intimate relationships (Doherty & Harkaway, 1990). My own recently published, integrative reviews of over 300 publications on a family systems perspective of cardiopulmonary rehabilitation suggest that Doherty's notions apply not only to specific health behaviors but to a range of issues relevant to risk factor modification and psychosocial adjustments important in cardiopulmonary rehabilitation (Sotile, Sotile, Ewen, & Sotile, 1993; Sotile, Sotile, Sotile, & Ewen, 1993):

- For male MI patients, having a supportive, optimistic mate leads to enhanced interpersonal efficacy, which results in more adaptive individual coping. In fact, a wife's perception of the male MI patient's efficacy is more predictive of the patient's recovery than is his own self-efficacy (Antonucci & Johnson, 1994).

- Having a smoking spouse has been found to significantly decrease the odds of a smoker's quitting (Hanson, Klesges, Eck, Cigrang, & Carle, 1990).

On the other hand, a supportive spouse, particularly one who is an ex-smoker, appears to influence quit attempts positively (Cohen & Lichtenstein, 1990).

• Reinforcement from a respected confidant has been found to be important in maintaining new eating behaviors (Pearce, LeBow, & Orchard, 1981).

• Marital and family factors have been shown alternately to stimulate and discourage drinking behavior in recovering alcoholics (O'Farrell, 1989).

• Hypertension treatment programs that incorporated a conscientious effort to promote marital or family support have been found to have a profound, positive effect on adherence to a hypertension treatment regimen, and such gains have been noted for periods of up to 5 years (Morisky et al., 1983; Storer, Frate, Johnson, & Greenberg, 1987).

• Research has shown that, independent of health status, a low-conflict marital relationship serves to promote a more positive sense of well-being for recovering Type A male MI patients (Waltz, Bandura, Pfaff, & Schott, 1988).

• The adherence literature supports the notion that a spouse's attitudes toward rehabilitation have a direct effect on the recovering cardiopulmonary patient's response to medical and rehabilitation interventions (Friis & Taff, 1986).

• High levels of spouse support have been found to enhance in-hospital recovery for male CABG patients (Kulik & Mahler, 1989). Marital attitudes, levels of marital intimacy, and levels of spouse support and communication have all been found to be crucial determiners of patient responses to outpatient cardiac rehabilitation (Bar-On & Cristal, 1987). Research has also documented that, when handled appropriately, the shock of rehabilitation from cardiopulmonary illness can actually lead to enhanced family functioning (Laerum, Johnsen, Smith, & Arnesen, 1991).

• Both retrospective and prospective studies have suggested that intimacy, and not just affiliation with a vaguely defined "social support network," is a crucial factor affecting well-being (Headey, Holmstron, & Wearing, 1984; Rook, 1984).

• The quality of a marriage has a direct effect on the individual stress status of the wife of a recovering heart patient (Croog & Fitzgerald, 1978).

• A prior or developing marital problem is more likely to precede depression than vice versa (Beach, Sandeen, & O'Leary, 1990).

• For decades, researchers have documented the importance of marital support in promoting adjustment to work-related stressors such as unemployment or retirement (Lowenthal & Haven, 1968).

In addition to this indisputable body of evidence that marital and family factors do matter in determining important rehabilitation outcomes, this literature also validates the notion that families are teams, in sickness and in health. The stresses of cardiopulmonary illness and rehabilitation have been found to have profound effects on both the recovering patient's spouse and children. For example, spouses of both cardiac and pulmonary patients suffer high incidences of stress, anxiety, depression, and somatic symptoms (e.g., Rabinowitz & Florian, 1992; Shanfield, 1990). In fact, any member of the family, including grown children, can evidence symptoms of psychological distress for up to 20 years following the onset of the parent's illness (Worby, Altrocchi, Veach, & Crosby, 1991). It is almost commonplace that family members hold themselves accountable for their loved one's illness and rehabilitation (Gilliss, 1984).

The importance of attending to marital and family factors in delivering clinical care was succinctly summarized by Coyne and Smith (1991) in their discussion of the interplay between marital dynamics and cardiac rehabilitation:

What needs to be done in coping with the infarction—the tasks or issues that coping entails—is shaped by what each partner does and how the other responds. To a large degree, such give and take, not just the couple's perception of the event, determines how the event unfolds and reverberates in these people's lives (Coyne, Ellard, & Smith, 1990). (Coyne & Smith, 1991, p. 405)

Unfortunately, it appears that the relationship between the patient's family system and the health care provider is most often either ignored or strained by the traditional practice of focusing exclusively on the identified medical patient. Wives of recovering cardiac patients frequently voice distress over being ignored by medical personnel during their husbands' hospitalization and aftercare (Thompson & Meddis, 1990), a factor that has been identified as one of the major stressors for this population (Coyne & Smith, 1991). Gillis (1984) and Coyne and Smith (1991) have cautioned that the failure of medical systems to provide guidance to the recovering patient's relationship system may account for many of the observed negative effects of the medical condition on both the patient and his or her spouse. In my aforementioned integrative reviews of literature, only one study was found (i.e., Papadopoulos et al., 1980) that addressed this issue. Clearly, the effective matching of interventions to patient concerns needs to begin with respect for the patient's family system. Many useful guidelines exist regarding ways to provide family-sensitive care to cardiac and pulmonary patients (Sotile, 1992, 1993). These will be discussed in the pages to follow.

INSIDE THE FAMILY'S TEAMWORK

A family-sensitive approach is crucial throughout the delivery of care to cardiac and pulmonary patients (Ries, 1990). Many factors need to be considered if you are to understand family-level reactions to illness.

HOW STRESSFUL IS THIS?

Dealing with illness is always stressful for a family, but the magnitude of the stressor varies tremendously, depending on six factors: the severity of the illness; the patient's age, gender, and roles within the family; the family's premorbid stress level; and the family's relationship with health care providers.

The Severity of Illness

Coyne and Smith (1991) remind us that:

> However important the couple's coping may be, it is not the only determinant of the outcomes they achieve, and it may not be the most crucial influence. In chronic and catastrophic illness, patients' medical conditions may largely determine both the range of possible outcomes and how well couples may adapt. Furthermore . . . lack of information and support from medical personnel . . . may hamper their adaptation . . . and create unnecessary distress. (p. 405)

On the other hand, ample research has suggested that medical diagnosis or degree of disability have only minimal effects in determining coping choice. In work with cardiovascular patients, Laffrey and Crabtree (1988) found that neither health behaviors nor health meanings were related to objective indices of physical limitations. Thus, coping choices in recovering cardiopulmonary patients are influenced not only by the diagnosis, but also by the appraisal of health and the family systems operations.

Age

The age of the patient and the family's developmental stage of life also have much to do with reactions to illness. More than their younger counterparts, older adults, when stressed, have been found to: aggressively attempt to alter the stressful situation (confrontive coping); acknowledge their own role in the problem and attempt to put things right (accepting responsibility); and attempt to create positive meaning by focusing on personal growth that can come in reacting to the stressor (positive reappraisal) (Folkman, Lazarus, Pimley, & Novacek, 1987).

For obvious reasons, older adults are more likely to accept the challenge of coping with illness as being an age-appropriate task and, in some instances, may welcome the structure and camaraderie that come with the "opportunity" the illness affords them to participate in a formal rehabilitation program (Sotile, 1993). Middle-aged adults, on the other hand, are beset with concerns with work or family issues (McCrae, 1984) and are much more likely to resist organizing their lives around rehabilitation procedures. More extensive discussion of psychosocial issues that face aged patients and the health care providers who treat them will be presented in chapter 13.

Gender

It is well documented that women have a more complicated convalescence from heart illness. The exact cause of this gender difference is only beginning to be researched. Preliminary studies have suggested that differences in referral patterns and in support systems may account for the relatively low numbers of female patients who have participated in formal cardiac rehabilitation programs (Lavie, Milani, & Littman, 1993; Ribisl et al., 1994). The fact that most female cardiac patients are aged and that many serve as caretakers for their dependent, equally, or more aged spouses has also been posed as an explanation for the relative absence of females in formal cardiac rehabilitation programs (Ades, Waldman, Polk, & Coflesky, 1992). The fact that the majority of COPD patients are aged males no doubt contributes to the relative lack of information regarding male/female differences in coping with this illness.

Regardless of the statistics about illness prevalence or participation in rehabilitation, there are important research-documented gender differences in reacting to stress. Indeed, in both healthy and chronically ill populations, men and women have been found to cope in somewhat different ways (Holahan & Moos, 1986). In general, it appears that men are more prone to attempt to regulate their own feelings and actions when stressed (self-control strategies) and to deliberately try to alter the stressor in a problem-solving, analytic way (planful problem-solving). Furthermore, men who evidence TYABP (especially if they show elevations on measures of speed and impatience) have been found to be particularly unlikely to seek social support when stressed (Hart, 1988). Stressed women, on the other hand, are more likely to resort to emotion-focused strategies, including seeking social support or engaging in wishful thinking, and behavioral efforts to escape or avoid the problem. More than Type B women or Type A men, women who elevate on measures of TYABP (especially those who elevate on measures of speed and impatience and hard-driving and competitive) are particularly likely to be self-blaming and self-critical when stressed and to struggle to maintain emotional control by employing cognitive-restructuring coping mechanisms (Hart, 1988).

When the stressor is cardiovascular disease, women have been found to be more resistant to implementing lifestyle changes than men (Badger, 1992). But preliminary research in this area has suggested that when they do participate, women generally evidence improvements during formal cardiac rehabilitation that are comparable to their male counterparts (Cannistra, Balady, O'Malley, Weiner, & Ryan, 1992). Interestingly, as individuals age, gender differences in coping styles diminish, as do responses to formal cardiac rehabilitation interventions.

Overall, only approximately 20% of subjects in investigations of cardiopulmonary rehabilitation interventions have been female. The individual and family-level coping challenges that face male and female cardiopulmonary patients need to be differentiated by future researchers. It has been noted that: "Given the demonstrably different relationship styles in reacting to stress in the general population of males and females . . . , it seems reasonable that a family might experience a differing psychosocial challenge and adaptive process during a father's versus a mother's cardiac rehabilitation" (Sotile, Sotile, Sotile, & Ewen, 1993, p. 231).

Family Roles

As already mentioned, families tend to assign and to assume roles to create homeostasis, or balance, in their overall teamwork. For example, one family member may become the system's emotional symptom bearer during stressful times, while another member blunts emotional expression in deference to showing logic and rationality (Satir, 1964). Depending on which member gets sick, a family's typical relational patterns will be more or less disrupted. It is possible that a family will experience less distress when a member who has historically evidenced health or behavioral problems gets sick than if the "wrong" family member (i.e., one who has been a source of strength and stability within the family) becomes ill.

Premorbid Levels of Stress

Finally, the extent to which a family is already stressed by developmental, financial, and emotional issues sets the stage for psychosocial struggles when cardiopulmonary illness strikes one of its members. For example, as mentioned above, many elderly cardiopulmonary patients have spouses who also are suffering from chronic illnesses. Younger patients may at once be dealing with managing a growing family and aiding aged parents who are themselves suffering from chronic illnesses. For such families, the magnitude of stress when facing cardiopulmonary illness is quite different than that faced by a financially secure family enjoying a relatively calm period of life when illness strikes.

DIAGNOSING FAMILY FUNCTIONING

Typically, if family functioning of recovering patients is assessed at all, it is assessed only once during the course of rehabilitation. In acute care settings, such cursory assessment might be justified; after all, contact with the patient and his or her loved ones will typically be brief, and the only imminent family issue at hand may be whether the family team is helping or hindering the patient's progression through hospitalization.

Fortunately, even the most disjointed families tend to band together and help each other cope during crisis. However, it is important to remember that the real work of family adjustment to illness begins after hospitalization.

Providers working in acute care settings need to prepare families for what they are likely to encounter as time unfolds and they continue to be impacted by the reality that cardiopulmonary illness is chronic in nature. In outpatient medical or rehabilitation settings, providers need to be attentive to indicators of family-level functioning throughout treatment and follow-up.

How can you accurately diagnose family-level patterns of adjustment? Details regarding healthy and unhealthy family patterns during rehabilitation were discussed extensively in Sotile (1992). Summaries of cogent points from this discussion are presented below.

Signs of Adaptive Family Functioning Following Illness

Clinical experience suggests that the majority of both healthy and unhealthy families respond to the crisis of illness in a similar fashion: differences are put aside, any ongoing arguments are at least momentarily suspended, and support and help are offered and reciprocated, all in deference to the need to endure through the stresses and fears that come with acute illness by a loved one (Sotile, 1992).

Families enter the intermediate phase of adjusting to illness filled with emotions and with questions. Here relatively brief, transient periods of grieving and/or depression associated with the stresses of the current bout of illness and its implications are commonplace. Members of the healthy family support each other during these periods of emotionality, remaining nonjudgmental and flexible in their support. During this phase, medical personnel are turned to for help in alleviating anxieties about the new and unknown territory the family will enter in the next stage of adjusting to illness. Despite good intentions, intrafamily differences in interpreting medical input are high during this stage of recovery. Care should be taken to ensure that individual family members (especially spouses) are hearing what is intended when medical input is delivered (Sotile, 1993).

Family teams develop certain roles and certain cognitive "sets" within the first several months following illness. These positions and their corresponding cognitive, behavioral, emotional, and interpersonal sequelae tend to persist for years and to resist efforts to change them. For example, wives' evaluations of their marriage after a husband's MI remain stable throughout the first year of recovery (Croog & Fitzgerald, 1978; Croog & Levine, 1977). In an ongoing study of relationship patterns after MI, Laerum and colleagues (Laerum et al., 1991; Laerum, Johnsen, Smith, & Larsen, 1987) have found that patient assessments of their total life situation and of their family life did not change significantly during evaluations performed 3 to 5 months post-MI and 2 to 4 years post-MI.

This and other research has documented the importance of early psychosocial intervention with recovering cardiopulmonary patients. For example, a study of 50 male patients regarding sexual functioning post-MI (Dhabuwala, Kumar, & Pierce, 1986) found that, although 80% of patients said they were afraid to resume sexual activity in the first 6 months following MI, only 40%

of these received any sexual counseling. But, of those patients who did receive such counseling, only 24% continued to display a fear of sexual activity in the first 6 months posthospitalization. Therefore, in treating recovering cardiopulmonary patients, it seems important to provide help regarding marital/family issues from the onset of the illness.

In preparing patients and their loved ones for hospital discharge, warn them of the likelihood and the normalcy of experiencing at least moderately intense periods of distress and family tension as they struggle to adjust to illness and to the demands and consequences of rehabilitation. Reassure them that no family copes perfectly smoothly with rehabilitation, and that they should not overreact to such struggles. Further guidelines for offering input to the family at this stage of adjustment will be presented at the end of this chapter.

Differentiating the healthy family from one that is struggling maladaptively is difficult during the initial and intermediate stages of coping. It is during long-range coping that families show what will prove to be their more lasting colors: some improve, and some get worse.

Healthy long-range family coping is signaled by the family's flexibility, openness, accurate understanding of what faces them, and ability to come to terms with the effects of the illness. It is characterized by three stages:

1. Initial Stage: Let's Get Together and Endure

2. Intermediate Stage: Developing a Game Plan

3. Long-Range Stage: Coping Together

Healthy families flexibly adjust their roles and rules to make room in the family process for rehabilitation, and they do so while adhering to a fundamental, two-part rule of thumb: No martyrs, and no spectators. No single family member is assigned or is allowed to assume the role of being overburdened by the implications of rehabilitation. In addition, the family works collectively to ensure that the ill member maintains an active as opposed to a spectator's role in the overall family process (Sotile, 1992).

On a purely practical level, healthy families respond to the challenges of rehabilitation by developing a realistic understanding of the medical and lifestyle implications of living with the illness. In absorbing the impact of the changes that come with illness, healthy families help each other to openly discuss the implications of the illness for each family member, and they freely offer help and understanding to each other as they grow resigned to incorporating the challenges of rehabilitation into the new reality of their life. In short, they:

- flexibly adjust family roles and rules,
- allow increased openness and honesty,
- seek accurate information about rehabilitation,

- set clear and realistic goals, and
- find peace with themselves and each other.

Signs of Maladaptive Family Functioning Following Illness

On the other hand, unhealthy family reactions to illness revolve around symptoms of struggle by one or more family members. There are 12 signs of unhealthy family reactions to illness:

1. Protracted depression
2. Failure to accept diagnosis
3. Denying the symptoms of illness
4. Remaining ignorant about the illness
5. Flights into activity
6. Persistent hostility
7. Prolonged exaggeration of typical personality traits
8. Discounting the possibility of coping
9. Old problems getting worse
10. Indirect battles for power
11. Children or teenagers showing signs of distress
12. Adult children of heart patients becoming triangulated and/or symptomatic

When assessing family functioning, it is important to remember that, from a systems perspective, any member of a distressed family—not only the cardiopulmonary patient—may become the symptom bearer for the team. Some symptoms of struggling adjustment may be obvious. For example, a family member may show symptoms of depression or exaggerated personality-based coping patterns (e.g., the orderly become compulsive; the grouchy become hostile; the careful become paranoid).

In other families, the signs of struggle show up in their relationships with each other, not in their individual coping patterns. The stresses of rehabilitation can stretch already-existing tensions to the breaking point. Complaints of long-standing struggles over trust, intimacy, nurturing, or communication are typical here. Other symptoms of family struggle may be less obvious. For example, refusal by some family members to accept the reality of the illness may lead to subtle proddings to doubt the validity of medical input; or family discounting of medical input may encourage "doctor shopping" or flights into a search for esoteric cures. Finally, some families flee into activities (e.g., travel, spending money, starting new projects) that serve to momentarily distract them from their fears.

Some symptoms of family struggling are quite subtle and easily missed unless the patient and his or her family are evaluated with an eye on family dynamics. Here illness behavior (again, on the part of any member of the family team, not only the diagnosed cardiopulmonary patient) becomes an integral part of the relationship process. This might mean that symptoms of illness become levers of power and influence in determining momentary relationship outcomes. In chapter 13, I will describe how symptoms such as chest tightness, breathlessness, dyspnea, or angina can regulate family activities and communication.

On the other hand, a loved one might assume a "one-down" position in the family power hierarchy in efforts to restore diminishing self-worth for the cardiopulmonary patient. The effect of showing their own symptoms of physical or emotional distress can serve the dual adaptive function of momentarily bolstering the cardiopulmonary patient's need to be needed and refocusing the family nurturing process onto a member other than the patient.

Other subtle signs of family struggle might involve the children or grand-children of the cardiopulmonary patient. As will also be discussed in chapter 13, middle-aged adults often are children of aged, ill patients. It is common-place for such grown children to be co-opted into the role of counselor and monitor of the ailing, aged parents whose resources and health may be failing. This caretaking comes at the expense of the grown child's own emotional or relationship health. Extended discussions of the dilemmas of adult children of cardiac patients are available in *Heart Illness and Intimacy: How Caring Relationships Aid Recovery* (Sotile, 1992).

The suffering of a parent or grandparent is painful to observe for children of any age, but it is important to remember that an elder's illness can terrify a young child. Most young children equate having a heart attack or heart surgery with dying. Unfortunately, children also tend to have difficulty expressing their feelings, and parents tend to fear that talking openly with children about upsetting topics will only frighten them. In my clinical experi-ence, young children are often the most subtle victims of an adult's illness. They are left to harbor unidentified fears and to hold in a storm of emotions—anxiety, anger, grief, embarrassment, guilt—in reacting to something they do not understand.

A child's way of dealing with the illness may be distressing not only to him or her; it can be heartbreaking for the patient. A frightened child may shy away from being alone with the ill parent or grandparent, fearing that strange thing called "cardiopulmonary illness" or the paraphernalia that accompany rehabilitation (such as the home oxygen machine).

In treating any cardiopulmonary patient, always inquire about the re-actions of children and/or grandchildren to the illness. Educate the patient to look for obvious as well as indirect signs that a child may need help in coping. Depending on his or her age, signs that a child may be struggling to cope with family-related stress might include any combination of the following symptoms:

- Decline in school performance
- Eating or sleeping problems
- Behavioral problems
- Outbursts of temper
- Vague or persistent physical problems
- Clinginess
- Excessive withdrawal or tiredness
- Drug or alcohol use
- Excessive efforts to please or "be good"
- Oppositional, rebellious behavior
- Refusal to discuss problems, especially feelings about the illness

Note. Sotile, Wayne M., *Heart Illness and Intimacy: How Caring Relationships Aid Recovery* (p. 45). The Johns Hopkins University Press, Baltimore/London, 1992.

As can be seen from this list, children can become emotionally, somatically, or behaviorally symptomatic. Most often, the symptoms will manifest in some important arena of life (e.g., school performance, family relationships, or physical functioning).

The following eight guidelines for discussing illness with children can be presented to parents and grandparents, paired with the advice to adjust input to make it age-appropriate for the children involved.

1. Talk about the illness. Begin by talking with your children about how you are reacting to your own fears and frustrations. Giving them a glimpse of how you are thinking, feeling, and coping with this illness will help children feel more normal and will model for them how they, too, might cope.

2. Ask if they have questions. Find out if they are worrying about what is happening or what will happen now that your family is coping with your illness.

3. If they have no questions, give them information anyway. Children often listen more than they let you know. Give them information that is appropriate to their age and that conveys hope and confidence that your family will endure this chapter of your life.

4. It's okay to admit that you don't know all the answers. Pretending to know answers to questions that boggle anyone's thinking just serves to confuse children. Sometimes, the best answer is, "That's a good question. But none of us knows the answer for sure."

5. At the same time, offer reassurance. It is especially important to reassure your children that you are receiving good medical care

and that you will continue to do all you can to recover. A good way to do this is to arrange for them to see you going through your rehabilitation routine. If applicable, just seeing how strong and hardy you are can soothe many of your children's fears.

6. Give your children permission to talk with others about their fears. Teenagers, especially, sometimes find brief counseling helpful in coping with their concerns. If you have only recently had surgery or a medical crisis, inform school guidance counselors to be especially attentive to your children.

7. Emphasize to your children that they had nothing to do with your illness. Children are self-centered in their insecurities, and they need explicit reassurance that their behavior did not cause the illness.

8. Keep communicating! As your rehabilitation progresses, talk openly and frequently about cardiopulmonary rehabilitation being a family affair. In these conversations, be sure to point out what you notice and appreciate about each another.

PRACTICAL APPLICATIONS OF FAMILY SYSTEMS THEORY IN TREATING CARDIAC AND PULMONARY PATIENTS

Delivering medical and rehabilitation interventions with heart or lung patients should always be done with sensitivity to the family factors outlined in this chapter. In closing, I offer the following ten keys for delivering family-sensitive care and sample scripts regarding how this might be done.

DURING HOSPITALIZATION, ENCOURAGE VISITATION BY FAMILY, AND MONITOR THE EFFECTS

A recent editorial by Dracup and Bryan-Brown (1992) pointed out that it is now considered barbaric that as recently as the 1950s, hospitalized children were allowed family visitations only twice per week. Family visitation policies for contemporary ICUs vary tremendously, but most allow recovering cardiopulmonary patients only 10-minute visits by loved ones, 4 to 12 times daily. Some researchers (e.g., Dracup & Bryan-Brown, 1992; Sickbert, 1989) claim that such restricted visiting deprives both patients and their loved ones of needed social support. Dracup and Bryan-Brown cite fascinating research (i.e., Fuller & Foster, 1982) documenting that, contrary to the popular notion that restricting family visitation is done to protect the patient from distress, staff/patient interactions are far more stressful for patients than family/patient interactions. The authors predicted that "sometime in the

21st century, critical care nurses and physicians may look back at our ICU visiting restrictions with the same amazement with which we view pediatric visiting restrictions of the 1950s. They may wonder at our motives and label our restrictions as arrogant. Perhaps we should be the first to question our practice" (p. 18).

Indeed, research has suggested that many recovering cardiopulmonary patients do benefit from family visitation. In reviewing the cardiovascular literature, Ell and Dunkel-Schetter (1994) point out that the effects of family visits are likely to be mediated by the quality of premorbid family relationships. However, this effect may not always be as one might assume. In a previously mentioned study by Kulik and Mahler (1989), CABG patients who received frequent visitations from their spouse were more quickly discharged from ICU and the hospital and took fewer pain medications than those who received low levels of spouse visitation. Interestingly, the patients who seemed to benefit most from such visitation were those with low levels of self-rated marital harmony. In another study, family visits that included the family member touching the patient and orienting the patient frequently to time and place led to reduction of postoperative delirium (Chatham, 1978).

Regarding visitation, information from a clinical report of questionnaires and interview data from 33 CHD patients and their spouses (Marsland & Logan, 1984) is worth noting: Spouses want to be more included in discussion of the patient's treatment and discharge planning, and they would like more privacy while visiting. Even minimal common courtesies—such as knocking on hospital room doors or announcing one's presence before opening bed drapes—can convey respect of the visiting loved one's right to at least moments of privacy with their recovering family member.

The issue of family visitation in ICU and CCU is not clear-cut. Kleman et al. (1993) presented an insightful discussion of this topic, pointing out that several investigations have found that recovering cardiopulmonary patients actually report only mild preference for visits from family (Forshee, 1988; Kleman et al., 1993) and that patients themselves do not favor changing current family visiting policies (Boykoff, 1986). Some surveys have found that patients prefer that family visits be limited to about 40 minutes (Simpson, 1991). Kleman and colleagues also reported data indicating that some patients might be especially reactive to family visits. Specifically, in the population studied in this investigation, patients who had experienced serious heart attacks (with ejection fractions of less than 40%) and who smoked (most of whom also were COPD patients) evidenced more pronounced changes in heart rate, blood pressure, S-T segment, and oxygen saturation during family visits. Interestingly, patients who reported a high preference for family visits evidenced the most pronounced physiological reactions to visitation.

It seems only prudent that here, too, the needs of the patient and the family be considered in making decisions regarding family visitation. Ideally, hospital environments should allow for flexibility that either restricts or loosens family visitation policies, depending upon the expressed desires of

the individual patient and the observed effects of such visits. You can determine your patient's preferences by asking something like:

 "Mr. Blakely, we want to do all that we can to help you cope with this
illness. Some patients find that frequent visits from their loved ones
can help soothe them during their recovery. Others simply want to be
left alone until they start feeling better. Within limits, we can arrange
visits from your family to your liking. What are your thoughts about this?
Do you think visits from your family will be more helpful or upsetting to
you during these next few days?"

COACH THE PATIENT'S FAMILY

It is important to prepare the family for what they are likely to experience
when visiting a hospitalized loved one. Upset by family members as they
react to the special circumstances encountered by recovering cardiopulmonary patients (e.g., seeing a loved one on a ventilator) can lead to increased
distress for the patient at a time when tranquillity is important to recovery.
For example, Doerr and Jones (1979) reported that visits by family members
who had no preparation for what they were to encounter upon entering the
coronary care unit led to increases in patient anxiety.

Give family members strong but supportive nursing management of visitation during intensive care stays (Boykoff, 1986). Family group conferences
delivered during hospitalization can serve the dual purpose of coaching
families in how to effectively provide support to patients and providing
emotional and information support to family members (Holub, Ecklund, &
Keenan, 1975).

 "I want to take a few minutes to describe to you what you will see
when you visit Mr. Blakely after his surgery. It's important to prepare
yourselves for this, because we want your reactions to be soothing
for Mr. Blakely. [Describe details of what is likely to be encountered.]

"I also want to give you a little bit of coaching about what you might
do and not do to soothe Mr. Blakely. It will be important for you to be
realistic about how much he will or will not be able to communicate
with you when you first see him. During your first visit, it will probably
be most helpful if you simply touch him gently and say soothing things
to him. He is not likely to be very communicative, given [explain further
details of the patient's likely condition]."

THINK "FAMILY" AND SPEAK TO THE FAMILY TEAM

Medical advice and feedback should be delivered at once to the patient and
his or her most significant other. Proponents of the rapidly-emerging trend

toward collaborative family health care underscores the importance of co-opting families into an individual patient's care by recommending that consultation for examination rooms in medical settings be built and furnished to accommodate the presence of one of the patient's loved ones when medical or rehabilitation feedback or prescriptions are offered. For many patients, it is wise to include their adult children in feedback sessions. During such sessions, you should offer not only medical input but also compassion about your appreciation of the fact that families function as teams and that rehabilitation is a family affair.

For example, when the patient faces vocational adjustments, a number of family-level issues should be addressed: the effects of family-level attention and concern regarding work return; the importance of marital communications and problem-solving capability in managing the stresses that come with this issue; and the importance of monitoring family stress reactions to changes in employment status of either patient or spouse (Sotile, Sotile, Sotile, & Ewen, 1993). Using simple analogies such as the following, educate the family to begin looking at themselves from a systems perspective.

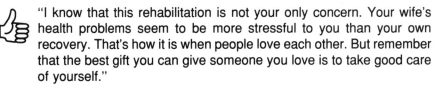 "When illness strikes your family, it's similar to what happens when you throw a big stone into a small pond: the 'shock waves' of the intruder roll on, and on, and on—affecting the whole pond, at least for a while. Same thing with your family. You are all going to feel the stress of this illness, and you will need each other's help in coping."

DISCUSS THE FAMILY'S COLLECTIVE CONDITION

As stated earlier, it is important to remember that every family copes with multiple stressors: the effects of aging, inner family dramas, external pressures, and now, the illness you are treating. Speaking briefly to this issue can further your rapport with any family:

"I know that this rehabilitation is not your only concern. Your wife's health problems seem to be more stressful to you than your own recovery. That's how it is when people love each other. But remember that the best gift you can give someone you love is to take good care of yourself."

NORMALIZE EMOTIONAL STRUGGLES

Let families know that it is normal to experience periods of anxiety, fear, anger, grief, and depression during the course of rehabilitation. Teach them the signs of clinical depression that were outlined in chapter 2 . Also encourage them to help each other bear through their awkwardness as they try to change in the many ways that rehabilitation will challenge them to change.

"In the months and years to come, you might notice that you sort of seem to be taking turns going through difficult emotional times. I don't think I have ever treated a family coping with this illness who did not go through periods of sadness, anxiety, grief, even depression and anger. Expect this to happen, and stay open to two things: (a) talking with each other about what you are feeling; and (b) the possibility of getting help in learning to cope, if need be. If you will let yourselves—individually and as a family—stay open and flexible, you will probably adjust well. But remember: no one goes through this without facing some hard-to-handle emotions.

"I also want to point out that, for all of us, changing is awkward. For most people, rehabilitation means changing a lot about the way they are living: what they eat; what they do; how they deal with their own and each other's emotions. Now here's the important point: Even if those changes are good, positive changes, they still force you to adjust to a new way of coping and a new way of living together. Change is stressful. Getting healthier means changing, which means bearing through the awkward feelings as you try to get used to this new way of dealing with your own emotions and with each other. It's sort of like when you're learning new steps in a dance that you're used to dancing: the new steps feel awkward until you get a lot of practice under your belt. You need each other's support and patience as you grow accustomed to these new steps in the 'dances' that go on in your family."

TEACH THE FAMILY HOW TO THINK ABOUT REHABILITATION

Tell families that they are at a crucial crossroads; a time when they can choose to either move closer to each other or further apart. More will be said about how to shape adaptive attitudes in recovering families in chapter 9. For now, I simply want to underscore the importance of encouraging families to see rehabilitation as the beginning of a healing or growing period in their close relationships. Such encouragement might be offered in this way:

"You know, you guys are facing an important choice. Crises like this one tend to get your attention, and I know that this is happening to you all. Facing this illness is scary and stressful. But I've learned from many of my patients that rehabilitation can also begin an important period of growth for families. This is a time for the angry to forgive; for the closed to become more open; for the cold to become warmer.

It's a time to forgive some of what you have to forgive, forget some of what you need to forget, begin doing what you have been putting off, and stop doing some stuff that you have known needs to stop for you all to love each other better. In a nutshell, this is a time for you all to work together to create a 'new normal' that can be even better than the way things have been between you."

EMPHASIZE THAT YOU EXPECT THE FAMILY TO BE PART OF REHABILITATION

In delivering cardiopulmonary care, health care providers often take it for granted that families understand that they are important to the rehabilitation process. It is crucial that you emphasize to loved ones—especially to spouses of married patients—your expectation that they will be actively involved in the rehabilitation process. Convey this expectation in front of the patient and couple it with acknowledgment that this does not mean that the spouse is responsible for the patient's rehabilitation; it simply means that patients who live in supportive environments rehabilitate better. This point might be made in this way:

"We recommend that you react to our recommendations about your rehabilitation just as you might react to the advice of an accountant that the two of you consulted because you wanted help in figuring out a family budget. Things won't work out so well if you leave the meeting and only one of you goes home and follows the budget. You both have to at least participate in the spirit of what you are trying to accomplish. The same goes for rehabilitation: It's not that both of you have to eat exactly the same foods, take the same medicines, exercise the same amount, and so on. One of you has this illness and the other doesn't. But the 'budget' you have to cooperate in following is committing yourselves to cooperate with each other and support each other as you each face your parts of the challenges that are going to come with living with this illness."

DESCRIBE HELPFUL AND UNHELPFUL BEHAVIORS

It may also be a mistake to assume that loved ones know how to support each other in ways that aid rehabilitation. In commonsense terms, the family needs to be taught what it means to provide each other with esteem and emotional, instrumental, and cognitive support (Ben-Sira & Eliezer, 1990; Shumaker & Czajkowski, 1994).

"Now let me clarify what I mean by cooperation and support. Families sometimes get confused here and do things that hurt rather than help each other's ability to cope during rehabilitation. There are a lot of ways to be supportive: (a) You can simply remind each other that you believe in each other and that you are important to each other; (b) you can show each other sincere concern, encouragement, understanding, love, and compassion; (c) you can encourage each other to gradually get on with your respective roles, inside and outside your family; (d) you can offer each other information and advice that helps each of you adjust; and (e) you can become an active participant in making the kinds of lifestyle changes that are important for healthy living.

"I encourage my patients and their families to remember my 'dos and don'ts' about being supportive [incorporate specific bits of advice from the following lists of helpful and unhelpful behaviors].

"In a nutshell, remember: Don't criticize, monitor, blame, shame, or ignore each other. Do cooperate with, participate in, and validate each other's efforts to change."

Spouse support has been operationalized as including eight factors (Hilbert, 1985):

- Expressions of positive affect, such as praise and encouragement;
- Supplying resources;
- Allowing participation in decision making;
- Use of behavior modification techniques;
- Providing physical assistance, such as sharing of tasks;
- Providing intimate interaction that allows expression of feelings and personal concerns;
- Facilitating social participation; and
- Sharing norms.

Marital helping behaviors that can serve to moderate the relationship between stress and well-being include:

- Open communication about problems and concerns;
- Cognizance of partner's helping needs and proactive action in responding to these needs;

- Minimal criticism and expressed satisfaction with the quality and quantity of the help received; and

- Confidence in the ability to be helpful to one another (Burke & Weir, 1977a, 1977b).

Cardiopulmonary patients especially need the following forms of support from loved ones:

- Reassurance from others of still being valued in their eyes, despite the present and possibly future difficulty in performing normal activities and in fulfilling usual roles;

- Sympathy and feedback regarding the medical condition;

- The mere presence of supportive others, which provides reassurance and calming of fears regarding whether or not help will be available should relapse occur (Fontana et al., 1989).

The importance of active family—especially marital—cooperation and participation in needed areas of health care management (such as smoking cessation, exercise, or dietary modification) should be pointed out. The recommended strategy below summarizes the "dos and don'ts" that might be emphasized in helping patients and their loved ones clarify this issue as they attempt to change some risk factor or manage the psychosocial adjustments they face.

Do:	Don't:
Help	Nag
Participate	Shun
Discuss	Police
Compliment	Criticize
Notice	Ignore
Encourage	Complain
Ask	Lecture
Share information	Compete
Respect differences	Expect similarity
Listen	
Reassure	
Empathize	
Sympathize	
Cherish	

(Aho, 1977; Brownell, Heckerman, Westlake, Hayes, & Monti, 1978; Cohen & Lichtenstein, 1990; Coyne & DeLongis, 1986; Ell & Dunkel-Schletter, 1994; Sotile & Sotile, 1991)

REPEATEDLY INQUIRE REGARDING FAMILY FUNCTIONING, AND, IF NEEDED, REFER FOR "FAMILY STRESS MANAGEMENT TRAINING"

As will be discussed more extensively in chapter 14, follow-up psychosocial assessment is important in providing long-term care to recovering cardiopulmonary patients. This is especially true in reference to family issues, where the salient family systems and marital issues change markedly with the passage of time, advancing age, and developmental struggles of different family members. Families that are having trouble coping or with managing such family issues should be referred for specialized help. Guidelines for structuring such referrals will also be discussed in chapter 14.

PROACTIVELY ADDRESS SEXUAL ASPECTS OF REHABILITATION

Finally, specific mention of the sexual consequences of the patient's illness and treatment should be addressed proactively, and reassurance and practical advice regarding this important area of adjustment should be offered. Guidelines for evaluating and intervening in this area will be discussed fully in chapter 11.

SUMMARY

It is clear that living with cardiopulmonary illness is a family affair. However, it is emphasized that, based upon existing literature and clinical experience, no definitive statements can be made regarding the likely course of family adjustment following illness. In contrast to the various problems highlighted in the foregoing chapter, a number of studies have suggested that recovering from cardiopulmonary illness correlates with enhanced rather than diminished family functioning (i.e., Jenkins et al., 1983; Jenkins, Stanton, Savageau, Denlinger, & Klein, 1983; Laerum et al., 1987; Laerum et al., 1991).

The foregoing information obviously focused on discussion of the functioning of traditional families and married couples. To my knowledge, empirical research has yet to focus on the operations of nontraditional family relationships and their relationship to cardiopulmonary rehabilitation. However, in prior work (i.e., Sotile, 1993), I proposed that the clinical advice that comes from a family systems perspective on cardiopulmonary rehabilitation can enhance the functioning of both traditional and nontraditional family relationships. In a similar vein, Ries (1990) and Connors and Hilling (1993) called for including the spouse, family members, and close friends of COPD patients in the screening process and throughout rehabilitation or treatment.

It remains for future researchers to determine when and why certain families band together adaptively while others struggle and complicate each others' lives following illness. In the interim, common sense and a wealth of research and clinical experience suggest that regardless of the biopsychosocial issue being addressed, it is prudent to attend to the relationship factors operative in the patient's life.

Clinical experience suggests that both personality and family dynamics interplay with a factor that determines much about how an individual copes with stress: cognitive habits. As will be shown in the next chapter, thinking patterns serve as the final common pathway between internal responses and behavioral and emotional coping patterns.

chapter 9

CONTROLLING COGNITIONS

An important part of brief counseling with cardiopulmonary patients is teaching both the patient and his or her loved ones adaptive ways to control their cognitions. This means teaching them to become aware of how their thoughts affect their feelings, their attitudes, and their behaviors. Intervention is targeted at having the patient replace maladaptive, demotivating, or distressing thinking patterns with more realistic or positive cognitions (Beck, 1979; Burns, 1980; Ellis, 1962).

How important is it to help patients control their cognitions? The importance of optimism in preserving health has now been well documented (Seligman, 1990). In addition, the stress hardiness research of Suzanne Kobassa and colleagues suggested that attitudinal factors differentiate stress-vulnerable from stress-hardy individuals (Kobasa, Maddi, Puccetti, & Zola, 1985). In her study of stress-hardy executives, Kobassa noted that, regardless of the objective magnitude of the stresses being faced, positive copers are distinguished by their ability to employ three specific cognitive frames of reference (the three Cs): They see the coping process as a *challenge* that they approach with a sense of *commitment*; and they maintain an attitude of willingness to learn and to implement what is necessary to develop a sense of *control* over the coping process.

The cognitive training component of EEM incorporates input from three related schools of thought: cognitive appraisal and its importance in controlling the stress response; cognitive theorists and their input regarding ways to treat adjustment problems; and the stress hardiness literature. The emphasis here is on helping patients recognize and control their tendencies to interpret or appraise situations in terms that exaggerate their sense of threat, harm, or fear. At minimum, EEM training should promote the notion that coping with the stresses at hand can be facilitated if the patient and his or her loved ones will cooperate in viewing their current situation from the perspectives of the three Cs of stress hardiness outlined above.

As was mentioned earlier, health care professionals should hold themselves accountable for being agents of stress hardiness in delivering their medical care. We need to help our patients frame their rehabilitation as a challenge to be addressed head-on. Through self- and family-enhancing support of positive self-esteem, we need to help them commit themselves to the lifelong process of living in more healthy ways. And we need to help them identify the skills and the supports necessary to maintain a comfortable sense of control in the process. Helping patients and their loved ones to embrace the collective tenets of the stress hardiness research not only leads to enhanced patient coping, it also facilitates the delivery of medical care. Specific strategies for pinpointing and retraining cognitive distortions and for structuring interventions that shape adaptive cognitive habits are presented below.

COGNITIONS AND EMOTIONS

Cognitive theorists have warned us that when stressed, it is human nature to think in distress-generating ways called "cognitive distortions." A number of specific cognitive distortions have been identified (e.g., Burns, 1980), and it has been proposed that six specific stress-generating thinking patterns tend to plague cardiopulmonary patients and their loved ones (Sotile, 1992). Following are definitions and examples of each of these patterns, from both the perspective of a recovering patient and that of his or her spouse. Examples of soothing thinking will also be presented.

ALL-OR-NOTHING THINKING

This is a perfectionistic, black-or-white mode of self-evaluation that makes it difficult to accept that one's experience is ever good enough.
    Patient:

 Stressful Thinking: "If I can't exercise regularly, I won't exercise at all."

 Soothing Thinking: "Any exercise is better than no exercise at all. I'll settle for what I can get done today, and feel good enough about that."

Family Member:

 Stressful Thinking: "Here we go again! First she commits herself to losing weight, so she exercises regularly for 2 weeks. Then she misses a few days and gives up. I know that she won't stick with this program."

Soothing Thinking: "No one does anything perfectly. At least she's paying more attention to her health these days."

OVERGENERALIZATION

Overgeneralization involves distressing oneself by concluding that something that happens occasionally will occur as a general rule.

Patient:

Stressful Thinking: "That was the last time I'll ever try to 'express myself'! I just said what was on my mind, and now I'm short of breath and my chest hurts like hell. From now on, I'll just keep my cool and keep my feelings to myself."

Soothing Thinking: "This upsets me. I expressed what I felt, and now I feel worse. I need to think about this; maybe I need to learn a different way of letting my family know what I feel when I am upset."

Family Member:

Stressful Thinking: "I have a friend who has a brother-in-law whose next-door neighbor died while trying to have sex a year after his heart attack. There's no way I'm going to take that risk!"

Soothing Thinking: "It makes me anxious to think what might happen if we have sex. But I remember the facts about sex not really straining the heart very much. It will probably help me if we just start out slowly and regain our confidence a little bit at a time."

SELECTIVE PERCEPTION

Selective perception involves mentally filtering out information with the result that only the distressing details of a situation are attended to.

Patient:

Stressful Thinking: "I feel like a slob. I broke my diet twice this week."

Soothing Thinking: "I feel badly about eating that junk food. But the truth is that during the past week, I have done a good overall job of managing my diet. Looking at my food diary, I see that I made two poor choices out of the 73 entries in the diary. That's not bad; I made a bunch of healthy choices."

Family Member:

 Stressful Thinking: "Since his diagnosis, all he ever does is sit around. He acts like this illness has killed him; he's already giving up."

 Soothing Thinking: "Since his diagnosis, he's been more quiet and less outgoing. He is still going to church and to his Rotary meetings, though. Plus, the truth is that we all have good and bad days. I guess that adjusting to this illness will take a while."

DISCOUNTING

Here the positive aspects of a situation are ignored, or neutral factors or positive experiences are changed into ones that are negative.
   Patient:

 Stressful Thinking: "My blood work today didn't show any improvement. All of this getting healthy stuff is for the birds. I'm not getting any better."

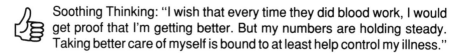 Soothing Thinking: "I wish that every time they did blood work, I would get proof that I'm getting better. But my numbers are holding steady. Taking better care of myself is bound to at least help control my illness."

Family Member:

Stressful Thinking: "All of a sudden she's wanting to act like 'Ms. Healthy.' Why didn't she decide to take care of herself before she got sick?"

Soothing Thinking: "I wish she had been this motivated to take care of herself before she developed this problem. But I guess it's better late than never."

MIND READING

Mind reading involves making upsetting assumptions about the intentions of others or about feared outcomes and jumping to conclusions without checking the facts when reacting to a stressor.
    Patient:

Stressful Thinking: "My doctor hasn't even asked me about my sex life since my surgery. I guess that means that I just need to forget about sex for now."

Soothing Thinking: "I'm worried about how my surgery has affected my sex life. My doctor hasn't talked with me about this, but I haven't let him know about my concerns. I need to call and schedule an appointment specifically to discuss this."

Family Member:

Stressful Thinking: "Whenever he gets quiet like this, I know it's because he's thinking about the fact that our sex life isn't so great these days. I just know that he's going to stop taking his medicine, and then this ordeal of going though surgery will have been for nothing."

Soothing Thinking: "It scares me when he gets quiet like this. I need to ask him what he's thinking, and tell him that I sometimes worry that he might quit taking care of himself. If he's worrying about our sex life, we need to talk about it."

CATASTROPHIZING

Catastrophizing is convincing oneself that the worst thing imaginable is actually happening or is about to happen.

Patient:

 Stressful Thinking: "Will this be my last chance to have a vacation with my family? I probably won't live long enough to ever do this again. I know that I'll never see my grandchildren enjoying themselves at the beach."

 Soothing Thinking: "Sometimes it takes loss to get you to appreciate your life. I love this family, and I am going to enjoy each of our days together, starting with this vacation."

Family Member:

 Stressful Thinking: "Here we are, spending all of this money to take what is supposed to be a nice family trip, and she's sitting over there moping. I know that this is going to be a catastrophe. We'll plow through a week of tension, and then I'll have to go back to the grindstone of work, exhausted and angry about her ruining this vacation by sitting there all week, worrying about her health."

Soothing Thinking: "I don't know what's wrong with her, but I do know that I want this trip to be relaxing and fun for us all. I need to find out what is bothering her. Maybe if we talk about it, she will feel better."

MAGNIFICATION AND MINIMIZATION

Focusing on faults, fears, and imperfections in a way that exaggerates their importance is called magnification. This usually corresponds with minimization, which involves shrinking awareness of the positives of the situation that is being dealt with.

Patient:

 Stressful Thinking: "Look at me: I'm old. I depend on this machine to breathe. I'm all used up. Why should I go on?"

Soothing Thinking: "Lord, I never thought I would end up needing a machine to breathe. I feel old. Hell, I am old. But at least I'm still here. Machine or not, I still have my mind and my sense of humor, and those grandkids. Plus, I'm still halfway good-looking!"

Family Member:

 Stressful Thinking: "We've been together for all of these years, and now he's so sick! He has to use that machine to breathe, he's not as strong as he used to be, and all I see in the future is medical bills and loneliness."

 Soothing Thinking: "If I let my imagination go, I get scared about the future. I hate that he's sick. But at least he's still here, quick wit, good looks, and all!"

EMOTIONAL REASONING

Here strong negative feelings are taken as proof of some bothersome, assumed truth.

Patient:

 Stressful Thinking: "If I feel this depressed since I stopped smoking and drinking, it must mean that I just can't function without cigarettes and alcohol. Maybe I'd be better off enjoying myself, even if it isn't such a healthy way to live."

Soothing Thinking: "Maybe my depression since I stopped smoking and drinking is part of nicotine and alcohol withdrawal. I need to ask my doctor about this. I also need to remember that depression can be treated and is less damaging to my health than drug addictions."

Family Member:

Stressful Thinking: "Every day I worry that she'll start drinking again. I know that this must mean that it's just a matter of time before she falls off the wagon again."

Soothing Thinking: "I guess my worries about whether or not she will stay sober are reasonable, given what we've been through in the past. But one thing I know is that I'm not in charge of her drinking. I need to enjoy what's good about right now, and take care of myself as well as I can. If she starts drinking again, we'll deal with it; we do have a lot of experience with this particular issue."

LABELING AND MISLABELING

Here negative self-evaluations are created by assuming an attitude of having failed as a person due to unfortunate outcomes that have occurred in a limited range of life experiences.

Patient:

Stressful Thinking: "What good did it do to work so hard in my life? I failed to take care of my health. I'm a failure as a father, as a husband, and as a human being."

Soothing Thinking: "Life is confusing. I did the best I could, given what I knew. But I do wish that I had taken better care of myself. I have succeeded in some areas and have failed in others."

Family Member:

Stressful Thinking: "Since my father's heart attack, my parents have been beside themselves with worries about their finances. If I had made enough money, they wouldn't be afraid right now. I failed them as a son, and I failed myself."

Soothing Thinking: "It breaks my heart to see my parents worried about money. I wish I could afford to support them now. I can't support them financially, but I have always been a loving son to them. I know that this counts, too."

PERSONALIZING BLAME

This involves unfairly assuming responsibility for negative events by blaming oneself for being the sole cause of some stressor.

Patient:

 Stressful Thinking: "The reason that I am in the shape that I'm in is that I am a lazy, unmotivated, selfish fool. I deserve what I've gotten."

 Soothing Thinking: "I wish that I had started being more truthful with myself and more responsible about my health years ago. But at least I have sense and courage enough to begin now."

Family Member:

 Stressful Thinking: "I should have forced him to take better care of himself before this happened. Now look where my foolishness has gotten us. He's in a mess, and I'm to blame."

 Soothing Thinking: "I wish I could keep everyone I love from suffering, but I can't. All I can do is be supportive and loving as I take care of myself and as my husband tries to take better care of himself."

THE RELATIONSHIP BETWEEN COGNITIONS, RECOVERY, AND REHABILITATION

Contemporary stress researchers have emphasized the crucial role that cognitions play in determining the stress response. The most universally accepted definitions of stress emphasize that, when stressed, human subjects naturally tend to think in ways that further distress themselves and that cognitive perceptions elicit physiological stress responses (Lazarus, 1966). The universality of the need for cognitive retraining in promoting stress management is suggested by cognitive theorists and researchers who have shown that controlling cognitive distortions is a key to coping with depression and anxiety (Burns, 1980). In addition, thinking in stress-generating ways can become habitual, and these cognitive habits can result in general attitudes (such as pessimism or cynicism) that interfere with adaptive coping.

Cognitive distortions of the sorts described above can become habitual responses to stress. These habitual ways of thinking then formulate overall cognitive sets or cognitive styles of explaining why stressful events happen (Seligman, 1990). Both individual and family-level definitions of the causes and the impact of illness can have profound effects on subsequent coping patterns, for patients as well as for their loved ones. Research has suggested that, in determining such rehabilitation outcomes as morale and return to work, a cardiopulmonary patient's perceptions of his or her health may be more important than the actual clinical severity of his or her condition (Blumenthal, 1985; Garrity, 1973a, 1973b). Furthermore, it has been shown that both patient and family perceptions may bear little relationship to actual severity of illness (Nagle, Gangola, Picton-Robinson, 1971). For example, following acute MI, patients frequently are limited more by inappropriate fear of exertion than by their actual medical status (Ewart, 1989). Research in this area has clearly demonstrated that cognitive frames of reference have much to do with the emotional reactions of recovering cardiopulmonary patients, and that these emotional reactions have behavioral consequences in the course of rehabilitation.

Such facts can be used to guide many practical psychosocial interventions with recovering cardiopulmonary patients. When counseling families, emphasize that the consequences of thinking habits go beyond the emotional; they have psychological, behavioral, interpersonal, and physical ramifications for the patient and family (Rejeski et al., 1985). In other words, emphasize that cognitions play a crucial role in determining not only situational coping responses, but also general beliefs and attitudes that shape multiple reactions and create overall coping patterns that can have profound effects on health and rehabilitation.

This point can be made by briefly elaborating the fundamental tenets of the Health Belief Model (Hochbaum, 1956; Kegeles, 1963). As mentioned earlier, an individual's health beliefs and expectations are seen as crucial factors that affect motivation to change a health behavior or to adhere to medical regimens. Further, this model poses that we are likely to change health behaviors depending upon two factors: the amount of perceived threat and the attractiveness of the change in question (Dracup & Meleis, 1982). The Health Belief Model will be discussed in more detail later. For now, it is emphasized that this model underscores the importance of the perceptions in determining health behaviors. For example, interactions of the following perceptions are deemed to be especially important in determining adherence to health-promoting advice:

1. Perceived susceptibility—the extent to which the individual believes he or she is likely to develop a particular illness or be affected by sequelae of an illness.

2. Perceived severity—the individual's assessment of the harmful or disruptive impact of having the illness.

3. Perceived benefits of a given intervention—the individual's assessment of the favorable results offered by the prescribed therapy.

4. Perceived costs—the individual's judgment of the discomfort, inconvenience, and other disadvantages (such as costs of money and time) of cooperating with the recommended intervention.

As was also mentioned earlier, landmark research has documented that overall cognitive frames of reference such as optimism and pessimism have health consequences. Patients can be motivated with a brief overview of fascinating research in this area. A 35-year longitudinal study begun by George Vaillant and continued by Martin Seligman and Christopher Peterson (Peterson, Seligman, & Vaillant, 1988) documented that mental attitudes clearly affect both susceptibility to disease and ability to recover from illness. Specifically, these researchers found that beginning around age 45, pessimistic individuals experienced significantly more health problems than did individuals who were optimistic in their outlook. Furthermore, it was reported that learning to control cognitive habits such as those outlined above can lead to shifts in overall frames of reference from pessimism to optimism (Seligman, 1990).

Exactly why optimism results in positive health outcomes remains to be explored by future researchers. Without question, however, cognitive frames of reference do relate directly to a crucial cognitive variable that has been shown to affect behavioral and health outcomes: self-efficacy. Borrowing from the school of social learning theory, self-efficacy refers to an individual's appraisal of his or her ability to perform a specific behavior or accomplish a certain task (Bandura, 1984). Self-efficacy is said to influence both the acquisition of new behaviors and the resumption or inhibition of prior behaviors (Oldridge & Rogowski, 1990). Furthermore, self-efficacy is thought to be task specific, not a global psychological trait.

Self-efficacy plays a crucial role in determining adherence to medical treatment recommendations, a fact that will be discussed extensively in chapter 14. Here it is emphasized that data are accumulating to suggest that self-efficacy expectations may also play a crucial role in determining overall behavioral and psychosocial adjustments to cardiopulmonary illness (Ewart, Taylor, Bandura, & DeBusk, 1980). Perceived physical and cardiac efficacy have been shown to be reliable predictors of post-MI activity, and research has demonstrated that such self-efficacy can be enhanced (O'Leary, 1985). For example, using treadmill performance and medical counseling, Ewart, Taylor, Reese, and DeBusk (1984) demonstrated that higher efficacy led to greater effort on the treadmill, which in turn led to higher attainment and further enhanced efficacy.

The effects of cognitive, behavioral, or cognitive-behavioral counseling on perceived self-efficacy for exercise by COPD patients have also been studied (Kaplan, Atkins, & Reinsch, 1984). In this study, self-efficacy for walking was raised maximally by the combined treatment condition, which incorporated goal-setting, behavioral contracting and contingency management, challenging of irrational beliefs concerning the effects of walking, and promotion of positive self-talk. Furthermore, changes in walking self-efficacy were significantly correlated with walking compliance at 3-month follow-up. Finally, Oldridge and Rogowski (1990) demonstrated that both a ward ambulation program and a dedicated exercise center program were effective in enhancing self-efficacy scores for walking time and overall exertion in a mixed group of recovering MI and CABG patients.

Other research findings suggest that self-efficacy may be a key aspect of the mind-body connection factor referred to in chapter 1. For example, Robert Kaplan and colleagues found that a simple, self-report rating of efficacy expectation was a significant univariate predictor of survival for patients with COPD (Kaplan, Ries, Prewitt, & Eakin, 1994). Kaplan's data are supported by the findings of other researchers (e.g., Mossey & Shapiro, 1982), who have reported that self-rated health is a reliable predictor of mortality, even when other measures of health status are statistically controlled.

In addition, fascinating research has demonstrated the circular interplay among cognitions, moods, and self-efficacy judgments. For example, inducing positive moods by having an individual recall a pleasant interpersonal experience has been shown to increase self-efficacy for a variety of tasks, including athletic performance (Kavanagh & Bower, 1985).

SPECIFIC COGNITIVE INTERVENTIONS WITH PATIENTS AND FAMILIES

Krantz (1980) emphasized the important role control mechanisms play in rehabilitative processes. When patients sense that the disease process is beyond effective personal control, they adopt a helpless posture, a mechanism that Rejeski et al. (1985) speculated may be a significant factor in noncompliance with rehabilitation. This notion is supported by a wealth of research suggesting that several cognitive factors are especially crucial in determining reactions to cardiopulmonary illness: general attitudes regarding the causes or effects of the illness; attitudes toward the rehabilitation team; and attitudes toward the rehabilitation tasks on the part of both the patient and his or her loved ones (Christopherson, 1968; Kline & Warren, 1983; Lipowski, 1977; Rejeski et al., 1985).

How can patients and their loved ones be helped to manage the cognitive aspect of their coping? Both formal and informal interventions can help reshape individual incidences of cognitive distortion and overall attitudes and explanatory styles.

ASK, LISTEN, AND CLARIFY

The simplest intervention is to ask. In discussing ways to evaluate self-efficacy and potential for adherence in treating COPD patients, Kaplan, Ries, Prewitt, & Eakin (1994) pointed out that a growing literature is documenting that "patients can provide meaningful information if they are asked the right questions" (p. 368). The authors noted that a newly developing trend in medicine emphasizes the importance of patient reports and that empirical research (e.g., Kaplan & Simon, 1990) has documented that simple ratings of expectation to comply with medical regimens are among the best predictors of adherence.

Specifically, in treating heart and lung patients, it is important to inquire as to how a patient and his or her loved ones are defining the stressors they face (Sotile, 1992). The same stressors can be seen quite differently by different people; one person may see a stressor as a punishment, whereas another sees the very same stressor as a relief. Another stressor may be interpreted either as proof of personal failure or simply as a surprise; as an enemy or as a friendly warning; as an irreparable loss or as a second chance; as a sign of weakness or as a challenge to grow; as an ending or as a beginning. Part of your job is to help your patients understand these stressors in the more positive light.

A point made in chapter 8 regarding family-level stress reactions also applies to individual cognitive coping reactions: When a stressor does not have clear consequences, coping patterns will be determined largely by cognitive-level interpretations of the implications of the stressor and its consequences. It is important to help recovering patients and their loved ones frame their illness and its implications in ways that will help promote physical and emotional management. Important information regarding cognitive frames of reference can be gotten simply by paying attention to what patients and their loved ones say in reacting to medical input or in response to pointed questions such as: "Why do you think this illness happened?" or "How do you suppose you will react to this advice?" or "What do you think will happen next?" In this manner, misinterpretations of medical advice or attitudes toward rehabilitation can be detected and corrected (Kline & Warren, 1983; Wishnie, Hackett, & Cassem, 1971). Such questioning also provides a vehicle for encouraging and coaching families to come to conceptual harmony regarding their understanding and interpretation of the meaning of rehabilitation recommendations (AACVPR, 1995; Rejeski, et al., 1985; Sotile, 1993).

In addition to informal discussions, a number of useful questionnaires and guidelines for structured interviewing are available for assessing individual and family perceptions of health status and altitudes toward rehabilitation. The reader is referred to chapter 3 for an overview of these instruments and to Rose and Robbins (1993) for more extensive discussion of this topic.

Here a simple example from Atkins et al. (1984) is offered as a demonstration of a cognitive retraining intervention:

Because exercise is uncomfortable for many COPD patients, they may . . . actually talk themselves out of walking. Patients (are) first encouraged to monitor their own self-statements that might interfere with walking (i.e., "I can't walk very far without getting short of breath, so what's the use?"). Then they (are) trained to substitute negative self-statements with more appropriate positive and goal-oriented self-statements (i.e., "This walking is uncomfortable, but I can handle it. Soon I will be able to walk farther."). (p. 594)

THOUGHT DIARIES

A more extensive intervention (Level IV, V, or VI from chapter 4) involves helping the individual learn to pay attention to habitual ways of thinking through the use of thought diaries (Burns, 1980) such as the one in Figure 9.1.

Following are instructions that can be used to coach patients in the use of a thought diary, including a brief case example of the sort that should be incorporated into such coaching.

"This is an exercise that is designed to help you recognize how your thinking habits complicate your stress reactions. By learning to 'talk back to' the bothersome ways of thinking outlined above, you can change a crucial 'domino' in your coping style—your tendency to think yourself into more distress when you are already stressed.

"For the next 2 weeks, I want you to keep a thought diary, or journal. This can be done by reproducing the following page or by copying this outline into a small notebook that you carry with you. Whenever you notice your stress 'red flag' [specified from information gleaned

---

Thought Diary

Time:

Situation:

Feelings:

Stressful thoughts:

Cognitive distortions:

Realistic thoughts:

Outcome:

Figure 9.1 Thought diary.

during an interview with the patient], or at some designated time, such as every hour, on the hour, throughout the day, take a minute to fill in your journal entries, as follows:

"Note your situation—what are you doing, or getting ready to do.

"Describe your feelings, and rate each feeling on a scale of 1-100, with 1 = very mild and 100 = terribly high.

"Describe in detail the stressful thoughts going through your mind. Remember that your thinking might take the form of pictures flashing in your mind or self-talk that you 'hear' in your mind.

"Identify which of the cognitive distortions are fueling this stressful thinking.

"Now take a moment to respond to your stressful thoughts by jotting down soothing or realistic thoughts about what is bothering you.

"Finally, notice the outcome of this exercise. Note both your behavior and what you are now feeling. Rate these feelings on a scale of 1-100 (1 = very mild; 100 = terribly high).

"Let me clarify what I mean with an example:

"I once treated a patient named Charley who really wanted to quit smoking. He was making nice progress—he had cut back to smoking only a few cigarettes a day. But one day Charley found himself lighting up a cigarette as he waited for his waitress to serve his lunch. Just as we had discussed in his counseling, Charley interpreted lighting the cigarette as a red flag that suggested to him that he must be stressed, so he filled out his thought journal. His journal read like this:

Time: 12:00 noon

Situation: At lunch, before 1:00 p.m. appointment with Mr. Smith at Ajax Corp.

Feelings (ratings): anxious (85); excited (75); scared (80); tired (70).

Stressful thoughts: This guy probably doesn't even want to meet with me. I bet I'm going to make a fool of myself; I'm not good at this. I hope I'm not late, like last time. This appointment is important; if I don't make this sale, I'll probably get my 'walking papers' and be proclaimed a failure, just like happened to Jim when his sales dipped.

Cognitive distortions: Catastrophizing. Selective perception. Mind reading. Labeling.

Realistic thoughts: This customer has always been friendly and reasonable. I was late last time, but never before when I've had an appointment with him. I do hope that I make this sale, but I also have other possibilities working. Jim had a history of problems with our company; I don't.

Outcome: Put out cigarette. Anxious (65); excited (75); scared (40); tired (70).

"Several points are obvious from Charley's journal. First, it is clear that keeping such a thought journal takes some time and effort. The good news is that most likely you will only have to do this exercise for a couple of weeks before you develop a new thinking habit that will occur automatically in response to stressful thinking, and that will serve you well for the rest of your life. Learning this technique is sort of like learning to ride a bicycle: once you 'get it,' you've 'got it' for life.

"Second, it is obvious that Charley responded to a typical sign of stress—lighting a cigarette—with the new behavior of writing out his thoughts and feelings. If you are willing to practice replacing old 'dominoes' with more soothing thoughts and behaviors, you will soon notice that your stressful thoughts and unhealthy behaviors actually begin to remind you to take more nurturing and healthy care of yourself, rather than serving as stimuli for unhealthy behaviors. Once learned, this technique automatically breaks up the habit of adding fuel to the fire when you are upset by thinking yourself into further distress.

"Finally, it is obvious from Charley's journal entry that his soothing thinking did not totally eliminate all of his anxiety and stress and did not change the fact that he was facing something that bothered him. After filling out his journal, he was still tired and moderately anxious about his upcoming business meeting, and he still had to go to the meeting. But at least he was able to disrupt his typical stress progression, a progression that usually resulted in his feeling anxious and smoking cigarettes.

"The point of this exercise is not to encourage you to try to think positively. Sometimes what you are facing is not positive, and positive thinking would be like lying to yourself.

"My point is that I want you to learn to stop another form of lying that we all automatically do: the negative, catastrophizing, distorting thinking patterns that automatically fill our heads during stressful times. Even when facing unwanted stressors, all is not dismal or lost. The point of this exercise is to help you learn to stop making your pain worse during stressful times and start developing the new habit of thinking realistically. This technique does not totally change your life, but it is an effective way to change your reactions to stressful moments in your life."

USE THE PATIENT'S EXPERIENCES TO PROMOTE SELF-EFFICACY

Bandura (1984) delineated four sources of efficacy information: enactive information, vicarious information, persuasive communication, and internal feedback. Information regarding the patient's cognitive tendencies can be used to enhance the positive benefits of exposure to each of these sources of self-efficacy.

Enactive information comes from the patient's actual performance. This is considered the most reliable and effective source of self-efficacy for a given activity and for those similar to it. Based on this principle, patients should be reminded that the best way to become comfortable with a new behavior is to begin engaging in that behavior (behavioral change), take note of one's progress in mastering the behavior (cognitive change), and bear through the awkwardness that comes with repeating the behavior until it starts to come more easily (emotional change).

Vicarious information can be obtained by observing others, a form of social modeling. In inpatient settings, the mere presence of others who have endured the ordeal being faced has been shown to have marked, positive effects on coping. For example, patients anticipating angiography who watched a film of another patient describing the experience and how he dealt with it reported and displayed less postsurgical distress than patients who did not receive this modeling intervention (Anderson & Masur, 1989). As was already mentioned, even simply having a patient awaiting surgery share a room with a postoperative patient, as opposed to a roommate also awaiting surgery, has been shown to lead to more postsurgical physical activity and shortened hospital stay (Kulik & Mahler, 1987). The touted benefits of support groups for spouses of hospitalized medical patients can also be seen as resulting from a form of vicarious modeling (e.g., Dracup, Meleis, Baker, & Edlefsen, 1984; Holub et al., 1975; McGann, 1976).

Posthospitalization, participation in a formal rehabilitation program can be a potent source of such vicarious information. In such settings, the patient should be explicitly encouraged to take cognitive note of information about the chances of achieving success through one's own efforts that come from observing the progress or failures of others with similar problems.

Persuasive communication about one's own efforts is a third source of efficacy information. Obviously, this is the form of efficacy influence most often used by health care providers in treating patients. A key factor that determines the effectiveness of such communication is the extent to which the patient believes what is being communicated.

Finally, *internal feedback* from one's physiological state affects efficacy regarding one's capabilities. In counseling patients, it is important to remember that the efficacy effect is most often specific to the activity being performed; if generalization of efficacy is desired, the patient must be helped to cognitively pair the demonstrated area of ability with a desired target of efficacy enhancement. The patient's treadmill testing experience can be a particularly potent tool for enhancing self-efficacy for exercise, and if counseled appropriately, patients can be helped to generalize their treadmill experiences to dissimilar activities (Ewart, Taylor, Reese, & DeBusk, 1983). Ewart et al.

(1983) showed that having patients who are inappropriately fearful of physical exertion undergo maximal treadmill exercise testing soon after suffering an MI resulted in improved self-efficacy gains. For example, a patient's lack of confidence in his or her ability to safely resume sexual activity might be bolstered by pairing already-existing self-efficacy regarding his or her ability to tolerate exercise exertion with the notion that, relatively speaking, sexual behavior is a nonstrenuous form of exercise. Examples of this cognitive intervention follow:

"Over the past 2 months you have learned that your body can comfortably and safely tolerate 45-60 minutes of pretty strenuous walking, and you just demonstrated great exercise tolerance on your treadmill test. You know what it feels like to get your heart rate and your breathing rate up, and to keep them up for quite a while. Bear this in mind when you consider your sex life: Sex is actually a much less intense form of exercise than you already are doing on a regular basis. And, hopefully, it's a lot more fun than walking!"

In a similar manner, cognitive framing can be used to enhance efficacy to return to work:

"Given your demonstrated exercise tolerance and what research has shown the cardiovascular workload to be for your particular job, it is clear that you are fit enough to return to work safely."

In fact, much empirical research has supported the notion that the likelihood of a patient returning to work is enhanced if the recommendation to return to work is based upon the results of exercise stress testing or other procedures that are integrated into the routine delivery of care in formal cardiopulmonary rehabilitation programs (Shanfield, 1990; Taylor, 1987). For example, Dennis et al. (1988), in a randomized clinical trial of post-MI patients, demonstrated that treadmill-tested patients given explicit instructions regarding prognosis, timing of work return, and treadmill results returned to work at a median of 51 days compared to 75 days in patients receiving less explicit instruction.

Exercise testing can also be useful in providing prophylactic relationship counseling for recovering cardiopulmonary patients and their mates. The aforementioned study by Taylor, Bandura, Ewart, Miller, & DeBusk (1985) demonstrated that both adjustment to illness and marital harmony can be enhanced by having a spouse not only observe but also participate in the patient's treadmill testing. Taylor and colleagues noted that having a spouse actually walk on the treadmill at the same speed and grade just completed by the patient promoted within-couple conceptual harmony regarding the patient's physical exertion capacity. Encouragement to generalize such tread-mill experiences to at-home behaviors can lessen marital tensions regarding the recovering patient's physical capabilities.

Finally, it must be underscored that inadvertent responses by health care providers can have the iatrogenic effect of shaping negative attitudes toward rehabilitation. Citing work by Garrity (1973a), Razin (1982) cautioned that "Patients may respond adversely to unintended, nonverbal or symbolic meanings of physicians' communications" (Razin, 1982, p. 376). Silence, skepticism, vague responses, or grave expressions can all serve as stimuli that will predictably stir cognitive reactions that distress patients and compli-cate their reactions to intervention.

SUMMARY OF INTERVENTION POSSIBILITIES

There are infinite potential applications of cognitive therapy with medical patients. For example, a patient who is facing cardiac surgery can be helped to cope with training in cognitive distraction techniques. This might involve coaching the patient to pay attention to the favorable aspects of the surgical experiences (such as the relaxing feeling of sedation) or to direct attention away from physical discomfort and onto other cognitive activities (such as pleasant fantasies or prayer). In addition, female patients who have under-gone Lamaze training in childbirth can be encouraged to recall the Lamaze strategies to effectively accomplish both cognitive distraction and relax-ation induction.

Reframing and relabeling have also been found to help patients think adaptively in responding to the stimuli they will encounter in the immediate rehabilitation milieu. For example, a patient who voices fear and intimidation in response to all of the machinery in the hospital can be soothed with simple statements to the effect that:

"These machines are like your guardian angels; they look over you and help take care of you. We know how to speak their 'language,' and we will interpret for you as we take care of you."

Or the patient can be helped to relabel his or her sense of failure at sticking with past resolutions to change some problematic health behavior with the reframe:

"What you are calling your past 'failures' I see as big steps you have already taken in the right direction. Most people only change after a number of false starts. You are well on your way to making an attempt that sticks. Let's talk about what you learned from these past expe-riences."

SUMMARY

The importance of promoting adaptive cognitive habits, frames of reference, and explanatory styles for recovering cardiopulmonary patients and their loved ones cannot be overemphasized. Support of this unqualified recommendation comes from a broad body of research. Typical of studies that support attending to the cognitive factor in promoting overall physical, behavioral, and emotional management for cardiopulmonary patients is the study of Gruen (1975), which showed that patients with an improved grasp of cognitive coping strategies spent less time in the hospital, were less likely to manifest arrhythmias, exhibited fewer signs of depression and anxiety, and were more able to return to work than a group of matched controls.

Each of the factors discussed thus far in Part II is important in promoting EEM. However, overall psychosocial adjustment also requires that a supportive "territory" be created and maintained. Part II ends with a discussion of practical ways to promote such positive coping environments.

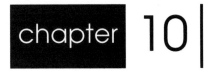

chapter 10

POSITIVE LIVING

- Understand the stress response.
- Learn to relax.
- Control family teamwork.
- Manage personality-based coping patterns.
- Control cognitions.

With these fundamentals of Effective Emotional Management in place, patients can better cope with various special challenges that fill the path of rehabilitation. Some of these, such as adhering to medical input and orchestrating social support, are of universal importance to this population. Other challenges, such as smoking cessation or managing anxieties about sexual functioning, affect many, but not all, recovering patients. The remaining chapters of this book will elaborate these topics.

The current chapter is devoted to discussing a crucial aspect of EEM: bolstering the support element in the patient's life. As mentioned in chapter 4, creating and living in nurturing, supportive "territory" is a key to the EEM process, and health care providers must at once provide such support and coach patients in how to establish and maintain their own supportive environments.

Interest in the relationship between health, illness, well-being, and social support is surging, spurred by several factors. First, as as mentioned before, the classic risk factors—hypertension, smoking, blood lipids, diabetes, and family history of illness—have been found to account for less than 50% of the variance in the occurrence of cardiovascular disease (Davidson & Shumaker, 1987). On the other hand, epidemiological research has repeatedly implicated social support (of one form or another) as playing a crucial role in the etiology of various illnesses (Seeman & Syme, 1987; Shumaker & Czajkowski, 1994). Finally, landmark investigations employing interventions containing strong elements of social support have reported a slowing of the progression of illnesses such as cancer (Spiegel et al., 1989) and cardiovascular disease (Frasure-Smith & Prince, 1985; Ornish et al., 1990). Such findings have led to an explosion of interest in bolstering the supportive component of medical care.

Discussion of this topic will borrow heavily from the broad and important literature on social support and will focus on two questions: Is social support important in promoting well-being, recovery, and rehabilitation for cardiopulmonary patients? and How can the social support factor for recovering cardiopulmonary patients be enhanced? For the most part, social support research with recovering cardiovascular patients has emphasized the importance of family support and support made available by health care providers in hospital and in posthospital medical settings (Gorkin et al., 1994). Both of these forms of support will be emphasized in the following discussion.

Two other factors must be mentioned in creating a backdrop for the discussion to follow. First, with reference to cardiopulmonary illness, the bulk of social support research has employed cardiac patient samples; to date, far less information has been published regarding social support and pulmonary patients. However, numerous researchers have emphasized the importance of overall psychosocial adaptation in promoting rehabilitation of patients suffering from COPD, and that social support—"being loved, feeling esteemed, being part of a mutual 'defense system' which in time of need one can utilize" (Dudley et al., 1980, p. 414)—is a primary psychosocial asset for the COPD patient (e.g., Connors & Hilling, 1993; Dudley et al., 1980; Ries, 1990).

Second, social support researchers have documented that—in addition to health status, standard of living, and spare-time activities—the most consistent predictors of well-being include such support factors as quality of family, community, and work involvements (Bharadwaj & Wilkening, 1977). Unfortunately, as their illness progresses, many cardiovascular patients and most COPD patients experience a narrowing of their range of activities and a diminishment in their vocational, social, recreational, and sexual activities. The result? Social isolation and diminished well-being (Dudley et al., 1980; Lustig, Haas, & Castillo, 1972). Commenting on clinical observations of a sample of COPD patients, Yellowlees et al., (1987) noted that:

"All patients who suffered from anxiety disorders hyperventilated at times, and many of them reported phobic avoidance of certain situations. Situations that were most often feared included taking a shower, shaving, going to the toilet, eating alone, going in lifts, or being outside home without an inhaler or a companion. . . . Phobic avoidance of these situations led to further anxiety and the development of a vicious circle of fear, hyperventilation, panic and avoidance. This behavior often led to significant handicaps with social and functional restriction." (p. 306)

In many ways, the issue of well-being is more complex for recovering pulmonary patients than for recovering heart patients (see chapter 14);

however, the overall adaptive tasks that face both pulmonary and cardiac patients overlap to a great degree. Since rehabilitation efforts for both populations essentially involve trying to enhance the patient's physical and psychosocial well-being, this chapter will intermingle discussions of both cardiac and pulmonary patients.

How can family, friends, and other social contacts (including health care providers) aid in the reduction of emotional distress and problems of living that can result from cardiopulmonary illness? It appears that social support may affect health and well-being in many ways, some positive and some negative. Understanding this issue begins with a clear definition of social support and how it works to enhance coping.

WHAT IS SOCIAL SUPPORT?

Social support can be defined as the emotional and material resources available to an individual through relationships with others (Friis & Taff, 1986). Either the actuality or the mere perception that others will be supportive can bolster an individual's overall levels of well-being and capacity to withstand and overcome frustrations and problem-solving challenges (Sarason et al., 1983; Wethington & Kessler, 1986).

In a recently published, definitive text on social support and cardiovascular disease, Shumaker and Czajkowski (1994) pointed out that this term is often used to describe both the structural and functional aspects of the social environment.

Structure includes the size, density, complexity, symmetry, and stability of an individual's family, friends, coworkers, and health professionals and community resources; it is usually referred to as one's "social network." The functional component of social support is defined as an individual's perception of the availability of support and of the resources provided, and is labeled "social support." (p. xi)

According to Amick and Ockene (1994), five factors are important in understanding the scope of social support:

1. Emotional support provides a sense of being cared for and loved and the sense that one has an opportunity for shared intimacy. Here one receives messages of empathy and concern from others.

2. Esteem support provides reminders that one is valued and esteemed and promotes a sense of personal worth. Here the individual receives messages of positive regard, encouragement, or agreement from others.

3. A sense of belonging comes from sharing mutual obligations, communication, and companionship with others.

4. Instrumental support comes from access to material or physical assistance. This form of support involves receiving direct assistance that reduces stress and provides tangible help to the individual.

5. Informational support comes from access to information, advice, appraisal, and guidance from others. Here the individual is given input, suggestions, directions, or feedback that is helpful in promoting adaptive coping.

THE BENEFITS OF SOCIAL SUPPORT

Exactly what are the mechanisms of change underlying the fact that social support affects physical and emotional well-being? Perhaps social support has the effect of buffering the individual from the harmful consequences of stress. Essentially, this perspective proposes that social support has a direct, positive effect on emotions, which, in turn, produce neuroendocrine and hemodynamic responses that provide protection against the consequences of exposure to stressful situations. The famous epidemiological researchers Berkman and Seeman (1986) gave clear voice to this perspective:

> We would like to propose something controversial for which there is little evidence at the present time—that social networks and support influence health status and longevity by influencing what longevity is most obviously related to—the rate of aging of the organism. Following this line of reasoning one would hypothesize that social isolation or lack of support is a chronically stressful situation to which the organism responds by aging faster. (p. 805)

On the other hand, the effect of social support may be psychological. Here high social support is said to lead to greater self-esteem and more adaptive subsequent coping. For example, close social ties can provide support and encouragement that the individual can cope during difficult times, thereby fueling a positive sense of hope.

Alternatively, the effect of support may be behavioral. Perhaps belongingness leads to a healthier lifestyle as friends and relatives offer advice or model prudent health habits (Reed, McGee, Katshuhiko, & Feinleib, 1983).

SOCIAL SUPPORT, WELL-BEING, AND INTIMACY

I propose that one form of support should be recognized as a primary factor in promoting well-being, stress resistance, and longevity: relationship intimacy. In cardiopulmonary rehabilitation, the intimacy factor has been defined as caring relationships with others that satisfy needs for affiliation, cooperation, and affection (Sotile, 1992, 1993). This proposal is based on a broad body of research.

As early as 1968, researchers (i.e., Lowenthal & Haven, 1968) called attention to the positive effects of intimacy in adapting to stress. In spurts, at first, and now in a steady cascade, the literature has supported this notion. Pearlin et al. (1981) reminded us that "support comes when people's engagement with one another extends to a level of involvement and concern, not when they merely touch at the surface of each other's lives" (p. 340). In a similar vein, Coyne and DeLongis (1986) cautioned that support from other relationships cannot compensate for an unsatisfactory marriage. In a review of the literature regarding subjective well-being, Diener (1984) stated that having a love relationship is the most important resource for happiness.

Key research studies have suggested that those who live accompanied by a spouse, a confidant, or a supportive family seem to enjoy enhanced well-being (Lowenthal & Haven, 1968). Specific attention has also been called to the importance of a supportive, intimate relationship in promoting recovery from cardiac illness. Noteworthy documentation of the importance of relationship intimacy in reducing both morbidity and mortality in cardiac populations has been published (see Indexed Bibliography). In a study of COPD patients (Jensen, 1983), high-risk patients with low social support were hospitalized significantly more frequently than low-risk patients or high-risk patients who were receiving increased social support. In a nutshell, the intimacy researchers have proposed that social embeddedness is not enough; for relationships to truly help mediate the effects of stress, they must contain healthy elements of solidarity, trust, intimate attachment, and helping behaviors (Burke & Weir, 1977a, 1977b; Headey, Holmstrom, & Wearing, 1984; Pearlin et al., 1981; Waltz, 1986). Furthermore, research has suggested that this intimate attachment may be provided by loving relationships of various sorts. For example, a study which documented that having a confidant significantly diminished the prevalence of depression in an aged population faced with the stresses of retirement also noted that the identities of the confidants of the subject sample were evenly distributed among spouse, child, and friend (Lowenthal & Haven, 1968). This finding is especially noteworthy given that many older cardiopulmonary patients depend upon their grown children for social support of various sorts (Campbell, 1986; Mayou, Foster, & Williamson, 1978a, 1978b).

Empirical investigations have shown that, when married, and especially for younger populations of recovering cardiopulmonary patients, a crucial form of social support is spouse support and marital intimacy (Campbell, 1986; Sotile, Sotile, Ewen, & Sotile, 1993; Sotile, Sotile, Sotile, & Ewen, 1993). Specifically what is meant by spouse support was discussed in chapter 8. For now, the emphasis is on what happens when a recovering patient receives adequate spouse support.

In an outstanding series of empirical investigations of well-being in a specific cardiac population, Mallard Waltz and colleagues found that marital intimacy plays a crucial role in increasing a patient's self-concept, enhancing confidence in the ability to cope with rehabilitation, fostering flexibility in coping, increasing use of social support, and promoting an overall sense of well-being. This was a 5-year, prospective study of 400 male cardiac patients and their spouses drawn from 200 German hospitals. The investigators found that, independent of degree of physical impairment, the presence or absence of emotional closeness in marriage was associated with substantial differences in the long-term subjective well-being of patients. While simply being married seemed to soothe coping in the hospital, the quality of marriage began to differentiate levels of well-being at 1-year follow-up (Waltz, 1986) and persisted through 3-year (Waltz et al., 1988) and 5-year (Waltz & Badura, 1988) follow-ups. Specifically, marital conflict was found to correlate significantly with patient levels of anxiety and depression (Waltz et al., 1988). Patients with low levels of marital conflict reported less anxiety than did patients with high levels of marital conflict, regardless of health status. On the other hand, high-intimacy subjects had lower ratings on objective measurements of depression (the Hopkins Depression Scale) than did low-intimacy subjects, regardless of health status.

THE NEGATIVE SIDE OF SOCIAL SUPPORT

Hackett and Cassem (1969) were among the first to call attention to the fact that, for some recovering cardiopulmonary patients, the family may not provide much-needed forms of support. One manifestation of this failure is the delay in seeking medical care that is often encouraged by family members. These authors noted, for example, that the delay between the onset of cardiac symptoms and seeking of medical care is three times longer when the individual is with a family member than when with a friend (12 hours compared to 4 hours). It appears that family members sometime inappropriately discount the significance of physical symptoms (Nyamathi, 1988).

Supposedly supportive relationships can also prove to be sources of disappointment in times of need. During a health crisis, most people expect their friends and family to help. If they do not, the lack of support proves to be a very significant stressor for the recovering person, one that increases the patient's experience of negative emotions (Davidson & Shumaker, 1987; Fiore, Becker, & Coppel, 1983). These findings apply throughout the continuum of recovery from cardiovascular illness.

Few things feel worse than not getting along with loved ones. The flip side of the "buffering hypothesis" regarding social support is that nonsupportive social relations make stress worse (Rook, 1984). Evidence exists that this phenomenon applies to both married and single individuals.

Coyne and DeLongis (1986) pointed out that family therapists often work to help individuals individuate or separate from troublesome overinvolvement in their families. The authors cite findings from a broad literature regarding the treatment of schizophrenics, depressed patients, those suffering from chronic pain, hemodialysis patients, and adolescents with asthma and diabetes or obesity which documents that for some people, positive adaptation means moving away from rather than toward others.

HOW HEALTH PROBLEMS AFFECT SUPPORT SYSTEMS

Support systems affect both health behaviors and health outcomes. In the best-case scenario, these effects are positive: illness or some other mode of distressed behavior mobilizes others to come to a person's aid (Cutrona, 1986; Gore, 1981), and shored up with such support, the individual copes more adaptively. However, the flip side of this process is also important: When illness strikes, the patient's support system is affected by the stresses of medical intervention, rehabilitation, and changes in the system that result from the effects of the illness. In turn, the patient's support system can become overwhelmed and symptomatic.

For example, during acute cardiac care, such as ICU stays, family members have been found to be more distressed than patients, more pessimistic and fearful of the patient's death, and more worried about the future (Speedling, 1982). Over one-third of spouses of post-MI patients (Skelton & Dominian, 1973) and comparable percentages of spouses of COPD patients report significant affective distress. An interesting study by Foxall, Ekbert, & Griffith (1987) assessed spouses of arthritics, COPD patients, and those suffering from peripheral vascular disease, CHD, and hypertension. Results indicated that the spouses, more so than the patients, reported debilitating levels of loneliness.

It appears that the stresses on support systems caused by the patient's illness may lead to a decrease in support of the patient (Fontana et al., 1989). This may occur because others feel ineffectual or uncomfortable in their efforts to help the recovering patient and therefore begin to avoid or shun the patient. Or the recovering patient may actually discourage others from offering support, causing supports to withdraw. Alternatively, the sick person's pessimism might simply diminish his or her perception of available supports, independent of the actual presence or absence of supportive others. Especially when dealing with a chronic illness, the stress of having a sick loved one might also simply lead to exhaustion of the capacity for the support system to continue providing aid.

SOCIAL SUPPORT AND WORK RETURN

Work return is an aspect of cardiopulmonary rehabilitation that epitomizes the interplay of the various factors discussed thus far: the importance of social support in the forms of family (especially marital) input in affecting a psychosocial outcome; the effect of this aspect of rehabilitation on well-being, both for the patient and for the loved ones; and the effects of the illness process on the very sources of support that are important in promoting adjustment in a given psychosocial domain. Research regarding work return in cardiopulmonary populations also underscores the importance of another form of social support—medical input.

SCOPE OF THE PROBLEM

A massive literature exists regarding this topic. Articles on vocational rehabilitation are second in number only to studies of the physical aspects of cardiac rehabilitation (Garrity, 1973b). Depending upon the study, the proportion of patients returning to work after an MI ranges from 49% to 93%, with the average return-to-work time being 60-90 days—a figure that has not changed appreciably during the past 15 years (Dennis et al., 1988). In treating COPD patients, work return is a less prevalent issue, mainly due to their relatively advanced age. However, when relevant, similar psychosocial issues impact work return for both CHD and COPD patients (Ries, 1990). Three facts underscore the importance of early intervention in this area:

• Most adults spend up to 50% of their time in work-related activities. Perhaps for this reason, employment status, in combination with other indicators such as health or family status, is one of the more powerful predictors of overall level of quality of life (Dafoe et al., 1993; Packa, 1989).

• If a recovering cardiopulmonary patient fails to return to work within 6 months of surgery or of an illness event, it is unlikely that he or she will ever do so (Wenger, 1987). In this regard, it has been said that "work is a habit which if allowed to lapse, is replaced by non-work" (Ross et al., 1978, p. 8).

• As will be shown in the following discussions, crucial determiners of work return or adjustment to decisions about no return or lessening of work involvement despite return are the patient's perceptions of the attitudes of significant others (especially health care providers and loved ones) regarding work return.

Discussion of work return must proceed with an important caveat. A number of writers have questioned the tradition of using return to work as a gold-standard indicator of improvement in the quality of life for a recovering cardiopulmonary patient. A large percentage of patients fail to return to work because of choosing early retirement following illness. Many others are already retired when illness strikes. But even in the population of younger, gainfully employed cardiopulmonary patients, the question of what constitutes a truly healthy work-related response to illness should be carefully evaluated (Lertzman & Cherniack, 1976; Shanfield, 1990).

Bear in mind that a given patient simply may not identify returning to work as a goal of rehabilitation. Here, as always, the patient's needs should be given due consideration in deciding how to structure interventions. Of course, no ethical health care provider will be supportive of unsubstantiated claims of vocational disability in order to be supportive of a patient's needs. However, many patients need emotional and informational support—not medical substantiation—as they grapple with this aspect of rehabilitation. Many physically fit patients grapple with the question of whether or not to return to preillness styles or places of work out of a healthy examination of their quality of life. In some cases, not returning to work may signal a positive, courageous decision on the patient's part to begin to clarify the "territory" of his or her life in order to live more healthily, a crucial factor in overall Effective Emotional Management.

This notion is supported by findings from a prospective study of CABG patients which documented that return to previous levels of work involvement was sometimes actually seen by the patients as a poor outcome, whereas for others, failure to return to work was seen as a positive outcome (Mayou & Bryant, 1987). In an excellent discussion of this topic, Garrity (1973b) pointed out that the issues of work and well-being in recovering cardiovascular patients need to be considered in terms of the quantity, quality, and self-satisfaction of work: how much will the patient work, how good will that work be, and how satisfied with this aspect of life will the patient be? Perhaps here, especially, we should heed the words of pioneer psychosocial researcher Richard Mayou: "Quality of life for any cardiac disorder should be defined in terms of what is important to patients and their families" (Mayou, 1990, p. 101), not solely in terms dictated by our own beliefs as health care providers.

FACTORS THAT AFFECT WORK RETURN

A multitude of factors have been found to affect work return in recovering cardiopulmonary patients.

Although many demographic factors have implications in this regard, overall this literature suggests that relatively young, male, white-collar, middle-class patients who have dependents are highly likely to return to work in short order (Smith & O'Rourke, 1988). Factors directly relevant to the patient's physical condition, including severity or extent of cardiopulmonary illness, number of previous episodes of illness, and the presence of other chronic medical disorders, affect work return (Garrity, 1973a, 1973b). However, the most important determinant of work return appears to be the patient's overall psychosocial status (Walter, 1985).

SUMMARY BOX

Determinants of Return to Work

Objective	Subjective
Medical • Severity and extent of illness **Psychological** • Pre- and postmorbid emotional state **Sociodemographic, economic, and cultural** • Gender • Age • Government services and legislation • Financial demands/assets • Cultural/national economic conditions • Local economic conditions • Insurance and disability coverage • Union policies and decision • Availability of job retraining **Individual's history** • Type of work • Self-employed • Physical demands of job • History of unemployment • Preillness work limitations • Educational level • Job autonomy	**Individual's perception of health and risk to life** • Severity of illness • Probability of progression of illness or disability • Attribution of cause of illness to previous job **Individual's perception of self** • Self-confidence • Self-efficacy • Role of work in overall life **Influence of social support and social networks** • Family's fear and altered dynamics • Employer's fear, liability • Community customs, work ethic, job offers • Personal physician and rehabilitation program **Individual's perception of prior work** • Stress • Satisfaction **Individual's expectations and predictions** • Of probability of return to work • Of intention to return to work

Important here are a number of factors that can be affected by social support, including the patient's perceptions of his or her own work capacity and self-efficacy regarding work; perceptions of health status; assessment of work safety; and overall emotional state and personality make-up (e.g., degree of work involvement manifested on standardized psychological testing) (Gundle, Reeves, & Tate, 1980). Vocational rehabilitation is especially problematic with any patient who believes that job stress contributed to the etiology of his or her illness or that the cause of the illness relates to factors beyond his or her control (Bar-On, 1987; Bar-On & Cristal, 1987).

Several other psychosocial factors demonstrate an integral interplay between work return patterns and individual and social system variables. For example, individuals who evidence Type A behavior pattern tend to return to work more quickly than their Type B counterparts, a fact that may either correlate with or cause marital tensions in the support system of such patients (Davidson, 1983; Sotile, Sotile, Sotile, & Ewen, 1993). Furthermore, a patient who evidences pessimism about his or her ability to return to work in-hospital is three times more likely to evidence delayed work return (Maeland & Havik, 1987). There also appears to be a stronger relationship between depression and failure to return to work than between anxiety and failure to return to work: Patients who evidence high levels of depression in early posthospital phases of recovery that continue into the next year are at particular risk of failing to return to work (Burgess, Lerner, C'Argostino, Vokonas, Hartman, & Gaccione, 1987; Malan, 1992). Tendencies toward hypochondriasis or exaggerated acceptance of the sick role have also been found to interfere with work return for recovering cardiopulmonary patients (Byrne, Whyte, & Butler, 1981; Hlatkey, Haney, & Barefoot, 1986).

Finally, as mentioned earlier, the patient's stage of life, stage of career development, and overall lifestyle are important psychosocial issues that need to be considered in structuring supportive interventions that might influence work return. For example, Dafoe et al. (1993) pointed out that when a cardiac event occurs between the ages of 45 and 50, it is likely to interfere with career advancement, and the specifics of cardiac rehabilitation are likely to conflict with the upwardly mobile lifestyle that is typical at that stage of life. Between the ages of 50 and 65, issues of career maintenance and stabilization or early retirement are impacted by the demands of rehabilitation. In obvious ways, adjustment to the work factor needs to be tailored according to the importance work has in the individual patient's life.

SOCIAL SUPPORT AND ADJUSTMENT TO CHANGES IN WORK STATUS

Since the 1930s many researchers have argued that social support is crucial in determining the psychological impact of planned or unanticipated unemployment. In a nutshell, it appears that social support can attenuate the severity of psychological and health-related responses to unemployment. This point was demonstrated in separate studies of the effects of an intimate relationship during an unexpected job loss. Gore (1978) found that a high level of social support during a 6-month period following job loss correlated with significant decrease in mean serum total cholesterol concentration, and Pearlin et al. (1981) reported that such support minimized the elevation of depression by dampening the loss of self-esteem in work-stressed subjects.

Lowenthal and Haven (1968) studied an aged population to determine what buffers some people against the effects of life events that typically yield social losses, such as widowhood and retirement. They found that having no confidant and retrenching one's social life following such a loss overwhelmingly increases the odds for depression. On the other hand, the retired person with a confidant—spouse, child, or friend—ranked the same with regard to morale as those still working who had no confidant. It appears that an intimate relationship may buffer depression that might result from life events that typically yield social losses.

SOCIAL SUPPORT AND WORK RETURN IN CARDIOPULMONARY PATIENTS

A multitude of social support factors have been found to affect work return and to be affected by work return patterns in recovering cardiopulmonary patients. For this population, the quality of the patient's relationships with family and significant others seems to be crucial in determining work return and in adjusting to the decisions made therein (Shanfield, 1990). Family fear and level of family concern about work return, and intrafamily patterns of overprotectiveness or conflict, have all been found to directly affect work return patterns for recovering cardiac patients (Mayou et al., 1978a, 1978b; Sotile, Sotile, Sotile, & Ewen, 1993). Specifically, patients who perceive that their families do not expect them to adjust fully to MI are less likely to return to work (Burgess et al., 1987; Garrity, 1973b). The patient's perception of the physician's expectations and the physician's actual attitude toward the patient's return to work have also been found to be crucial in this regard.

The attitudes and behaviors of employers and coworkers can also be significant social support factors affecting work return. Employers often discourage work return out of fear of liability, an attitude that may also be manifested by a patient's worker union. Even broad-based social institutions such as the government, through provision of disability services, may affect work return patterns (Dafoe et al., 1993; Davidson, 1983).

Several authors called attention to the fact that degree of work change following illness can have a profound effect on the quality of the social system within which the patient lives. Carter (1984) pointed out that, in addition to work return, the extent of marital conflict about work return and the quality of resolution of this conflict all must be considered in evaluating a recovering cardiac patient's overall level of well-being, especially as measured by the risk of marital separation/divorce postevent. The authors proposed that, compared to patients who return to work with no marital conflict, fail to return without conflict, or return but experience conflict with their mate, those who evidence a no return/poor conflict resolution pattern are at the greatest risk of separation or divorce.

Shanfield (1990) presented a thoughtful discussion of the psychosocial adjustments that revolve around issues of work for spouses of recovering

MI patients. Several predictive conclusions from this publication are worth underscoring. First, for the husband of a female MI patient with a prior history of working, it is overwhelmingly likely that his mate will not return to work, once heart illness is diagnosed. The wife of a male MI patient, on the other hand, will very likely increase her workload following her husband's illness. Shanfield claimed that one-half to two-thirds of wives of MI patients increase household chores, and half of working wives temporarily stop working to help their husbands during the early recovery period. At 1 year, many wives go to work for the first time, often due to the diminished family income subsequent to the husband's illness. These facts underscore the observation that, in many instances, spouses are perhaps impacted more by this work return factor than are patients.

Finlayson (1976) studied the ways that wives of recovering MI patients cope with such stressors and found that social support of the wife was crucial in determining positive versus negative adaptation patterns. Interestingly, support from husbands and nonrelatives appeared more important for wives whose husbands worked in nonmanual jobs, whereas support from adult children appeared most important for wives whose husbands worked as manual laborers.

SOCIAL SUPPORT INTERVENTIONS REGARDING WORK RETURN WITH CARDIOPULMONARY PATIENTS

Patients at high risk of experiencing work return problems should be flagged and provided additional assistance. As pointed out by Davidson (1983), frequently, the best way to learn something is to ask directly. As early as 3 weeks after their cardiac event, patients have been able to accurately predict when they will return to work. Inquiring as to the patient's attitude toward work return, and doing so early in the recovery process, can help flag at-risk patients. Of the many factors listed above that signal at-risk patients, Davidson cautions that those patients who have a gloomy prediction about their return to work and who have no obvious physical reasons on which to base this judgment are at special risk of not returning to work. Emphasizing the safety and wisdom of an early return to work is essential in treating such patients, and counseling regarding the factors underlying the resistance to work return is in order.

Evidence has accumulated that early intervention (i.e., psychosocial intervention delivered on the second or third day after admission to the CCU) leads to a significantly earlier return to work (Thockcloth, So, & Wright, 1973). In-hospital relaxation training and stress management has also been found to lead to better vocational adjustment at 6-month follow-up (Langosch et al., 1982). Providing additional staff and peer support to such patients has also been proven to promote more positive vocational rehabilitation. In a controlled comparison study, Naismith, Robinson, Shaw, and MacIntyre (1979) demonstrated the efficacy of a 6-month supportive-didactic rehabilitation counseling intervention in promoting earlier work return for recovering male MI patients. A number of studies (e.g., Pozen et al., 1977) have found that relatively simple, nurse-administered interventions can positively affect work return as well as other psychosocial adjustment issues in recovering MI patients. Participation in a formal pulmonary rehabilitation program, a process that is replete with social support, has been found to have profound positive effects on work return rates for COPD patients. For example, in a 5-year study of 252 COPD patients who participated in a formal pulmonary rehabilitation program, Haas and Cardon (1969) found that 25% of the participants maintained full-time employment 5 years after completion of the program, compared to only 3% of 50 control patients selected from an outpatient clinic. In addition, a significantly greater percentage of the rehabilitation patients evidenced independent self-care at follow-up (19% versus 5% of controls).

Clinical experience has also suggested the importance of providing immediate, accurate, and honest information to any patient who evidently anticipates that medical or rehabilitation personnel will support a claim for vocational disability when such is not the case. Such patients should be caringly forewarned of the low probability that his or her physical condition will justify declaration of disabled status, and rehabilitation should be framed as an opportunity for work-hardening or for gaining confidence in one's physical ability to return to work in some capacity. Involving state vocational rehabilitation counselors in serving such patients is highly recommended (Massey, 1994).

Clearly, work return is not a unitary phenomenon. Multiple determinants are operative (a) in the decision to return to work or not; (b) in the decision of how much to work following illness; and (c) in the effects of such decisions. In each instance, however, ample social support can enhance decision making and facilitate subsequent coping.

BOLSTERING SUPPORT

Designing interventions that bolster social support should begin with consideration of several general factors. Will interventions target individuals in the patient's personal life, intending to increase or decrease the density of the patient's social network or to change the behavior of the people within that network? Will interventions attempt to enhance the patient's ability to better create and maintain supportive relationships? On which level will intervention focus: broad-based social support or specific relationship intimacy? Will the treatment or rehabilitation setting itself be a source of social support?

Answers to these questions will structure specific interventions. In the remainder of this chapter, a number of issues relevant to the task of bolstering the social support factor for recovering cardiopulmonary patients will be explored.

WHAT DOES THIS PERSON NEED RIGHT NOW?

Patients and their families will have different coping needs at different times, depending on the nature of the stressful situation being faced. This fact should be kept in mind when designing social support interventions. Furthermore, we must remember that social support is a personal experience, and that an individual's subjective perceptions of well-being should be taken into consideration in addressing this factor (e.g., Dhooper, 1990; Packa, 1989). Research of the varying support needs of recovering cardiopulmonary patients and their loved ones has validated this observation. For example, as already discussed, the effectiveness of specific forms of support will vary, depending on the patient's stage of recovery, stage of life, and stage of changing.

ENCOURAGE GIVING AS WELL AS RECEIVING SUPPORT

Victor Frankle once said: "Health is escaping from an endless realm of servitude to that insatiable tyrant self and devoting oneself to higher ends, based on faith, hope, and love." In line with Frankle's wisdom, research is documenting the importance of reciprocity in giving and receiving support. Fundamentally, people seem to benefit from support in proportion to the extent of support they give to others. An individual who reciprocates the support received is less likely to feel guilty about being supported and is more likely to feel comfortable continuing to ask for help (Antonucci & Johnson, 1994; Dhooper, 1990). I therefore suggest that, in addition to encouraging individuals to give support, interventions should help clarify how each individual can be supportive of others. The importance of this issue can be demonstrated by simply questioning a patient and his or her loved ones, inquiring "What can your loved ones do to help you cope?" and "What can you do to help your loved ones cope?"

HELP IDENTIFY SOCIAL NETWORKS

Dhooper (1990) described a technique for mapping social networks borrowed from the work of Maguire (1983) and Gottlieb (1985) that can be modified for use with recovering cardiopulmonary patients. The individual is given a large piece of paper and asked to draw five concentric circles. The circles are then divided into five sections and labeled as indicated in Figure 10.1: (a) family and relatives, (b) friends, (c) neighbors, (d) work/school associates, and (e) health care providers. The central circle represents the patient and/ or family. (This technique can be used with reference to networks available to the couple or family as a system or to individual family members.) Next the couple or patient is asked to write the initials of those closest to them within each sphere of influence. Moving outward, the procedure is repeated and the initials of other network members in other circles are recorded, with

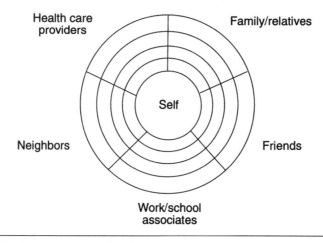

Figure 10.1 Mapping social networks.
Note. From "Social Network Mapping," by D. Todd. In *The Future Use of Social Network in Mental Health* (p. 143) by W.R. Curtis (Ed.), 1979, Boston: Social Matrix Research. Copyright 1979 by Social Matrix Research.

emotional closeness determining their distance from the center circle. When overlap occurs (e.g., one's friends may also be one's neighbors), each person is limited to one sphere.

Once the concentric areas in all spheres are charted, the individual is asked to connect with lines the initials of those who know each other. This illustrates the network, and the lines between and among the network members represent the network's density. Processing the information in the chart can clarify whether the individual finds the network too dense (e.g., smothering) or too disjointed.

The network can be further analyzed by having the individual list the types of support received from various network members and indicate whether or not that support is reciprocated. The final task is to help the individual specify those potential helpers who can provide the type of support needed. Here a form such as that depicted in Form 10.1 can be helpful.

Dhooper (1990) cautioned that it is important to help the individual decide how to approach the identified network members. This might require modeling or coaching regarding verbal and nonverbal communication skills. Role playing, rehearsal, and helping the individual reframe feelings of guilt associated with asking for help are recommended. Also recommended is helping the patient develop a backup plan to be implemented in the event that requests for support meet with frustration or disappointment.

WHERE POSSIBLE, IMPACT THE NETWORK ON THE PATIENT'S BEHALF

Dhooper (1990) proposed that a patient might also benefit from coaching his or her nonfamilial social network in effective support behaviors. This

Form 10.1   Identifying Supports

Name and phone no.	Relationship	Emotional closeness (high, medium, low)	Type of support	Perceived ability to help
1.				
2.				
3.				
4.				
5.				

Note. From *Understanding Social Networks* (p. 180), by L. Maguire, 1983, Beverly Hills, CA: Sage. Copyright 1983 by Sage Publications. Adapted with permission.

might mean taking the time and effort to speak to employers or co-workers on the patient's behalf. In this regard, Dhooper recommends the following guidelines:

- Prepare them for the patient's behavior.
- Reassure them about their attempts at being helpful.
- Provide them chances to discuss the problems they anticipate.
- Teach them how to manage and control their anxiety about interacting with the patient and family in need.
- Facilitate communication among the various participants.
- Support their efforts to help.

Burgess et al. (1987) demonstrated the importance of both providing staff support and directly working with a recovering heart patient's social network to affect adaptive work return. This study promoted work return in 89 acute MI patients by exposing them to a relatively simple 3-month psychosocial adjustment program run by masters-prepared nurse clinicians. The intervention emphasized four factors: *cognitive-behavioral interventions* for lessening psychological distress; *guidance* and *moral support* to patients and to a key member of each patient's primary social network; and *direct consultation* with the patients and their coworkers or supervisors to address mutual concerns about the patient's planned return to work. Routine telephone monitoring of patient's progress was also incorporated. Each patient received an average of six contacts.

Follow-up 13 months after hospitalization indicated that, compared to the control group, the intervention group evidenced overall enhanced psychological and social functioning, including enhanced vocational adjustment. There were no significant between-group differences in rates of work return, but the treatment group had significantly lower distress scores and less intense family supportiveness—an important factor, given the additional finding that the more moderate the degree of family support at first follow-up, the more rapid the return to work.

In a study conducted in the Wake Forest University cardiac rehabilitation program, Dominick et al. (1994) demonstrated that a combination of social support interventions can enhance the exercise behavior of recovering heart patients. Intervention consisted of two forms of social support: (a) enhanced staff support in the form of extra encouragement, attention, and monitoring of patients' exercise behavior; and (b) coaching a support person in the patient's home (usually a spouse) to be specifically supportive of the patient's exercise behavior. Compared to controls who received usual cardiac rehabilitation care (which, incidentally, is inherently quite rich in social support), intervention patients evidenced significant improvements in both at-home exercise behavior and in physiological measures of fitness at 3-month reevaluation.

Ways to Bolster Social Support
for Recovering Medical Patients and Their Loved Ones

In general:

- Attend to what the person needs right now.
- Modify support according to the stages of change.
- Provide staff support.

Specific in-hospital interventions:

- Offer support programs and groups.
- Support the patient's family.
- Encourage visitation by family, and monitor the effects.
- Coach the patient's family in what to expect and in how to be supportive.
- Flag patients and loved ones who are at risk of adjustment struggles.
- Prepare the patient and family for homecoming.

Specific outpatient interventions:

- Educate the patient and family regarding potential problematic interaction patterns.
- Operationalize positive supportive behaviors.

- Encourage giving as well as receiving support.
- Help identify the patient's social networks.
- When possible, impact the network on the patient's behalf.
- Refer to self-help or support groups.
- Refer to formal cardiac or pulmonary rehabilitation programs.
- Make the office or rehabilitation environment a supportive one.

SPIRITUAL CRISIS AND ILLNESS: IMPLICATIONS FOR SUPPORTIVE INTERVENTIONS

A special form of crisis impacts the lives of many cardiopulmonary patients, a crisis that warrants special discussion and special forms of supportive intervention. The North American Nursing Diagnosis Association (NANDA) defined spiritual distress as "a disruption in the life principle which pervades a person's entire being and which integrates and transcends biopsychosocial nature" (Hurley, 1986, p. 543). The recently published DSM-IV (American Psychiatric Association, 1994), cites religious and spiritual difficulties as a distinct disorder deserving treatment. In part, DSM-IV operationalizes this syndrome to include the circumstance in which distressing experiences lead to a loss or questioning of faith or a questioning of one's spiritual values.

It is clear that many medical patients experience such spiritual crisis during the course of rehabilitation. Illness may lead to the patient or the family's first examination of spiritual issues or to their first serious examination of the meaning and purpose of their lives (Colliton, 1981). Shaffer (1991) pointed out that spiritual crisis can take various forms during the course of coping with a critical illness:

1. Questioning or anger directed toward one's god
2. Urgent appeal to one's higher power for help in coping
3. Anxiety over being separated from one's spiritual support system

For many people, *spiritual* means involvement with organized religion, a factor that appears to have significant health-enhancing correlates. A number of investigations have documented the value of religion to the health and well-being of older adults (e.g., Koenig, Smiley, & Gonzales, 1988). In fact, religious groups are the third most important source of instrumental support to the aged, following support of families and the federal government (Blazer, 1991).

But spiritual well-being is a concept that goes beyond formal religious involvement. "Spiritual well-being is the affirmation of life in a relationship with a God, self, community, and environment that nurtures and celebrates wholeness" (National Interfaith Coalition on Aging, 1975, p. 4). The 1971 White House Conference on Aging identified six areas of spiritual need as deserving special attention by anyone working with elderly populations:

- Sociocultural sources of spiritual needs
- Relief from anxieties and fears
- Preparation for death
- Personality integration
- Personal dignity
- Philosophy of life (Moberg, 1971)

DEATH AND DYING

Of the many spiritual needs of patients and their family members that are often ignored in the delivery of routine medical and rehabilitation care, perhaps none is more obvious and more tragic than ignoring the need for help in preparing for death. Connors and Hilling (1993) reminded us that because many of the patients we treat have severe illnesses and limited life expectancy, we "must take an active role in helping all patients understand issues related to, and prepare for, death and dying" (Connors & Hilling, 1993, p. 53). Such needs of patients and loved ones are often attended to when death is imminent: the family is altered and responded to with compassion; religious counselors are called in; and the process of grieving begins.

But issues related to death and dying are most often avoided in treating patients in rehabilitation and outpatient settings, even when the participant's condition is seriously deteriorating. The ethics of our care should compel us to proactively counsel what often are the last psychosocial concerns of our patients and their loved ones: decisions about resuscitation, a living will, durable power of attorney for health care, and directives to medical personnel regarding the last stages of medical care (Nett & Petty, 1985).

PROVIDING HELP FOR SPIRITUAL DISTRESS

Excellent suggestions for assessing patients' spiritual needs have been offered by Stoll (1979) and Shaffer (1991). These authors recommend that a patient be questioned regarding his or her sources of hope and strength, religious practices, and beliefs in the relationship between spirituality and coping strength. In addition, the patient should be asked about his or her spiritual resources and whether or not the present illness has a particular meaning with regard to his or her spiritual beliefs.

Questions such as the following might be helpful in assessing the spiritual needs of a patient or family:

"Is belief in a higher power important to you?"

"Does this crisis have a special spiritual meaning for you?"

"Do you belong to a particular church community?" [if so] "Does this community offer support of a sort that would be helpful to you now?"

"When you have faced difficult times in the past, have you found that prayer has helped you to cope?"

"Would you like me to arrange any form of pastoral counseling for you at this time?"

By tactfully and sensitively posing questions of this sort, you can validate that spiritual concerns and use of spiritual resources are legitimate aspects of the whole-person medical treatment that you intend to offer. Such questioning should leave the patient feeling free to express his or her spirituality without fear of being judged.

Here, as in all areas of psychosocial intervention, the provider should pay attention to two guidelines in delivering care: (a) the intervention should meet the needs of the patient, not of the provider; and (b) the provider should not be coerced into doing anything that is excessively uncomfortable for him or her. Not every health care provider will be comfortable praying with or offering spiritual guidance to a spiritually distressed patient. However, it is important to convey respect and permission to the patient to acknowledge his or her spiritual needs and, if desired by the patient, a willingness to help the patient receive counseling in this area. Consultation from pastoral counselors or from the patient's own minister should be requested in such instances.

In their efforts to make sense of their suffering, both patients and their loved ones can benefit from brief spiritual counseling. Such counseling can provide much-needed and much-appreciated help in coping with the current crisis and in using the crisis to spur psychosocial growth. "We often claim that experience is a great teacher, but experience teaches us little if we do not reflect on it and learn from it" (Howe, 1983, p. 39). For many, spiritual integration is the ultimate form of reflection.

In summary, it is important to remember that few things change the meaning of life more abruptly than the death of a loved one or a brush with serious illness. Grieving the actual or anticipated loss of a loved one leads to a reflexive, close examination of the quality of the relationships that remain in our life. In many ways, grief serves as a magnifier and an amplifier: We feel more intensely, we see more clearly, we question more loudly. Part of our caring for heart and lung patients should be to help them and their families understand the normalcy of their struggles so that what they feel and see and hear in this last stage of their life together will lead to renewed appreciation and caring for each other.

SUMMARY

The EEM model can be used to structure interventions with cardiac or pulmonary patients treated in any setting. In addition to the individual components discussed in each of the preceding chapters in Part II, the creation of a supportive environment is essential to providing comprehensive EEM care. With such factors in place, the special topics discussed in Part III can be addressed more effectively.

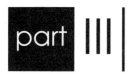

part IIII

SPECIAL TOPICS

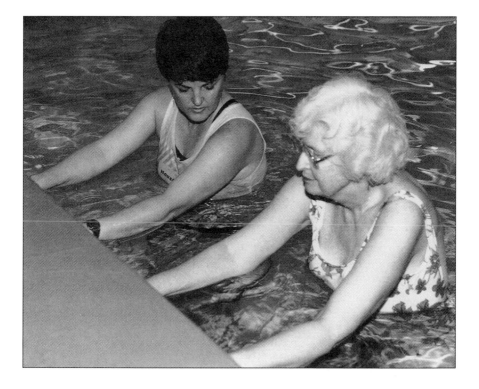

chapter 11

SEXUAL ASPECTS
OF HEART AND LUNG ILLNESSES

One of the most crucial aspects of Effective Emotional Management is the intimacy factor. Intimacy can mean many things, including cooperation, nonsexual affection, and specific variants of spouse support. Here attention will be directed to a topic that is often overlooked in the delivery of routine medical and rehabilitation care: the sexual aspects of living with heart and lung illnesses.

As in preceding chapters, the following discussion will focus predominantly on individuals living in traditional marital relationships. To my knowledge, specific information regarding the sexual rehabilitation issues faced by homosexual cardiopulmonary patients or by those living in nontraditional relationships is not available. In addition, research has basically ignored the sexual adjustment issues faced by single, elderly cardiopulmonary patients. However, as will be seen, much of the information contained in this chapter can be applied to the sexual adjustments faced by any cardiopulmonary patient.

WHAT IS "NORMAL" SEXUAL BEHAVIOR POST-CARDIOPULMONARY ILLNESS?

I begin this discussion by posing a question that has no answer. Researchers have estimated that somewhere between 25% and 40% of recovering cardiac patients and between 19% and 67% of recovering COPD patients report chronic sexual performance problems (Hanson, 1982; Schover & Jensen, 1988). However, as the following discussion will show, the meaning of these statistics in structuring interventions with recovering cardiopulmonary patients must be seriously questioned. The limitations of research regarding the sexual behaviors of both heart and lung patients, coupled with the infinite variety that characterizes human sexual expression, make it impossible to specify any "normal" post-cardiopulmonary illness sexual pattern.

LIMITATIONS OF RESEARCH IN THIS AREA

Research regarding the sexual aspects of cardiac rehabilitation has focused too exclusively on assessment of changes in sexual behaviors post-MI in male patients. This is especially unfortunate, given the well-documented sexual fears and concerns of female cardiac patients and of wives of recovering cardiac patients (Sotile, Sotile, Sotile, & Ewen, 1993).

Rabinowitz and Florian (1992) urged sexual counseling interventions in treating respiratory patients, especially in dealing with COPD patients, "because this is one area in which the patient can be assisted to regain some of his previous functioning" (p. 80). However, the sexual behavior of COPD patients is a grossly underresearched area, and here, too, those studies that have been published have almost exclusively involved male patients (Fletcher, 1984). Again, this limited focus of study is unfortunate, given that the sexual concerns of both male and female COPD patients have been documented and that younger patients suffering from such respiratory conditions as asthma and cystic fibrosis may have particular struggles with sexuality and sexual functioning due to the blows to self-esteem that can come from the psychological and physical consequences of a chronic illness begun in childhood (Kravetz, 1982; Kravetz & Pheatt, 1993; Walbroehl, 1992).

WHAT IS THE GOAL HERE, ANYWAY?

Several other facts cloud the picture when trying to define "normal" sexual patterns for recovering cardiopulmonary patients. It has been suggested that anxiety about sexual activity can lead to diminished quality of sexual and overall marital adjustment in recovering cardiopulmonary patients, and that resumption of sexual activity is an important correlate to enhanced marital functioning post-cardiac illness (Boone & Kelley, 1990; Papadopoulos et al., 1980). This implies that "healthy" couples resume sexual activity following illness. But how is it to be determined whether a given patient's pattern of sexual behavior following illness is "healthy" or not? Compared to others, what effect is the cardiopulmonary illness having on a given patient's resumption of sexual activity?

Unfortunately, and once again, available research offers only cloudy points of comparison in answering such questions. A broad international literature has documented that although more than 80% of recovering cardiopulmonary patients who are sexually active prior to illness onset will initially experience heightened anxieties regarding resumption of sexual activities, somewhere between 40% and 75% of these patients will resume sexual activity within the first year of recovery (Sotile, Sotile, Sotile, & Ewen, 1993). The limited research available on gender issues relative to this issue further suggests that a fairly similar pattern of return to sexual involvement occurs for both female and male cardiopulmonary patients. However, research has also indicated that the vast majority of these patients resume sexual activity at a decreased level of frequency compared to before their illness, and that this decreased level of sexual activity tends to persist in follow-up studies of up to 3-1/2 years (Kornfeld, Heller, Frank, Wilson, & Malm, 1982).

Further clouding the picture of the "optimal" pattern of resumption of sexual activity following illness is a small body of data suggesting that decreased post-MI sexual frequency during the initial stage of recovery correlates with better marital adjustment following illness (Michela, 1987). This observation suggests the possibility that, for some couples, healthy relationship adjustment involves responding to the crisis of illness by at least initially curtailing sexual activity.

WHICH COMES FIRST: ILLNESS OR SEXUAL FRUSTRATIONS?

Finally, the sexual behaviors of "normal" populations also add confusion to any reference data that might be used as a point of comparison in evaluating a given cardiopulmonary patient's postillness sexual behavior. General research on human sexual behavior argues strongly that cardiopulmonary illness is not a prerequisite for developing sexual performance concerns, dissatisfactions, or problems. Frank (1978) studied 100 happily married couples with a mean age of 37-42 years and found that 40% of the men suffered from either erectile or ejaculatory dysfunction. In a retrospective analysis, Wabrek and Burchell (1980) found that 66% of 131 male MI patients studied had sexual problems even before they suffered an MI. These data confirm numerous anecdotal reports of similar observations made by cardiopulmonary rehabilitation specialists who have observed that recovering patients often report a premorbid pattern of sexual dysfunction or sexual avoidance.

MOVING BEYOND STATISTICS

Based on such data, it is impossible to specify any optimal outcomes in promoting sexual adjustment post-cardiopulmonary illness. But the importance of this issue goes beyond mere statistics or fruitless attempts to specify general sexual adjustment patterns. It is important to remember that sexuality is tied to intimacy, and that intimacy is one of our most basic emotional needs (Sotile, 1992). Whether or not a patient is sexually active, it is highly likely that issues related to the patient's sexuality will have a strong bearing on levels of well-being and overall quality of life following illness (Sotile, 1993). At minimum, patients and their loved ones should be encouraged to recognize the importance of continuing (or beginning) steadfast attention to loving, caring interactions that validate each other's sex roles within overall family functioning.

A FRAMEWORK FOR SEXUAL COUNSELING WITH CARDIOPULMONARY PATIENTS

It is well documented that many sexual adjustment difficulties experienced during rehabilitation from heart and lung illnesses are contributed to by lack of information and by patient and spouse fears regarding the effects of sexual activity. Almost universally, researchers in this area call for brief sexual counseling delivered as part of comprehensive rehabilitation when the patient or spouse indicates a desire for information on this issue.

How should this education be structured? The multimodal behavior therapy framework of Lazarus (1976) can be useful in this regard. Accordingly, sexual counseling of recovering cardiopulmonary patients can be structured to incorporate information regarding the areas of adjustment outlined in "Issues to Address in Sexual Counseling With Heart and Lung Patients" on p. 211.

A detailed model for addressing relevant concerns in each of the areas specified in the Summary Box is available in *Heart Illness and Intimacy: How Caring Relationships Aid Recovery* (Sotile, 1992). For current purposes, detailed information regarding the biological factor will be presented, along with a brief overview of the gist of recommendations for intervening in each of the other areas of this model.

BIOLOGICAL FACTORS

Cardiopulmonary patients tend to worry about the potential physical consequences of sexual response. In addition, contrary to the antiquated notion that most sexual performance problems are psychogenic in nature, recent research has shown definitively that organic factors play the most prevalent etiological role in sexual performance problems (Schover & Jensen, 1988). These two facts suggest that it makes sense to start discussion of this issue by addressing five relevant biological factors:

1. The effects of the aging process on sexual functioning

2. Organic factors that occur secondary to cardiopulmonary illness that might affect sexual functioning

3. Facts about cardiac exertion experienced during sexual response

4. The sexual effects of medications frequently used in treating cardiopulmonary illness

5. Medical evaluations and medical treatments available for sexual dysfunctions

Sexual Response and the Aging Process

No two people respond sexually in exactly the same manner. However, a stage-specific conceptualization of sexual response that was originally

SUMMARY BOX

Issues to Address in Sexual Counseling
With Heart and Lung Patients

Biological issues
- Variations of sexual performance problems
- Effects of the aging process
- Sexual effects of organic factors related to the illness
- Is sexual activity safe?
- Effects of medications
- Evaluation and treatment options

Behavioral factors
- Setting the appropriate sexual context
- Specific sexual technique

Emotional factors
- Importance of relaxation and comfort
- Sexual effects of antierotic emotions

Cognitive factors
- Anxiety-provoking beliefs
- Myths versus realities

Personality factors
- Need for education, permission, or therapy

Relationship factors
- Issues that relate to overall intimacy
- Sex versus sexuality in context

Sensory factors
- Sensate focus as an antidote to anxiety
- Advisability of self-stimulation

---

popularized by the famous sex researchers, William Masters and Virginia Johnson, is quite useful in pinpointing specific sexual performance problems and in educating patients regarding this area of concern (Masters & Johnson, 1966).

Fueled by adequate biologically based sex drive, sexual response can be said to "normally" progress in this manner: Sexual stimulation and/or fantasy lead to arousal, signaled by vaginal lubrication and swelling for females and erection for males. Next, a plateau phase is entered, during which continued sexual stimulation is typically enjoyed and arousal is gradually heightened. Full sexual response culminates in orgasm, followed quickly (for men) and gradually (for women) by reversal of the vasocongestive phenomena that characterized prior stages of response. Difficulties in responding can occur at any point along the continuum of sexual response, from disturbances in sex drive to impairments of arousal or orgasm (Sotile, Killman, & Scovern, 1977; Zilbergeld, 1992).

With some modifications, the capacity for full sexual response persists well into the eighth decade of life if one is blessed with good health and a cooperative partner (Schover & Jensen, 1988). Basically, the sexual effects of aging can be simply explained as resulting in an elongation of the sexual response cycle: sex drive becomes less biologically driven; sexual arousal requires greater degrees of direct stimulation of erogenous zones; and orgasm becomes less intense (Masters & Johnson, 1966). However, as will be seen, many of the nonsexual concomitants that accompany the aging process (e.g., illnesses, menopause, or self-consciousness regarding aging) can have profound effects on the sexual behaviors of this population.

Organic Factors Secondary to Illness

In a superb academic discussion of sexuality and chronic illness, Schover and Jensen (1988) cautioned that sexual performance can be impaired by any organic or chemical factor that affects vascular, neurological, or hormonal functioning. These authors also summarized research regarding the various ways in which specific aspects of sexual response may be compromised by organic factors associated with particular cardiopulmonary diseases. For example, postmortem examinations have suggested that virtually all males over 38 years of age begin to show fibrous changes in small penile arteries (Ruzbarsky & Michal, 1977), a factor that is clearly related to sexual performance problems when these changes progress to create peripheral vascular disorders. Ischemia to the legs that leads to such symptoms as claudication during exercising has been found to impair erectile ability in 40% to 50% of male CHD patients (Leriche & Morel, 1948; Michal, 1982). As explained by Schover and Jensen, this may be due to the "stealing" of blood away from penile circulation to supply blood to the legs and buttocks, a syndrome frequently seen when the area where the aorta divides into the iliac arteries is partially blocked. Just as applies to major coronary arteries, the risk of pelvic atherosclerosis increases with age and in the presence of other risk factors such as cigarette smoking (Condra, Morales, Owen, Surridge, & Fenemore, 1986).

Schover and Jensen (1988) also caution that the hormonal balance between prolactin and free testosterone is crucial to various sexual functions, including sexual desire, arousal, and orgasm. Prolactin and free testosterone are related in an inverse manner: Anything that elevates prolactin tends to diminish levels of testosterone. Even mild elevations of prolactin can impair sexual function. This fact is important in treating cardiopulmonary patients because any medication that depletes brain dopamine can also cause mild hyperprolactinemia (De La Fuente & Rosenbaum, 1981). Medications that

deplete brain dopamine include many psychotropics (especially pheno-
thiazines and other agents used to treat psychosis) and antihypertensives
(especially reserpine and methyldopa).

Of course, hormonal changes associated with menopause can lead to
physiological alterations that have dramatic effects on sexual functioning
for any woman. Postmenopause, many women who are not on estrogen
replacement therapy experience vaginal dryness, thinning of the walls of
the vagina, and a general loss of vaginal elasticity—all of which can lead to
pain during intercourse (Semmens & Wagner, 1982). The effects of menopause on female sexual response are important to bear in mind in advising
the cardiopulmonary patient regarding his or her sexual functioning. Here,
as always, advice must be offered with respect for the fact that the patient's
regular sexual partner, too, may be experiencing diminished sexual performance secondary to the effects of his or her own medical conditions or aging
process (Sotile, 1993).

Different forms of cardiopulmonary illness carry certain illness-related
phenomena that can complicate or seriously compromise sexual response
in specific ways. For example, breathlessness or chest pain experienced
upon sexual exertion can occur in the presence of congestive heart failure,
rheumatic heart disease, CHD, and of course, COPD (Friedman, 1978;
Kolodny, Masters, & Johnson, 1979; LoPiccolo & LoPiccolo, 1978).

One frequent concomitant of CHD is diabetes, another illness that can
have marked effects on sexual functioning. Research has suggested that
as many as 55% of diabetic men evidence erectile dysfunction. Orgasmic
difficulties have been reported in samples of diabetic women, but this finding
has yet to be replicated in a wealth of research. The fact that diabetes can lead
to peripheral neuropathy has been implicated in observations of impaired
erection in male diabetics and decreased vaginal lubrication in female diabetics (Jensen, 1986). However, the exact relationship between diabetic neu-
ropathies and sexual response remains unclear. Schover and Jensen (1988)
emphasized that evidence of neurological factors in diabetic women's sexual
problems is unconvincing and that, even in the case of advanced peripheral
neuropathy, most male and female diabetics maintain the ability to experience orgasm. The role of vascular pathology in the sexual response of diabetics is also unclear. For example, research has found that diabetic men
with erectile dysfunction do not differ on measures of penile blood flow
from diabetic men with normal erections (Buvat et al., 1985). Here, too,
compounding risk factors multiplies the risk of experiencing sexual impairment. For example, higher incidences of erection problems have been reported in diabetic males who abuse alcohol or are heavy smokers (Jensen,
1986; McCulloch, Young, Prescott, Campbell, & Clark, 1984).

Early studies suggested that respiratory illness rarely interferes with sexual
functioning except in advanced stages (e.g., Kass, Updegraff, & Muffly,
1972); however, more recent research has suggested that the various chronic
respiratory illnesses can each complicate sexual response in some way. A

much-cited study by Fletcher and Martin (1982) found evidence that COPD may directly affect erectile function independent of age, peripheral vascular disease, or hormonal abnormalities.

In clinical practice, it appears certain that the mechanism underlying sexual performance difficulties for some pulmonary patients is the psycho-physiological nature of breathlessness and its relationship to sexual arousal. Pietropinto and Arora (1989) reminded us that "hyperventilation is so typical of human sexual response that men and women who feign orgasm, actors who simulate sexual activity, and even animated cartoon characters who are caught in the throes of comic passion rely on rapid breathing to convey the impression of sexual arousal" (p. 78). Indeed, such breathlessness during sexual arousal is not just an act. In fact, deeper breathing accompanies the plateau phase of sexual response. The average normal respiratory rate may triple to about 40 breaths/min during orgasm (Masters & Johnson, 1966). For any patient with respiratory impairment, the possibility of having to double or triple normal respiratory patterns can make sexual response a distressing and threatening experience (Pietropinto & Arora, 1989).

In a related fashion, sexual response can be a particular problem for those prone to exercise-induced bronchospasm. Sexual arousal triggers a vasocongestive phenomenon that sometimes involves the nasal membranes. As a result, excitement can impair an asthmatic's already compromised breathing capacity (Pietropinto & Arora, 1989).

Once a patient experiences shortness of breath, dyspnea, chest pain, or other symptoms associated with cardiopulmonary illness during sex, he or she is likely to develop anticipatory anxiety that interferes with further sexual activities. This anticipatory anxiety may lead to gradual reductions in sexual activity levels and to disturbances in arousal or orgasm.

Young adults with cystic fibrosis may experience sexual inhibitions due to self-consciousness about physical effects of the illness: short stature, thinness, stained teeth, and clubbed fingers (Coffman, Levine, Althof, & Stern, 1984). Kravetz and Pheatt (1993) pointed out that, in a society that ascribes great significance to the attractiveness of the chest area, a man with broad shoulders and a woman with large breasts is considered desirable. This factor can impair the development of positive sexual self-image in pulmonary patients of all ages, many of whom have compromised chest profiles secondary to the chronicity of their illness. On the other hand, it has also been proposed that the very chronicity of their conditions affords many asthma and cystic fibrosis patients enough time to learn to master anxieties about sexual performance, unlike the situation that faces the COPD patient who develops lung obstruction later in life (Pietropinto & Arora, 1989).

The very physiology of COPD may compromise sexual functioning in many ways. It has been reported that chronic hypoxemia lowers serum testosterone levels in male COPD patients. Other researchers have found that COPD patients evidence normal hormonal levels but abnormal bulbo-cavernosus reflex latencies, the crucial vascular event that mediates erection.

Recent studies of nocturnal penile tumescence suggested that disturbance in peripheral nerve functioning may cause impotence in male COPD patients (Fletcher & Martin, 1982; Semple, Beastall, Watson, & Hume, 1980).

Regardless of the physiological factors that mediate the effects of COPD on sexual functioning, it is clear that patients with advanced COPD suffer certain physical sequelae to the illness that can impair sexual enjoyment. Physical correlates of COPD that can have negative sexual consequences include general weariness, loss of physical strength, and interruptions in lovemaking due to bronchospasms that produce coughing. In addition, the fact that approximately 83% of COPD patients are 60 years old or older heightens the likelihood that multiple etiological factors might be at play in determining a given patient's sexual response patterns (Rabinowitz & Florian, 1992).

Facts About Cardiac Exertion During Sexual Response

Few cardiopulmonary patients (and perhaps even fewer of their spouses) escape at least transitory fears of the cardiac effects of sexual exertion. Even though it is a very rare occurrence, the fear of coital coronary is very real in the privacy of the bedrooms of the patients we treat (Boone & Kelley, 1990; Ueno, 1963). Patients should be soothed with the facts regarding the minimal cardiac strain caused by typical sexual behaviors:

• The average heart rate experienced during sexual relations is 85 beats/min (2 min before and 2 min after orgasm). Heart rates peak at 117 beats/min at orgasm, with a range of 90 to 144 beats/min (Hellerstein & Friedman, 1969; Stein, 1975). The peak coital heart rate lessens in cardiac patients who engage in regular exercise programs (Douglas & Wilkes, 1975).

• Blood pressure during sexual intercourse peaks at approximately 162/89 mmHg (Nemec, Mansfield, & Kennedy, 1976).

• The energy cost of sexual foreplay and afterplay has been found to be 3.5 metabolic equivalents (METs); and for orgasm, 4.7-5.5 METs. This fact tends to especially soothe fears of sexual performance if it is paired with the information that the average patient who has recovered from an uncomplicated MI has a metabolic capacity of 8-9 METs (Eliot & Miles, 1973).

Contrary to popular mythology, sexual position has not been found to account for any significant variability in heart rate or blood pressure when sexual behaviors are studied in the privacy of patients' own homes (Nemec et al., 1976). Approximately 7% to 14% of cardiac patients do report arrhythmias during sex, but researchers tend to attribute these more to the general emotional arousal and sympathetic reactions that come with sexual response than to any cardiac compromise (Derogatis & King, 1981). In general, patients can be assured that having sex with one's partner in a sensible circumstance is no more stressful than walking five level blocks or climbing two flights of stairs (Hellerstein & Friedman, 1970; Larson, McNaughton, Kennedy, & Mansfield, 1980).

Medications

In addition to issues of aging, organicity, and cardiac strain, the biological aspect of the sexual functioning of a cardiovascular patient must be evaluated with an eye toward the sexual effects of medications. Given the well-documented fact that patient expectations have much to do with side-effect profiles when taking medications, definitive, predictive statements about this topic cannot be made. Clinical experience suggests that it is fairly impossible to predict which patients will have which sexual side effects from any given medication taken at any given dosage (Fuentes, Rosenberg, & Marks, 1983). With this caveat in mind, tentative guidelines regarding counseling patients in this area are offered.

At high dosages, antihypertensive medications have been found to cause sexual dysfunction in both sexes (Weiss, 1991). An overview of documented side effects of various antihypertensives was presented in Sotile (1992) and is reproduced in Table 11.1.

In counseling patients who take hypertensive medications, several points are worthy of emphasis. First, most patients do not experience negative side effects from medications taken at low to moderate dosages; if they are to occur, problems come when taking higher dosages of medicine. For example, Kolodny et al. (1979) summarized research which showed that, when taking 1.0 g per day of alpha-methyldopa (Aldomet), only 10% to 15% of male and female subjects experienced decreased libido and/or impaired arousal. However, this percentage of sexual impairment rose to 20% to 25% when dosage levels were raised to between 1.0 and 1.5 g per day and skyrocketed to an approximately 50% incidence of sexual impairment when raised to 2 g per day or more.

Patients should also be reassured that, contrary to the frequent assumption of laypeople, hypertensive medications do not actually lower the heart's ability to pump enough blood to the pelvis to facilitate sexual arousal. The fact that the effect of antihypertensive medicine is neurological, not literally vascular, and that interference with the neural arc response that mediates sexual arousal is what causes the sexual side effects of these medicines should be explained (Weiss, 1991).

Finally, any hypertensive patient who requires antihypertensive medications to control blood pressure should be clearly warned of the dangers of discontinuing his or her medicines in an effort to enhance sexual performance. Peak intraarterial blood pressures as high as 237/138 mm/Hg have been observed during orgasm in hypertensive patients who were not taking their medications (Mann, Craig, Gould, Melville, & Raftery, 1982). Advise patients that a much more prudent approach to addressing sexual concerns about any antihypertensive treatment regimen is to consult his or her physician about the possibility of trying an alternative hypertensive agent. Further

Table 11.1   Sexual Side Effects of Antihypertensive Medications

Medication type	Brand names	Possible sexual side effects
Diuretics	Aldactone Dyazide Enduron Esidrex Hydro-Diuril Hygroton Lasix Maxzide Naqua Oretic	Minimal or none, except Aldactone, which may cause impotence and loss of sex drive
Sympathetic blockers	Aldomet Blocadren Catapres Corgard Inderal Ismelin Lopressor Reserpine Serpasil Tenormin Trandate	At high dosages, problems include decreased sex drive, erection and ejaculation problems (for men), and impaired orgasm (for women); fewest sexual side effects are from Corgard, Tenormin, and Trandate
Vasodilators	Apresoline Minipress	None
Calcium channel blockers	Calan Cardizem Isoptin Procardia	None
ACE inhibitors	Capoten Vasotec	None

Note. Reprinted by permission of The Putnam Publishing Group/Jeremy P. Tarcher, Inc. from *Sex Over Forty* by Saul H. Rosenthal. Copyright (©) 1987 by Saul H. Rosenthal.

guidelines for counseling patients regarding the effects of antihypertensives can be gotten from Weiss (1991).

It is also important to bear in mind that several medications commonly used in treating respiratory patients may have adverse effects on sexual functioning. Corticosteroids often yield cushingoid side effects (such as hirsutism, weight gain, and changes in physique) that can negatively affect the sexual self-image, promote depression, and lower libido for both female and male patients. Antihistamines have been found to reduce vaginal secretions in some women. In addition, theophylline and epinephrine derivatives, which have no direct effect on sexual functioning, can produce tremulous-ness and aggravate anxiety, which in turn may inhibit arousal (Fletcher, 1984; Pietropinto & Arora, 1989).

Finally, it must be emphasized that many psychotropic medications impair sexual response. The reader is referred to excellent discussions of this issue by Fuentes et al. (1983), Rosenthal (1987), and Zilbergeld (1992).

Medical Evaluations and Treatments of Sexual Concerns

Exhaustive discussion of medical evaluation and treatment procedures for sexual concerns are available elsewhere (i.e., Kaplan, 1983; Kolodny et al., 1979; LoPiccolo & LoPiccolo, 1978; Mohr & Beutler, 1990; Schover & Jensen, 1988). This discussion will be limited to an overview of several issues that are especially pertinent to structuring brief sexual counseling interventions with cardiopulmonary patients. In this regard, perhaps the most important information to remember to convey to patients is that further information regarding medical aspects of their sexual functioning is available, if desired. The patient should be reminded that if strategies outlined in brief counseling do not lead to reversal of sexual performance problems, evaluation by a urologist or gynecologist should be pursued in conjunction with referral for formal sexual therapy.

A number of diagnostic procedures can help clarify the etiology of male sexual dysfunctions. These include nocturnal penile tumescence monitoring, either in laboratory or home settings; and noninvasive vascular assessments such as Doppler ultrasound to assess blood pressure and flow in each of the four penile arteries or cavernography to detect venous leakage. Unfortu-nately, noninvasive techniques such as Doppler analysis have been found to misdiagnose vascular problems in as many as 54% of men suffering from vasculogenic impotence (Mellinger, Vaughan, Thompson, & Goldstein, 1987). Invasive diagnostic procedures include use of intracorporeal injections of papaverine, saline, or radiographic contrast medium to assess erectile capacity; and use of stimulating electrodes or sacral electromyogram to assess sensory nervous system functions. Finally, hormonal functions that affect sexual response can be evaluated through serum testosterone and serum prolactin assays (Schover & Jensen, 1988; Indexed Bibliography).

Far fewer medical evaluation procedures are available for assessing sexual dysfunction in females. Changes in vaginal blood flow can be monitored, but fewer procedures for doing so are available and the validity and reliability of such studies is in question. The most common procedure here is use of the vaginal photoplethysmograph, a tampon-shaped probe inserted into the vagina. In addition, heated oxygen electrodes can be used to measure changes in vaginal temperature and surface oxygen during sexual arousal. As yet, no universally accepted methods for measuring sensory nerve functions of the female genitals have been developed (Schover & Jensen, 1988). Assess-ment of hormonal functions in women is commonplace, but this well-developed technology does not necessarily shed light on issues relevant to female sexual response: "At our current state of knowledge, knowing precise levels of serum estrogen, androgens, and progesterone does not help a clinician understand the cause of a woman's sexual problem" (Schover & Jensen, 1988, p. 147).

A variety of medical treatments for sexual performance problems are available for men; far fewer are available for women. In each case, treatments carry certain advantages and disadvantages. Hormone replacement therapy is available for both sexes, and both the benefits and risks of this treatment have been well documented (American Council of Science and Health, 1983). Revascularization, which is essentially an arterial bypass operation intended to aid erection, has been employed, but this method has generally met with disappointing outcomes (Goldstein, 1987). Popular in the treatment of impotence is the use of a surgically implanted penile prosthesis, several varieties of which are currently available. In addition, erection can be aided by intracavernous injections of vasodilators such as papaverine or phentolamine (Regitine). However, research has indicated that frequent penile injections can cause bruising, scarring and the development of nodules and fibrosis in the penis, priapism, and abnormal liver function. Use of prostaglandin E1 in place of papaverine supposedly avoids many of these negative side effects (Mohr & Beutler, 1990).

The vacuum construction device, a noninvasive aid for erection, is also gaining wide acceptance. Finally, oral medications such as yohimbine, an alpha-adrenergic antagonist, as well as various orally administered vasodilators are sometimes administered in efforts to enhance erection, despite any convincing evidence of their efficacy (Nadig, Ware, & Blumoff, 1986; Schover & Jensen, 1988; Zilbergeld, 1992).

For decades, it has been argued that relationship factors should be given due consideration in evaluating the appropriateness and the effects of surgical and medical treatments of sexual problems. This caution is based on the observation that a man's unilateral decision to (re)introduce erectile functioning into the marriage can have a negative effect (Mohr & Beutler, 1990; Sotile, 1979a).

Sexual Advice Based on Biological Factors

Based on implications of various of the biological factors discussed above, a number of practical recommendations for enhancing sexual performance can be offered to cardiopulmonary patients.

 • Warn respiratory patients that proximity to a partner's perfume, cologne, body lotion, or hair styling agents during sex may trigger respiratory distress.

• Also advise respiratory patients that use of an inhaled beta-agonist bronchodilator before sexual relations may be helpful, especially if the patient has had a history of experiencing episodes of respiratory distress during sexual relations (Pietropinto & Arora, 1989; Wal-broehl, 1992).

• The use of a metered dose inhaler approximately 1 hr before engaging in sexual activities or during sexual relations might also be recommended (Curgian & Gronkiewicz, 1988).

• Patients can also be advised to inhale oxygen during intercourse via nasal prongs connected to a supply tank with a tube. However, Fletcher (1984) cautioned against the liberal use of home oxygen supplementation during sexual activity, stating that research does not document that enhanced sexual functioning comes from such therapy and warning that the possibility of psychological dependence on such devices is real. Other authors (e.g., Pietropinto & Arora, 1989) advise that such treatment should only be employed in the case of low arterial blood levels, polycythemia, or cor pulmonale.

• Both pulmonary and cardiac patients might be encouraged to learn that participation in a formal rehabilitation program can lead to enhanced sexual functioning. The rationale here is that formal rehabilitation might enhance sexual functioning through improvements in overall physical strength; boosts to confidence and efficacy for tolerating physical exertion; and training in such essentials as breathing techniques. Although this recommendation makes common sense, no definitive data regarding the sexual consequences of formal rehabilitation exist (Miller et al., 1990; Sotile, Sotile, Sotile, & Ewen, 1993).

• Several issues should be particularly noted when counseling younger cardiopulmonary patients. Walbroehl (1992) noted that young patients suffering from such chronic pulmonary conditions as asthma or cystic fibrosis sometimes rebel against their seemingly dismal fate by a flight into promiscuous, unsafe sex. Kravetz and Pheatt (1993) also pointed out that because young asthmatics and cystic fibrosis patients have had lung disease all of their lives, they may never have had the opportunity to accumulate psychosexually maturing experiences that were not warped by the presence of their illness. For example, from an early age, females with cystic fibrosis are warned of the dangers of pregnancy due to their already impaired pulmonary system (Hodson, 1989). My own clinical experiences with young cardiac patients has led to similar observations.

Acknowledgment of these issues in a compassionate manner that matches the age-appropriate concerns of the patient is important. Younger patients (especially those with asthma or cystic fibrosis) can be reassured that their illnesses will tend to have intermittent flare-ups but that they will also likely experience lengthy periods of relatively symptom-free functioning during which the capacity for sexual performance should be unencumbered (Walbroehl, 1992).

BEHAVIORAL FACTORS

Patients should be reassured that, if done in the appropriate context, sexual behavior can be a safe, fun form of exercise. Experimenting with various forms of sexual pleasuring that can be given and received with a comfortable degree of physical exertion should be encouraged. This may mean trying new sexual positions or noncoital, mutual forms of sexual stimulation. For some patients, specific advice regarding effective sexual technique might also be appropriate. In this regard, excellent self-help materials are available (e.g., Barbach, 1984; Gochros & Fisher, 1986; Heiman, LoPiccolo, & LoPiccolo, 1976; Rosenthal, 1987; Zilbergeld, 1992).

It is also important to advise the patient and his or her partner to pay attention to the context in which sexual relations occur. It is generally wise to remind patients to orchestrate sexual "exercising" using guidelines similar to those that structure their other forms of exercise: choose activities that are physically comfortable to perform and interesting to do; rest before and after; choose times when feeling fresh and relaxed; abstain from heavy eating or drinking immediately before; and, with medical direction, prophylactically use medications or oxygen to diminish chest or pulmonary discomfort (Sotile, 1992).

Special care should be taken to educate CABG patients and their spouses regarding the anticipated rates of healing of wounds to the sternum and leg at the sites from which the vein or veins for the bypass graft were harvested (Weisberger, 1985). Emphasize the importance of not engaging in forms of sexual activity that will stress the sternum and cause separation or that will aggravate the healing leg wounds.

In addition, clinical experience suggests that it is important to proactively address the likelihood that, posthospitalization, the patient may at first be hesitant about appearing nude in front of his or her partner due to self-consciousness about the scars that result from surgery. Encourage patients to accept such shyness as a normal part of adjusting to surgery, and encourage loved ones to be patient and reassuring regarding this issue. Coach such couples to gradually approximate interacting while nude. The patient may at first feel more comfortable remaining partially clothed when in the partner's presence, even during physical interactions. This, too, should be normalized. The anxiety associated with this issue can be desensitized by encouraging the patient to allow his or her mate (if acceptable to the mate) to see and touch the surgery scar, perhaps by having the mate apply soothing ointments or lotions to the scar. Although anxieties of these sorts are common, even more common in clinical practice is desensitization of this issue within the first several months postsurgery.

EMOTIONAL FACTORS

Patients often benefit from the reassuring reminder that effective sexual response tends to occur reflexively if two prerequisites are met: relaxation and effective sexual stimulation. Any antierotic emotion—fear, apprehension, anger, or anxiety about one's sexual performance or appearance—can shut down the sexual response cycle. In addition, depression or grief predictably lead to loss of libido and impaired sexual response. Encourage patients and their loved ones to attend to the many factors relevant to overall EEM in approaching this particular area of sexual rehabilitation.

COGNITIVE FACTORS

Unrealistic or anxiety-provoking beliefs about sexual functioning should be corrected with accurate information. In addition, patients and their partners should be encouraged to share supportive input regarding their continued love for each other and their patience in establishing or reestablishing affectionate, mutually pleasurable sexual relations.

PERSONALITY FACTORS

Some sexual performance problems in recovering cardiopulmonary patients are simply due to misinformation, transitory stress reactions, or fears. In such cases, brief education, support, and permission to resume or implement sexual pleasuring can be effective treatment (Annon & Robinson, 1978). Others experience sexual dysfunction as part of complex, personality-based struggles with intimacy and/or with sexuality (Kaplan, 1974). For some, exaggerations of their typical style of coping with stress can interfere with the relaxed, open attitude that is most effective in soothing anxieties about sexual performance. For example, Sjogren (1983) cautioned that the Type A's competitive, time-urgent, pressured attitudes about performance and competition can foster an anxiety-generating performance orientation to sexuality following illness and thus may interfere with the willingness to resume sex, even when illness has had no lasting organic effects on sexual functioning. Here, as in every area of psychosocial concern, patients who do not respond to brief counseling interventions should be referred for more specialized treatment.

RELATIONSHIP FACTORS

The importance of relationship factors in coping with any medical issue, including sexual performance anxieties or the sexual consequences of illness, cannot be overemphasized. Even in the presence of organic pathology, a supportive and loving relationship can make a crucial difference in determining sexual behavior or satisfaction with sexual performance. For example, Schover and Jensen (1988) reviewed data indicating that the ability of both partners to cope with illness is also predictive of sexual functioning in couples when one partner has diabetes. In interviews of 51 couples where one member was diabetic, only 15% of couples with good "disease acceptance" reported a sexual dysfunction. Disease acceptance was assessed largely by ratings of both partners' success in managing the crisis of the diagnosis, complying with medical treatments, and maintaining supportive social networks. In contrast, 57% of those with moderate or poor disease acceptance reported sexual performance problems.

Any of the many family system factors discussed in preceding pages can contaminate the sexual aspect of a patient's intimate relationship. As per the family systems perspective of illness, it is important to remember that sexual concerns seldom occur in solo. As mentioned before, spouses of patients often experience even more general distress and specific anxiety regarding sexual relations following illness than do cardiopulmonary patients (Appleton, 1982; Shanfield, 1990). In addition, patients and their loved ones should be reminded that for both partners, periods of fear, anger, and guilt are normal in the course of adjusting to illness. Coaching the couple in ways to communicate about such issues can serve an important prophylactic function (Sotile, 1992, 1993).

SENSORY FACTORS

"Get out of your mind, and into your senses" (Sotile, 1992, p. 137). This bit of advice regarding an effective way to combat sexual performance anxiety post-cardiopulmonary illness was borrowed from the work of the father of Gestalt psychotherapy, Fritz Perls, who cautioned that thinking too much and experiencing too little during the moments of one's life is the source of much distress (Perls, 1969). As Perls stated it:

> Anxiety is the gap between the now and the then. If you are in the now, you can't be anxious, because the excitement flows immediately into ongoing spontaneous activity. If you are in the now, you are creative, you are inventive. If you have your senses ready, if you have your eyes and ears open . . . you find a solution. (Perls, 1969, p. 3)

Sexual performance can be enhanced by a combination of relaxation training and guided imagery or instructions to tune into sexual activity from multisensory perspectives (Sotile, 1992; Sotile & Kilmann, 1977; Sotile & Kilmann, 1978; Sotile, Kilmann, & Follingstad, 1977). The relaxation exercises recommended in chapter 6 in the description of the EEM model can be quite helpful in coaching the patient regarding sexual reconditioning experiences. Cardiopulmonary patients might benefit from support, permission, and guidance in structuring self-pleasuring and masturbation experiences. Such experiences can serve as nonthreatening vehicles for regaining confidence in the ability to physically tolerate sexual response. Masturbation is also a viable sexual outlet for the large numbers of aged patients who have no available sexual partner, a fact that should be normalized by health care providers who care for this population (Hobson, 1984).

For couples, sensate focus pleasuring (Masters & Johnson, 1970) can serve as a foundation for developing relaxed sensual and affectionate interactions that move beyond the constrictions of anxiety-provoking, intercourse-focused sex. Such experiences can be expanded to remind patients that "mutual masturbation, oral sex, and simply fondling can be rewarding sexually" (Walbroehl, 1992, p. 458).

A TIME FRAME FOR SEXUAL COUNSELING

In practice, many patients report having received no information about sexual functioning upon being discharged from the hospital after treatment of an acute cardiopulmonary event. Clinical experience suggests that the reason for this is often that, although sexual information was offered, it was presented at a time when the patient was preoccupied with more pressing rehabilitation concerns that preempted focusing on information regarding sexual activity. Cole, Levin, Whitley, and Young (1979) advised that the second-month follow-up visit, the time when a stress tolerance assessment is typically conducted to determine the patient's functional capacity, is an opportune time to again address this issue. It is again underscored that discussing the patient's sexual concerns and capabilities in light of the results of stress tolerance testing can be quite effective.

SUMMARY

A number of specific guidelines for counseling recovering patients about sexual issues have been offered. These guidelines can serve as a summary of the information in this chapter and can be helpful in structuring interventions in both hospital and outpatient treatment settings.

---

1. Take a sexual history. Formally or informally, ask whether the patient and/or his or her regular sexual partner have concerns about past, current, or future sexual functioning. Incorporate this questioning into the general history that is taken as part of the delivery of routine care. In this way, sexual concerns can be established as being legitimate and important in overall rehabilitation.

2. Be respectful of the patient's needs. Not all recovering cardiopulmonary patients care to change their existing sexual patterns.

This is a matter of intense personal preference. Two specific mistakes should be avoided in this area: failure to validate sexual concerns as an acceptable aspect of medical care; and forcing the issue, despite the patient's indication of no interest in making sex an aspect of his or her rehabilitation.

3. Normalize concerns regarding sex. Emphasize that all people, and especially recovering cardiopulmonary patients, tend to harbor fears and anxieties regarding sexual functioning. Specifically allay unsupported fears regarding the dangers associated with sexual activity.

4. Emphasize that for many patients, sexual adjustment is a relationship, not an individual, matter. Just as it is important for the patient to become comfortable with returning to sexual activities, it is essential that his or her regular sexual partner, too, learn that it is safe to do so.

5. Don't discriminate against aged or unmarried patients. In clinical practice, it is often erroneously assumed that aged or single patients—and especially those many patients who are both aged and single—do not need or want information about sexual functioning. This can be a cruel omission of an important aspect of care. Throughout the life cycle, sexuality is a core-level psychological factor for every individual, and for many, sexual expression remains important regardless of marital status, age, or sexual orientation.

6. Discuss sex in a clear and concise manner: Don't be vague, and don't use slang. The best way to gain a patient's confidence and to ensure that accurate information is being gleaned during sexual counseling is to avoid the use of vague statements such as: "Things will get back to normal soon enough" or "Just go at your own pace." Rather, it is helpful to offer specific guidelines regarding when, how, and where sex can safely be resumed and detailed information regarding what to expect once this occurs.

7. Give information about an expected time frame for sexual recovery. Generally, experts agree that an individual who has been impacted by cardiopulmonary illness can safely return to intercourse within 8 to 12 weeks. However, emphasize that individual sexual recovery rates may vary, just as they do in other aspects of rehabilitation, and that medical clearance should be gotten before resuming sexual relations.

8. Forewarn that some of the symptoms of sexual arousal (e.g., elevated heart rate, shallow breathing) mimic certain symptoms of cardiopulmonary illness. The patient can be helped to discriminate between these two syndromes through experience and by learning

to view sexual response as a special form of exercise. In fact, the same guidelines for safely structuring exercise can be used to safely orchestrate sexual involvements for recovering cardiopulmonary patients: "Don't have sex in excessive heat or cold; rest before and after sex; use naturally high-energy times and comfortable activities to have sex; and so on." (Review the points made in the "Sexual Advice Based on Biological Factors" section of the preceding pages.)

9. Emphasize the importance of nonsexual affection and communication. Explain sexual response as being a psychosomatic one; the more comfortable one feels, the more likely it is that a comfortable sexual response will occur.

10. Emphasize that sexual functioning can be enhanced by overall good physical conditioning and psychosocial adjustment. This fact can serve as an extra source of motivation to participate in multifaceted rehabilitation.

11. Encourage patients to go slowly. Reassure the patient that pacing, patience, and open communication with one's regular sexual partner are keys to developing more comfort with physical affection and with sex.

12. Repeat the discussion. It is a mistake to assume that once this topic has been addressed, it is forever resolved. Periodically inquiring about sexual adjustment and concerns is a respectful and important aspect of providing comprehensive cardiopulmonary care.

Useful, practical tools for educating lung patients regarding sexual aspects of recovery are available from Herb Kravetz, M.D., and colleagues in the form of three slide/tape educational programs: one targets sexual concerns of males (Kravetz, 1982a); one targets concerns of females (Kravetz, 1982b); and one advises health care professionals about how to implement sexual counseling (Kravetz, Weiss, & Meadows, 1980). These materials can be ordered from the Pulmonary Foundation, 1150 Smoki Avenue, Prescott, AZ 86303. My own series of videotaped educational programs, *Coping with Heart Illness*, includes segments that address sexual issues for individual patients, couples, and the aged. This series of three videotapes is available from Human Kinetics, 1607 North Market Street, P.O. Box 5076, Champaign, IL 61825-5076 (1-800-747-4457). In addition, audiotapes of my presentations, *Sex After Heart Illness* and *Thriving, Not Just Surviving: Healthy Living Is a Family Affair*, contain specific advice for couples regarding ways to manage sexual behavior and intimacy following illness. These tapes are available from Sotile Psychological Associates, 1396 Old Mill Circle, Winston-Salem, NC 27103 (910-765-3032).

chapter 12

HELPING PATIENTS STOP SMOKING

Approximately 30% of the population with established cardiopulmonary illness will be smoking at the time of a cardiac event, and this percentage is even higher for patients diagnosed with COPD. Smoking accounts for 82% of all deaths from COPD and 21% of all deaths from CHD (Centers for Disease Control, 1989). The importance of smoking cessation for anyone with obstructive lung disease is obvious. Not so obvious to the lay population is the fact that the rates of reinfarction and subsequent death are as much as twice as high in cardiac patients who continue to smoke as in those who abstain (Burling, Singleton, Bigelow, Baile, & Gottlieb, 1984; Rosenberg, Kaufman, Helmrich, & Shapiro, 1985; Taylor, Miller, Haskell, & DeBusk, 1988). Smoking cessation is generally considered the "single most important lifestyle change to reduce subsequent morbidity and mortality" in both cardiac and pulmonary rehabilitation populations (Houston-Miller et al., 1990, p. 199).

IS INTERVENTION NECESSARY?

In truth, one of the most successful smoking cessation interventions is delivery of the diagnosis of CHD. In comparison to the general population, recently diagnosed cardiac patients report a tremendously high rate of cessation, a fact that, in my opinion, is not given enough attention in the literature. While the general population cessation rates are only approximately 8% (Ockene et al., 1985), cessation rates of between 20% and 60% have consistently been reported in studies of chronic smokers subsequent to diagnosis of an acute MI, with some studies reporting cessation rates as high as 70% to 79% (Higgins & Schweiger 1983; Mulcahy, 1983). An international literature regarding smoking cessation patterns indicates cessation rates of 30% to 50% in recovering MI populations, suggesting that the relatively high rate of cessation post-MI is a cross-cultural phenomenon (Burt et al., 1974). Unfortunately, there is a negative side to this picture: Only about one-third to one-half of the total CHD patient population quits smoking (Burling et al., 1984; Perkins, 1988). Especially likely to quit are those CHD patients who are younger, better educated professionals; those who believe there is a link between smoking and CHD; and those who have family members who disapprove of continued smoking (Conroy, Mulcahy, Graham, Reid, & Cahill, 1986; Giannetti, Reynolds, & Rihn, 1985; Sotile, Sotile, Ewen, & Sotile, 1993).

Relapse is also a problem, both in the general population and in recovering cardiopulmonary populations. In the general population, approximately 75% of people who do stop smoking relapse (Hanson, Isacsson, & Janzon, 1990; Ockene, Benfari, Nuttall, Hurwitz, & Ockene, 1982). In comparison, overall long-term cessation rates remain impressive for CHD populations, but published 1-year or beyond quit rates still seldom exceed 51% (Taylor, Houston-Miller, Killen, & DeBusk, 1990). Given the absolute importance of smoking cessation, the posthospitalization relapse rates for these populations remain a concern (Ockene et al., 1985).

Smoking cessation can be a particularly complex topic for any COPD patient who smokes. The report of an abnormal finding from a lung function test can put a dent in any smoker's psyche. This alarm at least momentarily heightens an almost universal phenomenon among smokers—the desire to quit. National statistics show that in the general population, over 70% of smokers report an interest in quitting and that they endure repeated failures in their attempts to quit. Interest in quitting and motivation to quit is renewed when the patient is confronted with personalized data indicating that smoking is harming his or her health. However, this reaction can take unique twists for the COPD patient. If there is any history of smoking, both the COPD patient and his or her family will tend to assume that the patient has caused the illness. This blame is particularly unfortunate, given that many COPD patients started smoking before it was widely known that smoking is seriously dangerous to one's health (Yellowlees, 1987; Yellowlees et al., 1987). Furthermore, many uninformed COPD patients believe that the only treatment for lung disease is to stop smoking, and their subsequent failure to stop may lead them to avoid seeking medical care (Dudley et al., 1980; Dudley, Wermuth, & Hague, 1973).

Unfortunately, relatively few smoking cessation intervention studies have been published that used COPD patient samples (Crowley, MacDonald, Zerbe, & Petty, 1991). Many of those that have been published have indicated relatively poor long-term cessation rates. According to Yellowlees et al. (1987), a complicating factor in smoking cessation for COPD patients is the quandary caused by the relationship between anxiety, dyspnea, and the antianxiety effect of smoking reported by many COPD patients. For some patients, smoking reduces anxiety; at times of stress, a cigarette seems to "calm the nerves." For such patients, the fear of breathlessness seems to heighten throughout the early stages of cessation, a factor that needs to be compassionately addressed by providing the patient with ancillary help with anxiety management during quit attempts.

WHAT CAN BE DONE TO HELP?

It is true that a significant number of individuals quit smoking following an MI or diagnosis of some form of cardiopulmonary illness without receiving formal antismoking treatment (Marlatt, Curry, & Gordon, 1988); it also seems to be the case that even brief interventions can greatly improve long-term cessation rates. The massive literature on smoking cessation in the general population, coupled with the growing literature on smoking cessation interventions with cardiopulmonary populations, offers a number of useful guidelines for structuring this important component of overall cardiopulmonary care.

The remainder of this chapter will describe various components of effective smoking cessation interventions. These components can be combined either to formulate brief office-based or bedside nicotine counseling interventions or to structure long-term, comprehensive smoke-stopping treatments. Although the discussion will focus on smoking cessation, many of the concepts and techniques described in this chapter can be adapted to help structure interventions for modifying a variety of health behaviors. For example, the behavioral techniques to be described can be modified to match a target behavior such as compulsive eating or dysfunctional use of alcohol. In addition, as will be apparent, certain scales to be described (e.g., the Self-Efficacy Questionnaire, the "Why Do You Smoke?" Questionnaire) could easily be modified to apply to other targeted behaviors. An overview of recommended smoking cessation intervention strategies follows.

SEIZE TEACHABLE MOMENTS, START INTERVENTION EARLY, AND, IF NECESSARY, REPEAT IT

As mentioned earlier, medical crisis creates opportune teachable moments that can be used to therapeutic advantage. In addition, the routine delivery of medical or rehabilitation care can provide many, mini-opportunities to pair medical advice with motivating input regarding needed areas of health behavior change. Any hospitalized cardiopulmonary patient who smokes is involved in an ongoing episode of smoking cessation. Given the recent mandate for smoke-free hospitals that was delivered by the Joint Commission on Accreditation of Health Care Organizations, patients are forced to take what could be construed as the first—and often the most painful—step in smoking cessation: quitting and enduring the initial smoke-free days. The struggle of this first step is often soothed by a number of factors that typically correspond with hospitalization: distractions that come with the medical crisis that brought on hospitalization; frequent supportive/monitoring contact with medical personnel; the use of sedating medications; and a momentary respite from at-home stressors.

The advisability of taking advantage of such smoking-stopping circumstances was clearly demonstrated by Taylor et al. (1990), who employed nurses to provide a brief, in-hospital behavioral intervention followed by telephone-administered relapse prevention interventions administered to 86 post-MI patients. Treated patients were also given self-help manuals and audiotaped information and relaxation training instructions. Telephone follow-up consisted of weekly calls for the first 2 or 3 weeks posthospitaliza-tion and then monthly calls for the next 4 months. At 12-month follow-up, the researchers reported a biochemically confirmed cessation rate of 61% in a treatment group compared to a 32% cessation rate in a usual care control group.

Kottke and Solbert (1993) pointed out that rehabilitation specialists who have daily contact with patients—both in inpatient and outpatient settings—are the most effective persons to deliver smoking cessation interventions. These authors support the notion proposed throughout this book that effec-tive interventions can be delivered in a few minutes and can be worked into the delivery of typical medical care. In this sense, every contact with a patient can be viewed as a potential time for further inquiry, coaching, reinforcement of progress, and support for smoking cessation or for modification of other important health behaviors.

In reality, however, many such teachable moments for promoting smoking cessation are missed. In some instances, lack of attention to the patient's smoking actually promotes smoking continuation. A wealth of anecdotal clinical experiences suggest that medical personnel working in outpatient settings often underestimate the extent to which patients and their loved ones silently attend to whether or not the consulting physician, nurse, or rehabilitation specialist focuses on smoking cessation as being necessary. Patients often leave the physician's office or the rehabilitation setting inter-preting messages such as "You're in good health" or "Your lungs are clear" as permission to continue smoking (Rimer & Orleans, 1993).

Physician and smoking cessation researcher Michael Fiore, of the Univer-sity of Wisconsin Medical School, advises that assessment of nicotine depen-dence should be considered a new vital sign to be routinely monitored along with the monitoring of blood pressure, pulse, temperature, and respiratory rate (Fiore, 1991). Fiore's research documented the frequent omission of assessment or input regarding smoking cessation during the delivery of medical care. Exit interviews with smokers following routine visits to their doctors' offices indicated that only 45% of patients who smoked reported that their clinician had asked them if they smoke and that less than 15% reported that their clinician provided specific advice on how to quit smoking. To remedy this error of omission in delivering medical care, Fiore recom-mends that a Vital Sign Stamp such as that depicted on page 231 be attached to the front of every patient's medical chart. The stamp can effectively serve as a reminder to question, advise, and/or encourage the patients regarding smoking behavior or ongoing quit attempts.

Anecdotal reports also indicate that health care providers often do take note of the patient's smoking status but remain silent out of fear that they will appear to be nagging or shaming a smoker if cessation is repeatedly emphasized. No intervention should be delivered in a manner that blames, shames, or embarrasses the patient. But, given the documented dangers of continued smoking and the demonstrated effectiveness of brief, firm medical

Form 12.1   The Vital Sign Stamp

Blood pressure: _____

Pulse: _____

Temperature: _____

Respiratory rate: _____

Smoking status (circle):   Current   Former   Never

Note. From "The New Vital Sign: Assessing and Documenting Smoking Status," by M. Fiore, 1991, *Journal of the American Medical Association,* **266**(22), pp. 3183-3184. Copyright 1991 by the Journal of the American Medical Association. Reprinted with permission.

input in promoting cessation, the ethics of not continuing to recommend cessation to a smoking patient must be questioned. According to the aforementioned research by Prochaska, DiClemente, and colleagues regarding the stages of change (Prochaska & DiClemente, 1984), it is likely that even if the patient does not respond immediately to input by stopping smoking, much potential value comes from repeatedly offering advice, encouragement, and information regarding cessation. Such persistence can accomplish several things: the patient's consciousness level regarding this issue may be elevated; the fact that help is available to aid cessation can be underscored; positive social support for quitting is provided; positive peer (especially family) pressure to quit can be elicited; and, it is hoped, all of the forgoing will serve to nudge the patient to the next stage of change.

GIVE STRONG, COMPASSIONATE, AND PERSONALIZED MEDICAL ADVICE TO QUIT

Most simply, and perhaps most importantly, every recovering cardiopulmonary patient should receive strong yet compassionate advice to stop smoking. Framing this advice as a medical recommendation, and especially having a physician deliver the advice, can significantly enhance its impact. Edward Lichtenstein and colleagues (Hollis et al., 1993) reported that a 30-second, physician-delivered message of the sort described below served to motivate 87% of patients to attend at least one nurse-delivered smoking cessation counseling session. The message used was some variant of the following:

 "The best thing you can do for your health is to immediately stop smoking. I am advising you to stop as soon as possible. I know that this may be difficult to do. Many people try several times before they finally make it. You may or may not want to stop smoking right now,

> but I do want you to talk at least briefly with our health counselor. She (or he) will give you many tips that will make stopping easier when you decide the time is right."

In a similar vein, Burt et al. (1974) reported a 62% abstinence rate 1 to 3 years after MI for a group of men who received firm medical advice to stop smoking, detailed information regarding why they should stop, and brief, follow-up support delivered to them and their spouses. The antismoking advice offered in that study was unequivocal: "Never smoke again in any form as long as you live if you wish to give yourself the best chance." The 62% quit rate for the treatment group far exceeded the only 28% quit rate for the group of patients who received routine medical advice about smoking cessation [e.g., "You really should stop smoking"].

It is emphasized that such input should be delivered with compassion and empathy. In addition to emphasizing the negative effects of continued smoking, you should acknowledge that smoking cessation is made difficult by the fact that most smokers derive much pleasure from smoking and that nicotine withdrawal can be a complex, distressing experience. Take special care to bear in mind the aforementioned statement that many COPD patients who are currently smoking or who smoked in the past may feel guilty about smoking and should be dealt with compassionately.

Continuing to smoke postdiagnosis leads to further guilt, shame, and tensions between the smoker and his or her family and attending medical staff (Yellowlees et al., 1987). Such tensions should not be fueled by insensitively delivered medical comments such as:

"Of course your lung functions are not improving. What do you expect when you are still bent on killing yourself with those damned cigarettes?" Or "If you ever decide to care enough about yourself and your family to find the strength to quit smoking, you'll probably start to feel better." Or "Sometimes I think that we're wasting our time here. Are you ever going to put those cigarettes down?"

There are many ways to offer strong medical advice and compassion at the same time:

"I know that you are discouraged about the test results. You are making many important changes, and I think that these will pay off for you. I know that this is complicated, but your smoking is probably working against all of your other good efforts."

Or: "As much as you care about your family and your own health, I know that it's confusing to you that you still smoke. Don't give up hope; everyone has to change a complicated behavior at their own pace.

> I've worked with people who smoked for 30 years, quit and relapsed many times, but eventually got it right. I believe that you will deal with this at your own pace. Of course, I do hope that you will stop smoking soon."

However it is done, it is important to convey to the patient a combination of advice to stop smoking, compassion that this may be difficult advice to follow, and input regarding ways to succeed in a quit attempt. Equally important is to make clear your willingness to continue treating the patient, even if he or she does not immediately stop smoking.

EMPLOY MULTIPLE INTERVENTIONS

Depending upon the desired level of intervention (see chapter 4), any or all of the following strategies might be incorporated into a smoking cessation intervention.

Educate the Patient and His or Her Family

Most smokers know that they should stop smoking, but not all know exactly why. It is important to incorporate commonsense explanations of the physical facts about smoking and smoking cessation into the delivery of routine medical and rehabilitation care. This information should be presented in a tone that at once conveys the seriousness of continued smoking and the optimistic message that, in many cases, stopping smoking leads to slowing of disease progression or return to baseline levels of risk within 1 year.

At minimum, the following information should be emphasized.

1. Nicotine acts directly on the sympathetic nervous system. As such, it elevates heart rate and both systolic and diastolic blood pressures and can increase the likelihood of silent ischemia and anginal episodes.

2. Because nicotine increases circulating free fatty acids and platelet aggregation, it makes clotting in the cardiovascular system worse.

3. The average cigarette contains approximately 2,500 chemicals. When the cigarette is lit, however, the combustion multiplies the number of chemicals beyond 4,000. These chemicals have been found to cause cancers of various sorts, including lung cancer.

4. One of the toxins in cigarette smoke is carbon monoxide, a chemical that is a particular culprit in promoting heart illness. Carbon monoxide damages the intima of the coronary arteries, which sets the stage for lipid infiltration and plaque development. In addition, both carbon monoxide and nicotine have been found to raise low-density lipoprotein (LDL) cholesterol levels and decrease high-density lipoprotein (HDL) cholesterol levels.

5. The good news: The body begins to purify toxins within 24 hr of quitting smoking. The relative risk for CHD is halved in 1 year and approaches the

risk for a nonsmoker 2 to 3 years after quitting, and the risk for cancer decreases beyond 5 to 10 years after quitting. Plus, mortality from CHD declines once smoking is stopped. Approximately 10 years following cessation, the CHD death rate for ex-smokers who consumed less than a pack of cigarettes per day is virtually identical to that of lifelong nonsmokers.

Prepare the Patient for the Ordeal of Nicotine Withdrawal

As a way of preparing for the ordeal of nicotine withdrawal, have the patient chart evidence of nicotine addiction. In clinical practice, the tool most often used to assess the extent of nicotine addiction is the Fagerstrom Tolerance Questionnaire. Developed in 1978 (Fagerstrom, 1978), the test has received much research attention. Criticism of its psychometric properties (Lichtenstein & Mermelstein, 1986) led to a recent revision of this instrument. The new instrument is called the Fagerstrom Test for Nicotine Dependence (FTND). The FTND consists of six of the original eight items from the Fagerstrom Tolerance Questionnaire, with revised scoring for two of the items. This test, which is described in Heatherton, Kozlowski, Frecker, & Fagerstrom (1991), can be used to assess the probability that quitting smoking may be accompanied by withdrawal symptoms.

Before quitting, many patients either under- or overestimate the withdrawal ordeal. Either case can sabotage a quit attempt, as routine, transient symptoms of nicotine withdrawal get misinterpreted as indication that one's physical system cannot tolerate smoking cessation, and this misguided panic fuels a return to smoking. Such sabotaging can be aborted by educating the patient as to the worst-case withdrawal scenario and prophylactically offering advice about how to minimize and cope with such symptoms, if they do occur. Most importantly, the patient should be reassured that even in the worst case, the acute symptoms of withdrawal seldom persist beyond several weeks. Symptoms that may accompany nicotine withdrawal and commonsense antidotes to these symptoms are listed in Table 12.1.

Two points of clarification regarding the information presented in this table are in order. First, many of these symptoms can be significantly circumvented with the use of nicotine replacement therapy, a treatment strategy to be discussed fully below. Second, the issue of increased appetite and possible weight gain following smoking cessation deserves special mention. Hatsukami and Lando (1993) offered a noteworthy analysis and thoughtful discussion of behavioral treatments for smoking cessation. The authors pointed out that gaining weight is an almost universal experience after stopping smoking. Smokers typically gain somewhere between 5 and 8 pounds (Kleges & Shumaker, 1992), and clinical experience suggests that a return to prior weight levels is often quite difficult to achieve. This weight gain may be due either to increased caloric intake (especially likely during the first month of cessation) or to slight decreases in metabolism that occur with smoking cessation. In either case, it appears that it is extremely difficult to avoid gaining weight, either immediately during a quit attempt or within

Table 12.1   Keys to Coping With Nicotine Withdrawal

Symptom	Antidotes
Anxiety/irritability	Relax, manage stress, decrease stimulants, exercise, nicotine gum or patch
Headaches	Reduce caffeine, use analgesics (with doctor's advice)
Sleep disturbance	Relax, exercise, reduce caffeine, modify dosage if nicotine replacement is being used
Fatigue, drowsiness, decreased concentration	Exercise, relax, eliminate depressants; for a few weeks: increase self-nurturance, decrease activity, don't start new projects
Cough	Accept as body's way of cleansing, use cough drops, drink water or warm liquids
Appetite increase	Increase water intake, expect and accept a weight gain of 5 to 8 lb
Stomach gnawing/nausea	Eat low-calorie snacks or chew sugar-free gum
Constipation	Increase fluids and dietary fiber
Overall syndrome	Use nicotine replacement therapy

Note. From "Facilitating Smoking Cessation" by K. McKool, 1987, *Journal of Cardiovascular Nursing, 1*(4), p. 36. Copyright 1987 by Aspen Publishers, Inc. Adapted with permission.

1 to 2 years after quitting. Most noteworthy is the fact that minimal short-term but no long-term positive effects on weight management have been noted from interventions such as behavioral therapy or use of medications such as serotonergic agents, phenylpropanolamine, or nicotine gum (Hatsukami & Lando, 1993) during smoking cessation. In addition, both animal and human studies have shown that reduced caloric intake may actually increase the likelihood of relapse use of any drug (Carroll & Melsch, 1984; Carroll, Stitzer, & Strain, 1990).

For these reasons, Hatsukami and Lando (1993) underscored the sentiments of many experts in this field who believe that in lieu of unrealistically challenging patients to avoid weight gain during quit attempts, they should be helped to accept a degree of weight gain subsequent to smoking cessation. Advice regarding management of cravings for sweets and foods high in carbohydrates during the active phases of withdrawal is certainly prudent. But, in light of the facts outlined above, implying or stating that appropriate self-management will result in no weight gain is quite unfair; doing so simply promotes a sense of failure for most patients, and such distress can compel return to smoking. Particular care should be taken to flag any patient who evidences extreme weight consciousness. Such patients should be forewarned that extraordinary effort to control a modest weight gain may simply increase the odds of a smoking relapse.

In anticipation of withdrawal symptoms, it is often helpful to instruct the patient and his or her loved ones that the patient should plan on experiencing a 2- to 3-week period of flulike symptoms upon quitting. The patient should be advised that, just as in the case of suffering through the flu, it will be important to take and to receive extra nurturing during this time. This care should include frequent reminders (from self and from supportive others) that even though the symptoms of withdrawal are painful, they are not damaging. Advise that when they do occur, such symptoms are signs that "the body is healing," or "coming back into balance," or is "moving toward recovery." Armed with these frames of reference, the patient will likely be more able to make sense of the suffering that comes with withdrawal and maintain motivation for continued quitting.

Use Self-Assessment Strategies to Help the Smoker Know How to Approach the Problem

A useful way to begin any program of change is to enhance the patient's awareness of their particular version of the problem being addressed. In this regard, smoking cessation is aided by helping the patient to accurately conceptualize his or her smoking history. Compassionately phrased questions in a variety of areas can help the patient begin to see his or her smoking habit in context. Questions might include the following:

- At what age did you begin smoking?
- How many cigarettes do you smoke each day, on average?
- How many times in the past have you tried to quit? What worked best? What worked least? (Here remind the patient that smokers who eventually stop smoking only do so after an average of three to seven quit attempts, a fact that can be used to normalize the patient's experiences in this regard.)
- What kinds of smoking-related symptoms are you having?
- Do you believe that smoking had anything to do with your illness or that smoking cessation is an important part of your rehabilitation?
- How confident are you that you can quit smoking at this time?
- Who among your family or friends will be most supportive of your quitting smoking?
- Who among your family or friends will have the most difficulty with your stopping smoking?

In addition, it might be helpful to have the patient respond to a "Why Do You Smoke?" questionnaire such as the one outlined in Form 12.2.

This questionnaire is a useful tool for specifying the factors that underlie the smoking habit. Using the guidelines for scoring presented in Form 12.3,

Form 12.2   "Why Do You Smoke?" Questionnaire

Why Do You Smoke?

Here are some statements made by people to describe what they get out of smoking cigarettes. How often do you feel this way when smoking them? Circle one number for each statement.

Important: Answer every question.

	Always	Frequently	Occasionally	Seldom	Never
1. I smoke cigarettes to keep myself from slowing down.	5	4	3	2	1
2. Handling a cigarette is part of the enjoyment of smoking it.	5	4	3	2	1
3. Smoking cigarettes is pleasant and relaxing.	5	4	3	2	1
4. I light up a cigarette when I feel angry about something.	5	4	3	2	1
5. When I run out of cigarettes, I find it almost unbearable until I can get them.	5	4	3	2	1
6. I smoke cigarettes automatically without even being aware of it.	5	4	3	2	1
7. I smoke cigarettes to stimulate myself to perk myself up.	5	4	3	2	1
8. Part of the enjoyment of smoking a cigarette comes from the steps I take to light up.	5	4	3	2	1
9. I find cigarettes pleasurable.	5	4	3	2	1
10. When I feel uncomfortable or upset about something, I light up a cigarette.	5	4	3	2	1
11. I am very much aware of when I am not smoking a cigarette.	5	4	3	2	1
12. I light up a cigarette without realizing I still have one burning in the ashtray.	5	4	3	2	1
13. I smoke cigarettes to give myself a "lift."	5	4	3	2	1
14. When I smoke a cigarette, part of the enjoyment is watching the smoke as I exhale it.	5	4	3	2	1

Form 12.2 "Why Do You Smoke?" Questionnaire (continued)

	Always	Frequently	Occasionally	Seldom	Never
15. I want a cigarette most when I am comfortable and relaxed.	5	4	3	2	1
16. When I feel "blue" or want to take my mind off cares and worries, I smoke cigarettes.	5	4	3	2	1
17. I get a real gnawing hunger for a cigarette when I haven't smoked for a while.	5	4	3	2	1
18. I've found a cigarette in my mouth and didn't remember putting it there.	5	4	3	2	1

Form 12.3 Scoring for "Why Do You Smoke?" Questionnaire

How to score:

1. Enter the numbers you have circled to the questions in the spaces below, putting the number you have circled for Question 1 over line 1, for Question 2 over line 2, etc.

2. Add the three scores on each line to get your totals. For example, the sum of your scores over lines 1, 7, and 13 gives your score on Stimulation, the sum of your scores over lines 2, 8, and 14 give your score on Handling, etc.

19. _____ + _____ + _____ = _____
      1   7   13   Stimulation

20. _____ + _____ + _____ = _____
      2   8   14   Handling

21. _____ + _____ + _____ = _____
      3   9   15   Pleasurable relaxation

22. _____ + _____ + _____ = _____
      4   10   16   Crutch: tension reduction

23. _____ + _____ + _____ = _____
      5   11   17   Craving: psychological addictions

24. _____ + _____ + _____ = _____
      6   12   18   Habit

Scores can vary from 3 to 15. A score of 11 or above is high; a score of 7 or below is low.

the smoker can determine the extent to which smoking is associated with the following factors: stimulation, handling, pleasurable relaxation, tension reduction, cravings associated with psychological addiction, or habit.

Analyses such as the one outlined above can have a surprising effect: The patient may consciously realize how many different functions smoking serves in his or her life, and insecurities about the inability to quit smoking may heighten. It is important to remember that most smokers harbor secret doubts and fears about their ability to quit, fears that may be masked with bravado ("I know that I could quit if I wanted to; I just haven't made up my mind yet."). Refusing to try is often a way to avoid failure. Such patients can be helped by input that normalizes fear about the ability to quit and normalizes the fact that perhaps a number of past quit attempts have met with failure. Research has shown that 40% of adult smokers have made three or more attempts to quit (McKool, 1987). Smokers need help in framing each past attempt as having taken them one step closer to the attempt at cessation that will work.

Coach the Patient in Alternative Need-Fulfillment Strategies

It is also important to help the patient devise alternative ways of satisfying the needs that underlie smoking that were identified in the foregoing exercises. New coping strategies can be structured into the cessation attempt. For example, the patient might be coached in these alternative strategies:

Coping Strategies During Smoking Cessation

Factor	Coping strategy
Stimulation	Carry entertaining reading material. Work crossword or jigsaw puzzles. Distract oneself: go to a movie, take a walk, ask for support from loved ones or friends to bear through.
Handling	To satisfy needs for fiddling, carry a "worry stone" or other small object, doodle, or squeeze a ball.
Pleasurable relaxation	Take regular self-nurturing breaks in daily activities. Give yourself extra permission to self-nurture throughout the quitting ordeal. Remind yourself of the pleasures that will come with being a nonsmoker.
Tension reduction	Learn and practice a relaxation technique; exercise; distract yourself.
Cravings	Use cognitive distraction and supportive interactions. Change the environment (e.g., take a walk around the office or block; move to another room; take a drive). Clean and floss your teeth. Do something that is impossible to do while smoking. Avoid alcohol or coffee. Eat fresh vegetables or low-fat snacks.

Habit	Learn to monitor when cigarettes are reached for. Notice the "hidden" stimuli that tend to generate the smoking response.

Next, it is helpful to have the patient pinpoint high-risk situations. This can be done with the aid of a Smoking Cessation Self-Efficacy Questionnaire of the sort presented in Form 12.4. This questionnaire helps specify circumstances in which the smoker is confident of the ability to avoid smoking and those in which confidence for cessation is low. Ratings of 4 or above

---

Form 12.4   Smoking Cessation Self-Efficacy Questionnaire

Self-Efficacy Questionnaire

INSTRUCTIONS: Rate each of the items on the right-hand scale to indicate how sure you are that you would be able to resist smoking in that situation. Circle the appropriate response.

Item	Completely unsure						Completely sure
1. When you feel impatient	1	2	3	4	5	6	7
2. When you are waiting for someone or something	1	2	3	4	5	6	7
3. When you feel frustrated	1	2	3	4	5	6	7
4. When you are worried	1	2	3	4	5	6	7
5. When you want something in your mouth	1	2	3	4	5	6	7
6. When you want to cheer up	1	2	3	4	5	6	7
7. When you want to keep yourself busy	1	2	3	4	5	6	7
8. When you are trying to pass time	1	2	3	4	5	6	7
9. When someone offers you a cigarette	1	2	3	4	5	6	7
10. When you are drinking an alcoholic beverage	1	2	3	4	5	6	7
11. When you feel uncomfortable	1	2	3	4	5	6	7
12. When you feel embarrassed	1	2	3	4	5	6	7
13. When you are in a situation in which you feel smoking is a part of your self-image	1	2	3	4	5	6	7
14. When you want to feel more mature and sophisticated	1	2	3	4	5	6	7

indicate high-risk situations. The patient should be encouraged to employ extra prudence in approaching such circumstances.

Help the Patient Verbalize His or Her Reasons for Wanting to Quit Smoking

It is also helpful to have a smoker specify exactly why he or she wants to quit smoking. Reviewing these reasons can serve as a potent source of motivation throughout the quitting ordeal. Encourage the patient to write out as many reasons as can be identified. Many patients think only in global or in narrow terms and might need help identifying various reasons for quitting. Frequently cited motivators for smoking cessation include:

- I want to improve my health.
- It will please me to make my family proud of me.
- My teeth will look whiter and my breath will smell fresher.
- I'll save money.
- I'm embarrassed about being a smoker. If I stop, I'll have nothing to be embarrassed about.
- My house, car, and clothes will smell cleaner and fresher.
- I'll stop wasting so much time.
- I'll be able to enjoy being with people who don't smoke.
- I will feel more similar to other people.
- I won't have to hide and sneak around to smoke anymore.

Encourage the patient to get personal in listing reasons for quitting smoking. The motivations of others (i.e., a loved one or a health care provider) in encouraging quitting smoking may be well intended, but actually quitting is aided by personal motivation. In fact, quit attempts begun under coercion from others seldom succeed. Instruct the patient to list his or her reasons for wanting to quit on a 3-by-5-in. card, and to carry the card throughout the quitting ordeal. The card should be referred to frequently, especially during times of craving.

Use Monitoring Strategies to Motivate

To motivate smoking cessation, both the patient's physiology and smoking behavior can be monitored. In each instance, relatively simple procedures can be employed.

Assessing Expired Air Carbon Monoxide and Serum Thiocyanate Levels

Assessing expired air carbon monoxide (CO) and/or monitoring serum thiocyanate can serve to motivate quit attempts and as means of evaluating continued progress and providing positive reinforcement for continued cessation (Butts, Kucheman, & Widdowson, 1974; McKool, 1987; Taylor et al.,

1990). Expired air CO can be measured with a simple procedure that involves collecting the expired air of a smoker in a plastic bag or balloon that is attached to a pump that draws the air through a filter and registers the amount of CO in the expired air (McKool, 1987). Patients are typically classified as nonsmokers if their CO measure is less than 10 parts per million (Taylor et al., 1990). A frequently used CO analyzer is the Carbon Monoxide Ecolyzer system, which is manufactured by National Draeger of Pittsburgh, PA. Another system is the Ecolyzer manufactured by Energetics Science, Inc., New York, NY.

Serum thiocyanate can be analyzed using a method developed by Butts et al. (1974). A serum thiocyanate level of less than 110 umo/L is typically indicative of a smoke-free system (Taylor et al., 1990).

These two techniques are ways to provide the patient with concrete evidence of the effects of smoking and of smoking cessation. Periodic reevaluations of these parameters should be incorporated into routine medical or rehabilitation care. Such follow-up assessment will either serve to underscore the need for the patient to once again consider stopping smoking or to provide much-appreciated reinforcement for the fact that cessation has occurred.

Pack Wrap Training

A simple way to slow the smoking habit is to keep track of each cigarette smoked (Kilmann, Wagner, & Sotile, 1977). The goal here is to raise into consciousness the many aspects of the smoking habit and to call attention to the fact that many cigarettes are smoked sheerly out of a stimulus-response habit, not due to physiological craving. This can be accomplished by instructing the patient in the use of a pack wrap—a piece of paper wrapped around a pack of cigarettes, designed to help the smoker assess his or her smoking habit. Form 12.5 is an example of a pack wrap.

The patient should be encouraged to reproduce many copies of this form, always wrapping a copy around any pack of cigarettes being carried. Instructions in the use of the pack wrap follow.

"For the next week, I recommend that you smoke as you regularly do. Don't worry yet about changing anything but this: I want you to become more aware of the different 'flavors' of cigarette smoking you do. Like most people, you probably smoke for many different reasons. We want to bring these into your conscious awareness.

"To do this, I recommend that you use this pack wrap. Always wrap a copy of this sheet around the pack of cigarettes that you are carrying. As you notice yourself reaching for a cigarette and before you light up, take a moment to fill in information about that particular cigarette. First, note your circumstance (eating, relaxing, at work, etc.). Next, note how you are feeling (anxious, bored, angry, etc.). Finally, note your degree of craving for that particular cigarette. Rate your craving using a scale of 1-3, with 1 indicating 'I don't really feel like smoking this cigarette' and 3 indicating 'My body is craving this cigarette.' Once you've filled out the form, if you want to, smoke the cigarette."

In follow-up consultation sessions, it is helpful to process with the patient the information presented in the pack wraps. Recommend that the patient bring the week's pack wraps in to the session. Informally analyze how many cigarettes fell into each category, noting any particularly high-risk situational or emotional cues. Also note how many cigarettes were rated low (i.e., scored a 1 or 2) on the craving scale. Increasing awareness of the triggers or cues that lead to smoking is an important step in helping the smoker disrupt the habit. As will be discussed below, an approximation to cessation is first eliminating those cigarettes that are not really craved, a step that can be aided by use of the pack wrap.

Form 12.5 "Pack Wrap Form"

Inv. _____ Pt. No. _____ Pt. Initials _____

Date _____ Day of Week _____

Time	Food and/or alcohol	Relaxation	Work	Social/recreational	Driving	Other (please describe)	Angry	Anxious	Bored	Depressed	Frustrated	Happy	Relaxed	Tired	Need rating Most Least
1															1 2 3
2															1 2 3
3															1 2 3
4															1 2 3
5															1 2 3
6															1 2 3
7															1 2 3
8															1 2 3
9															1 2 3
10															1 2 3

Wrap this Daily Cigarette Count around your pack of cigarettes and hold it fast with a rubber band. When you are about to take a cigarette, but before you actually put it in your mouth and light up: (1) enter the time of day; (2) check the activity you are doing; (3) check the word or words that best describe your feeling at the time; and (4) indicate how important that particular cigarette is to you at the time (1 = most important, 2 = above average, 3 = least important).

Teach the Patient About Stimulus Control

Once the patient develops a basic understanding of the patterns that comprise his or her smoking habit, intervention should shift to coaching in ways to reduce or control exposure or reaction to high-risk cues or stimuli. Interventions here can take many forms. For example, support can be bolstered during upcoming high-risk situations that cannot be avoided (e.g., social gatherings or lunch breaks), or cigarettes can be made inaccessible by placing them in the trunk of one's car or in an inconvenient place in one's residence. Alternatively, the patient can be coached to systematically limit his or her smoking by eliminating smoking in an increasingly greater number of situations (Smith & Leon, 1992), or by eliminating "unnecessary" cigarettes— those that are not associated with true nicotine cravings. A related approach is coaching the patient to substitute alternative behaviors when experiencing an urge to smoke. Here such strategies as partner support, exercise, relaxation, or psychomotor distraction techniques can be helpful.

Use a Contract

From the outset of this stage of treatment, a smoking cessation contract should be used. An example of such a contract is presented in Form 12.6. Such a contract should contain several elements: the exact date on which the last cigarette will be smoked (preferably no later than 2 weeks from the date of signing the contract); a reiteration of the patient's reasons for stopping; and the specific steps to be used to stop.

Continue to Provide Support After the Patient Has Quit

Once the last cigarette has been smoked, and periodically throughout the first several months of living smoke-free, it is especially important to proactively provide support to the patient about his or her withdrawal ordeal. Information from the Shiffman Withdrawal Questionnaire in Form 12.7 on p. 244 can be used to facilitate discussion and education through this period.

It is important to emphasize compassionately to patients and their loved ones that for most people, smoking is a combination of addiction to nicotine and a very complex behavioral habit. For these reasons, quitting requires a wealth of willpower, courage, wisdom, and support. Quitting should never be dismissed as something that is easy to accomplish. Forewarn that cravings for cigarettes may persist for years. Clinical experience suggests that emphasizing this point helps frame quit attempts as indications of bravery and courage, perspectives that promote self-efficacy for quitting. It is also important to emphasize the importance of maintaining hope in one's ability to quit and faith that if behaviors are controlled (i.e., smoking is avoided), nicotine cravings will soon lessen and eventually cease.

Use Nicotine Replacement Therapy When Appropriate

Given that as many as 80% of smokers experience signs of withdrawal (Benowitz, 1988), nicotine replacement therapy (NRT) should be seriously

Form 12.6   Stop Smoking Contract

After careful consideration, I have decided to stop smoking cigarettes on

_____.
(Date)

I am responsible for this decision and understand that my own commitment to stop smoking is of primary importance.

My reasons for stopping are:

_____

_____

_____

_____

Steps I will take to achieve stopping are:

_____

_____

_____

_____

_____   _____
My signature   Today's date

_____
Therapist's signature

We recommend posting a copy of this contract in a prominent location at home and/or at the office.

considered for any patient undergoing smoking cessation. Nicotine replacement therapy should especially be considered in treating older smokers (aged 50 to 74), who tend to have long-term smoking habits and to be heavier smokers (Rimer & Orleans, 1993). Unfortunately, this consideration is often omitted during the delivery of medical care. Over 50% of NRT is begun at the request of the patient, not upon the recommendation of informed health care providers. Furthermore, despite convincing evidence that even brief coaching in behavioral strategies for smoking cessation greatly enhances the effectiveness of NRT (P. Glover, 1993), in practice, the bulk of NRT is implemented with no accompanying behavioral modification advice.

Nicotine replacement can be implemented either through use of nicotine gum (polacrilex) or the transdermal nicotine patch. A review of research

Form 12.7   "Shiffman Withdrawal Questionnaire"

☐ If not done, enter an X in this box.

Circle the number to the right of each question that most accurately reflects how you feel *at this moment.*

	Definitely not					**Definitely**	
1. If you could smoke freely, would you like a cigarette this minute?	1	2	3	4	5	6	7
2. Is your heart beating faster than usual?	1	2	3	4	5	6	7
3. Do you feel more calm than usual?	1	2	3	4	5	6	7
4. Are you able to concentrate as well as usual?	1	2	3	4	5	6	7
5. Do you feel wide awake?	1	2	3	4	5	6	7
6. Do you feel content?	1	2	3	4	5	6	7
7. Are you thinking of cigarettes more than usual?	1	2	3	4	5	6	7
8. Do you have fluttery feelings in your chest?	1	2	3	4	5	6	7
9. Do you feel hungrier than usual for this time of day?	1	2	3	4	5	6	7
10. If you were permitted to smoke, would you refuse a cigarette right now?	1	2	3	4	5	6	7
11. Do you feel more tense than usual?	1	2	3	4	5	6	7
12. Do you miss a cigarette?	1	2	3	4	5	6	7
13. Do you have an urge to smoke a cigarette right now?	1	2	3	4	5	6	7
14. Are you feeling irritable?	1	2	3	4	5	6	7
15. Are your hands shaky?	1	2	3	4	5	6	7

literature and very helpful guidelines for using each of these forms of NRT is available in a special issue of *Health Values: The Journal of Health Behavior, Education & Promotion* (E.D. Glover, 1993) and from product manufacturers. Despite several publications to the contrary, recent research (e.g., Renard et al., 1991) has suggested that NRT is medically safe in treating most cardiac and pulmonary patients.

Nicotine Gum

Nicotine gum has been available since 1984 in 2-mg dosage. As of 1993, a 4-mg dosage has been made available. The 2-mg nicotine gum provides one-third of the plasma nicotine of cigarettes, whereas the 4-mg dosage provides two-thirds of the plasma nicotine of cigarettes.

Effective use of nicotine gum requires coaching the patient in the peculiarities of this product. The gum must be chewed in a particular manner, often referred to as "chewing and parking." Instruct the patient to chew slowly and to place the gum next to the cheek for a moment between bites. This allows the nicotine to be absorbed through the buccal mucosa. Absorption is usually signaled by a slight tingling in the mouth or tongue. The patient should also be forewarned that, because absorption of the nicotine from the gum is enhanced by an alkaline pH and is decreased by acidic pH in the mouth, low pH beverages such as coffee, cola drinks, and citrus juices should be avoided. Patients should also be advised that annoying side effects of nicotine gum occur in 10% to 25% of patients (Cox, 1993). These can include: bad taste, throat irritation, mouth ulcers, hiccups, vomiting, nausea, and palpitations (McKenna, 1992). It is also essential to emphasize the importance of remaining smoke-free while using any form of NRT. Research suggests that somewhere between 7% and 41% of smokers concurrently use cigarettes and nicotine gum, at least during the initial stages of quit attempts (Hughes, 1989).

It is generally recommended that nicotine gum be used at a fixed dosage of 1 piece per hour (Killen et al., 1990), with 10-16 pieces per day recommended for the average pack-per-day smoker. Usage should not exceed 30 pieces per day for the 2-mg gum or 20 pieces per day for the 4-mg gum (Cox, 1993). Other, ad lib methods of use have also been reported, such as replacing cigarettes with a formula of 1 mg of gum for each cigarette smoked. However, as pointed out in an excellent review by Cox (1993), there is some evidence to suggest that ad lib schedules for gum usage promotes behavioral and physical dependence. In either case, it is recommended that weaning from gum usage occur over a 6-month period by decreasing daily usage by 1 piece each week (e.g., during week 10 of gum use, chew 12 pieces per day; during week 11, chew 11 pieces per day; and so on). The typical patient who successfully uses nicotine gum chews six to eight boxes over a 12- to 15-week period.

Research on the effectiveness of nicotine gum suggests very high 6-month cessation rates but less impressive 1-year cessation rates. Contraindications for use of nicotine polacrilex include use in the immediate post-MI period for smokers with a history of life-threatening dysrhythmias or those with unstable angina (Cox, 1993). Reliance upon behavioral strategies is recommended for such patients.

Transdermal Nicotine Patch

The nicotine patch has been available since 1985 but only received its first Food and Drug Administration (FDA) approval in 1991. The transdermal patch offers many advantages over nicotine gum, including a steady concentration of nicotine, the ability to sustain nicotine levels during sleep, and the ability to be used by hospitalized smokers (McKenna, 1992). In addition, the patch has minimal side effects. Possible side effects include allergic reactions to the adhesive on the patch, skin rash, and sleep problems, but less than 5% of patients have to stop using the nicotine patch due to side effects (Hughes & Glaser, 1993). Perhaps most noteworthy is that the simplicity of using a nicotine patch fosters increased treatment compliance.

A few commonsense suggestions should always be made to any patient using the transdermal nicotine patch. Remind the patient that he or she is not to smoke while wearing the patch. Emphasize that the patch must be replaced, not added to, each day. There are many anecdotal reports of patients discovered during medical consultation to be wearing multiple patches, attributing this fact to their interpretation of the advice to "wear one patch each day" as meaning to "add one patch each day." Emphasize that each day at the same time, the old patch should be removed and discarded and a new patch applied to a different area of hairless (or shaved) skin on the upper body. A patch can be safely reapplied to an already used body area after 1 week.

Generally, the patch provides one-half the nicotine of that from smoking, depending upon the dosage. Patches from various pharmaceutical companies range in strengths from 5 mg to 21 mg. Both 16- and 24-hr patches are available. (The interested reader is referred to E. D. Glover [1993] for a discussion of the relative merits of the 16- and 24-hr patches.) The most frequently used patches are Nicoderm and Habitrol, both of which come in 7-mg, 14-mg, and 21-mg dosages. Typical treatment with a transdermal nicotine patch progresses over a 6- to 18-week period. The 21-mg patch is used for 4-6 weeks, followed by 2-4 weeks' use of the 14-mg patch and 2-4 weeks' use of the 7-mg patch. Use of lower strength patches is recommended with any patient who weighs less than 100 lb, has CHD, or smokes less than one-half pack of cigarettes per day.

Outcome studies have indicated that the nicotine patch is approximately twice as effective in promoting long-term cessation as placebo but not necessarily better than nicotine gum (Hughes & Glaser, 1993). Clinical experience suggests that, although effective for most patients at typical dosages, individualization of treatment is often necessary for specific patients. For example, even the maximal dosage patch may not prevent withdrawal for heavy smokers. One sign of this problem may be early-morning awakening due to withdrawal experienced during sleep. For others, even minimal patch doses may promote insomnia due to overmedication.

In reference to this fact, E.D. Glover (1993) recommended that patients who need additional nicotine replacement can benefit from supplementing the 21-mg patch with a 7-mg patch or with use of nicotine polacrilex on a fixed schedule. In this later regard, it is helpful to note that 6 2-mg pieces of gum are approximately equivalent to one 7-mg patch, whereas 16 to 20 pieces of gum provide an amount of plasma nicotine equivalent to one 21-mg patch. In the case of overstimulation from patch use, some clinicians have reported advantages from cutting patches in half. Adjustments of this sort need to be monitored closely, given that such treatment strategies have not been FDA-approved.

Whether or not use of the transdermal nicotine patch is safe for recovering cardiopulmonary patients is debatable. Questions have been raised regarding its safety for patients who suffer unstable angina (Benowitz, 1991; Hughes & Glaser, 1993). However, given that the patch simply contains nicotine, and none of the toxic gases that fill cigarette smoke and that are known to have disastrous cardiopulmonary effects, use of this product needs to be seriously considered in aiding smoking cessation with heart and lung patients. Nicotine in cigarettes does appear to worsen some risk factors for myocardial infarction, but evidence also exists that short-term, gradual, low doses of nicotine from the transdermal nicotine patch does not increase the risk for infarction (Rennard et al., 1991). In their thoughtful review of relevant literature, Hughes and Glaser (1993) concluded that there is no solid evidence that transdermal nicotine replacement therapy is dangerous, either for recovering cardiac patients or for the aged.

As mentioned, NRT is especially effective if presented in conjunction with brief behavioral counseling. Marion Merrell Dow, Inc., has made readily available a noteworthy program of assistance for smokers who are attempting to quit with the aid of NRT. The COMMITTED QUITTER'S PROGRAM Personal Support Plan integrates cutting-edge techniques (Campbell et al., 1994) for using computer-based algorithms that incorporate patients' motives, barriers, and interest in changing their smoking habit into personalized letters and phone-call interventions. A series of supportive phone calls and postal-delivered calendars provide day-by-day guidelines for smoking cessation. The communication is tailored to the individual smoker's needs, based upon a brief telephone interview conducted at the program's outset. Telephone and written advice is provided for 6 weeks of intervention, and continued reinforcement for quitting is provided through periodic newsletters addressing the importance of quitting. Information regarding this program can be obtained from any Marion Merrell Dow representative or by calling 1-800-NICODERM.

Gradual Cigarette Reduction and Nicotine Fading

Although quitting cold turkey is considered the most effective method of smoking cessation, two techniques often attempted by smokers are gradual reduction in the number of cigarettes smoked and nicotine fading (Hatsukami & Lando, 1993). The gradual reduction method involves systematically decreasing the number of cigarettes smoked in a given day by increasing the time interval between cigarettes. Limiting the places in which smoking is allowed to very few is an aid to this strategy. Hatsukami and Lando (1993) cautioned that research has documented that this method is considered unsuccessful because each remaining cigarette becomes more reinforcing and smokers tend to compensate for the reduced nicotine intake by inhaling more deeply and taking greater numbers of puffs.

Nicotine fading is accomplished by systematically switching to brands of cigarettes that contain progressively less nicotine or by using commercial filters that gradually reduce nicotine intake over the course of several weeks. Nicotine fading for several weeks prior to quitting can help counter the effects of nicotine withdrawal and increase a sense of self-control (McKool, 1987). Particular success has been noted from interventions that combine nicotine fading with other methods of smoking cessation (Hatsukami & Lando, 1993).

Aversive Procedures

Several other interventions are sometimes employed by smoking cessation experts working in specialized settings. These techniques involve use of aversive procedures that either punish cigarette smoking behavior or, through classical conditioning, establish a link between smoking stimuli and some aversive response. Aversive treatment strategies that have been reported include electric shock, covert sensitization (using negative imagery), breath-holding, overexposure to stale smoke, and satiation by increasing the number and rate of cigarettes smoked (Hatsukami & Lando, 1993).

A variation of this last aversive technique is rapid smoking. Here the patient is instructed to smoke much more quickly than is pleasant, typically one puff every 6 seconds. This is continued until the patient becomes ill. Research has demonstrated the effectiveness and safety of this procedure in treating a group of CHD patients. No adverse effects on cardiovascular functions and no increases in myocardial ischemia or cardiac arrhythmias were noted in CHD patients while engaging in rapid smoking, and compared to no-treatment controls, this procedure led to greater cessation rates (Hall, Sachs, Hall, & Benowitz, 1984).

In practice, these techniques are used rarely due to patient resistance, concerns about safety of these procedures, humanistic considerations, and the fact that nicotine replacement therapy appears to produce more effective results with less therapeutic effort (Hatsukami & Lando, 1993). Again, only smoking cessation experts should consider using these aversive techniques.

Coach Regarding the Importance of Family Support and Participation in Cessation Attempts

Marital dynamics have been documented to have definite effects on the outcome of smoking cessation attempts. Compared to nonquitters, successful quitters are more likely to have partners who make useful self-help suggestions and who are perceived as being reinforcing, confident, and actively interested and involved in the smoker's quitting efforts (Hatsukami & Lando, 1993). Nonquitters, on the other hand, tend to have an unhealthy reliance on the partner for both supporting and assuming responsibility for the smoker's quitting efforts (Ginsberg, Hall, Rosinski, 1991). Particularly ineffective seems to be a partner's criticism or complaining about the smoker's behavior (Mermelstein et al., 1983).

An extensive review of relevant family systems literature (Sotile, Sotile, Ewen, & Sotile, 1993) found only four studies that investigated marital factors in smoking cessation attempts either by recovering cardiac patients or by patients diagnosed at high risk for cardiac illness. Three of these studies (Gianetti, Reynolds, & Rihn, 1985; Higgins & Schweiger, 1983; Ockene et al., 1982) documented the importance of spouse and family support and encouragement in promoting and maintaining smoking cessation in this population. Another study found that although a group of 205 male MI patients maintained a drastic drop in cigarette consumption throughout the first year of recovery, their spouses, as a group, did not decrease and in many cases actually increased their cigarette consumption (Croog & Richards, 1977).

Researchers in this area emphasize the importance of coaching family members and loved ones specifically on how their behaviors can either help or harm the smoker's quitting attempt. The information below, drawn largely from the work of Cohen and Lichtenstein (1990), can be used to structure such coaching.

 Negative Partner Behaviors

1. Asking you to quit smoking
2. Commenting that smoking is a dirty habit
3. Talking you out of smoking a cigarette
4. Commenting on your lack of willpower
5. Commenting that the house (or car) smells of smoke
6. Refusing to let you smoke in the house (or car)
7. Mentioning being bothered by smoke
8. Criticizing your smoking
9. Expressing doubt about your ability to quit/stay quit
10. Refusing to clean up your cigarette butts

Positive Partner Behaviors

1. Complimenting you on not smoking
2. Congratulating you for your decision to quit smoking
3. Helping you think of substitutes for smoking
4. Celebrating your quitting with you
5. Helping to calm you down when you are feeling stressed or irritable
6. Telling you to stick with it

7. Expressing confidence in your ability to quit/remain quit

8. Helping you to use substitutes for cigarettes

9. Expressing pleasure at your efforts to quit

10. Participating in an activity with you that keeps you from smoking (e.g., going for a walk instead of smoking)

Note. From "Partner Behaviors That Support Quitting Smoking" by S. Cohen & E. Lichtenstein, 1990, *Journal of Consulting and Clinical Psychology, 58,* pp. 304-309. Copyright 1990 by American Psychological Association. Adapted with permission.

Coach Regarding Cognitive/Behavioral Strategies

In chapter 9, I discussed how powerful it can be to help a patient change his or her way of thinking. Cognitive intervention is an important part of effective smoking cessation, especially when it comes to challenging many of the myths about smoking cessation that tend to predominate the thinking of smokers (McKool, 1987). For example, the smoker may hold misconceptions such as the following:

• Quitting is easy or impossible.

• Cravings for nicotine last forever.

• Quitting just takes willpower—no expertise is required.

• Quitting needs to happen spontaneously.

The smoker should be reminded that the facts are quite different from such myths:

• Reactions to quitting vary tremendously.

• Cravings decrease in frequency but may remain intense.

• Knowing about and employing specific skills and coping strategies can aid quitting.

• Quitting needs to be planned and systematically implemented.

Use Relapse Prevention Strategies

Perhaps the most important component of smoking cessation is what happens once it is supposedly accomplished. As mentioned previously, relapse rates for smokers are alarmingly high. Efforts here should focus on helping patients develop coping strategies for high-risk situations and on helping them avoid full-blown relapses in the wake of lapses or slips (Hatsukami & Lando, 1993).

First, it is important to forewarn of the potential of relapse, especially during the first 3 months after quitting (Hunt, Barrett, & Branch, 1971). The patient should be advised to exercise special prudence in reacting to the following:

- Environmental cues such as drinking alcohol or encountering old high-risk situations.

- Social pressure from others' smoking or during special occasions.

- Interpersonal conflict.

- Negative emotional states, especially stress, loneliness, or depression.

- Maladaptive attitudes such as: "Given all that I've been through, I deserve a cigarette."

- Times of physiological discomfort such as fatigue, hunger, nicotine cravings, nicotine withdrawal, or frustration with weight gain.

Research has clearly shown that the more coping strategies used by the individual during such times, the more likely smoking will be resisted (Hatsukami & Lando, 1993). In this regard, the wealth of coping strategies outlined throughout this book, and the specific strategies outlined as part of overall Effective Emotional Management, are recommended.

While conveying confidence in the patient's ability to ultimately maintain cessation, it is also helpful to prepare for the possibility that a slip may occur. The patient should be advised that any slip will be used as a learning opportunity. Here discussion of Marlatt and Gordon's (1980) Abstinence Violation Effect is particularly relevant. In their study of smokers who had lapsed, Marlatt and Gordon found that those who stumbled into full-blown relapse tended to chastise themselves as failures and convince themselves that they were unable to quit smoking successfully. They recommend that the quitter be taught ways to deal with slips. Helping the patient reframe a slip by seeing how few cigarettes have actually been smoked in recent days or weeks compared to a comparable period of time during precessation days is recommended. Further, the patient should be coached to focus on previous successes and benefits from quitting rather than on failures. The relapse prevention literature also emphasizes that quitters need ongoing support from health care providers. Even brief telephone contacts have been found to be effective aids to continued cessation and to increased overall quit rates (Hollis et al., 1993; Lando, Hellerstedt, Pirie, & McGovern, 1992).

SUMMARY

There is no doubt that treatment programs combining various of the strategies outlined in this chapter can be effective in promoting smoking cessation. At minimum, in inpatient settings, intervention should focus on education, discussion of high-risk situations the patient anticipates encountering post-hospitalization, and support and advice regarding ways to handle symptoms of withdrawal. Implementation of nicotine replacement therapy or, at minimum, education regarding this important aid to long-term cessation should also be incorporated into bedside nicotine counseling (Nett, 1992). In outpatient settings, patients should, at minimum, be offered assistance in completing a detailed assessment of their smoking habit, education regarding nicotine replacement therapy, an overview of the cessation protocol described in this chapter, and an offer to provide either ongoing smoking cessation assistance or referral for the same. In both inpatient and outpatient settings, the importance of smoking cessation to overall rehabilitation should be strongly emphasized.

Much additional information regarding brief and comprehensive smoking cessation treatment programs is available (e.g., P. Glover, 1993; Hatsukami & Lando, 1993). Especially helpful are guides for structuring brief, office-based cessation interventions available from the National Cancer Institute (Glynn & Manley, 1992) and the American Academy of Family Physicians (American Academy of Family Physicians, 1987). Helpful information for laypersons is available from the American Lung Association and from the aforementioned COMMITTED QUITTER'S PROGRAM from Marion Merrell Dow, Inc., and the other manufacturers listed in the Indexed Bibliography.

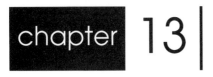

chapter 13

COPD AND AGED CARDIOPULMONARY PATIENTS

This chapter is devoted to discussion of two topics that deserve special mention in designing and implementing care of coronary and pulmonary patients. First, certain unique psychosocial challenges that confront the COPD patient will be discussed, along with implications for delivering psychosocial interventions. Subsequent discussion will be devoted to understanding the developmental dramas encountered by aged patients.

SPECIAL CONSIDERATIONS FOR COPD PATIENTS

Every illness brings with it certain unique adaptive challenges. Although the rehabilitative tasks of various cardiac and pulmonary illnesses are similar in many ways, it is also clear that COPD patients face certain biopsychosocial stressors that distinguish them and bring complexity to their treatment.

UNIQUE PROBLEMS OF TREATING COPD PATIENTS

It is impossible to characterize the "typical" COPD patient. However, certain descriptions of this population have been offered that call attention to the relatively unique combination of factors that shape the challenges associated with treating any individual with COPD.

In a study of 50 consecutive patients hospitalized for chronic airflow obstruction, Yellowlees et al. (1987) found a high incidence of psychiatric disorders, particularly anxiety states, which were often undiagnosed and untreated. These researchers also noted that the psychologically distressed patients tended to stay in the hospital twice as long as other respiratory patients (16 days compared to 7 days). The "typical" patient in the Yellowlees et al. (1987) study depicts the complex of factors that are often encountered when treating a patient suffering from COPD:

The patient is likely to be a married elderly man who has been chronically ill for between 5 and 10 years and has markedly impaired respiratory function test results. He has been admitted to hospital at least five times with chronic airflow obstruction— twice in the past year—and has at least one other major medical condition that requires concurrent treatment. He takes about five different medications each day and has a smoking history of approximately 60 pack-years but has now stopped, or reduced markedly, his smoking. He is likely to hyperventilate and to have a formal psychiatric disorder but is unlikely to have an obvious cognitive deficit. If he is showing signs of anxiety or depression then he is likely to ingest alcohol. (Yellowlees et al., 1987, p. 306)

Various aspects of this description of the plight of the COPD patient are supported in the literature regarding this condition. Indeed, it does appear that the majority of diagnosed COPD patients are males and that the vast majority (over 80%) are 60 years old or older (Rabinowitz & Florian, 1992). The high incidence of anxiety disorders and general emotional distress in the COPD population has also been amply documented in this literature, a fact that has been discussed throughout this book. Gift and McCrone (1993) observed that, although relatively few COPD patients meet diagnostic criteria for major depression, perhaps even fewer fail to meet diagnostic criteria for dysthymia. As explained in chapter 2, dysthymia is characterized by chronically depressed or irritable mood for most of the day, more days than not; symptoms present for at least 2 years and involve at least two of the following: poor appetite or overeating, insomnia or hypersomnia, low energy or fatigue, low self-esteem, poor concentration or difficulty making decisions, and feelings of hopelessness.

The psychosocial impact differs from stage to stage of COPD, but it appears that at all stages, the predominant psychological experiences of the COPD patient are anxiety and depression. A number of researchers (e.g., Foxall et al., 1987; Gift & McCrone, 1993) have pointed out that COPD involves more role losses than living with other chronic illnesses such as peripheral vascular disease. Effects can include more feelings of uselessness, poorer mental health, lower life satisfaction, loss of more social roles, and increased sexual difficulties, including decreased libido or inability to achieve erection. As mentioned earlier, COPD patients also often become remorseful with self-blame over the perception of having caused their illness through smoking (Yellowlees, 1987).

Studies of the personality factors evidenced by COPD patients also suggest unique adjustment patterns for this population (Gift & McCrone, 1993). Specifically, comparative standardized personality testing of individuals with various chronic illnesses has found that COPD patients tend to evidence lower self-esteem, lower self-confidence, and less spontaneity during the course of daily living (Covino, Dirks, Kinsman, & Seidel, 1982). Variations of this finding are present throughout the COPD literature. Often patients with obstructive lung disease have been found to be pessimistic and to harbor feelings of hopelessness and worthlessness (DeCenio, Leshner, & Leshner, 1968). A glimpse at the inner workings of coping with COPD across the life span begins to shed light on why this might be.

THE "STRAIGHT JACKET" OF COPD

COPD is a gradual, progressive, chronic illness. This statement contains both the good news and the bad news about this malady. As with many illnesses, the progression of COPD often occurs in relative "silence"; the condition frequently goes undiagnosed until it results in moderate to severe disability and respiratory insufficiency (Dudley et al., 1980). This means that many patients with early-stage respiratory illnesses live unaffected by their condition in obvious ways, even though their daily activities may be subtly shaped by the beginning stages of respiratory limitations.

Once diagnosed, the bad news hits for most patients: They must face the fact that their illness cannot be reversed; it is a chronic condition that will progress. Many patients live in denial regarding what this progression will be like; others seek detailed information about what will happen to them as their illness advances.

Dudley et al. (1980) classified five levels of functioning of COPD patients. A look at these levels provides a glimpse of the progression of this illness.

Level I: At the mildest level in this categorization, the patient has recognized disease but has not yet suffered restrictions in daily living. Able to do what peers can do, the patient continues normal patterns of daily living.

Level II: Here the patient's illness leads to minimal or moderately restricted activity. He or she is able to do productive work, but difficulty keeping up with peers results in the beginning stages of modifying patterns of daily living.

Level III: Once the patient's illness has markedly restricted his or her activity, Level III is entered. Here the patient is still able to care for him- or herself and is not homebound, but he or she may be unable to do productive work.

Level IV: At this level, the patient's activity has become severely restricted by the illness. He or she is homebound and is unable to do productive work. However, the patient is still able to care for most of his or her own needs in daily living.

Level V: In this advanced stage, the patient's illness severely restricts activities of daily living. The patient has become homebound or is living in an institutional setting and is no longer capable of effective self-care.

As COPD progresses, biological and psychosocial factors combine to affect overall psychological and social functioning. For example, blood gas changes that accompany COPD, such as hypoxia and hypercapnia, can result in various cognitive alterations and neurophysiologic changes (Gift & McCrone, 1993). As the illness advances, the patient may also become embarrassed as the result of cough and sputum production (Dudley et al., 1980). Depression in this population has been found to be related to dyspnea and a loss of energy that increases the time necessary to perform even simple activities of daily living (Gift & McCrone, 1993; Hodgkin, Connors, & Bell, 1993).

A variety of psychological and social phenomena can stem from these physical changes, some in reaction to and some in anticipation of the changes. Even before these symptoms begin to manifest, many COPD patients experience grief, depression, and demoralization at the specter of such an existence and its impact on loved ones. For others, the slow course of the illness may delay any conscious mourning until some event (e.g., the onset of need for home ventilation) clearly demarcates entry into the next stage of debilitation. Unfortunately, such patients then tend to withhold expression of their feelings for fear of the effect that displaying emotions might have on their breathing (Post & Collins, 1981). They then can become progressively more anxious, isolated, and depressed in misguided efforts to ward off emotional or social stresses that can complicate the physical manifestations of COPD. Agle and Baum (1977) described the COPD patient as living in an "emotional straight jacket": Fearful of the pulmonary consequences of any sudden emotional shift, the patient attempts to protect him- or herself by using the defense mechanisms of denial, repression, suppression, projection and displacement.

Donald Dudley and colleagues elaborated on this notion. The narrow range of emotions and behaviors that many COPD patients seem compelled to maintain may be based on the catch-22 of their respiratory reactions to any strong emotion. These researchers note that any extreme emotional state may increase symptoms in the COPD patient. Significant degrees of activating emotions such as anxiety, anger, or euphoria increase energy expenditure and elevate ventilation, oxygen consumption, and skeletal muscle tension; whereas nonactivating emotional states such as apathy, depression, and deep relaxation reduce energy expenditure, decrease ventilation, lower oxygen consumption, and relax skeletal musculature. Thus, in reacting to extreme emotions in either category—action or nonaction—the COPD patient with already compromised ventilation and borderline blood gas values may experience serious pulmonary distress.

A patient whose ventilation is already being severely taxed may not be able to increase ventilation to meet greater psychological and physiological demands. Thus, the patient with severe COPD may become hypoxic, hypercarbic, and dyspneic because of

> the increased metabolic load and the failure of ventilation to compensate by increasing the oxygen supply. The patient with moderate COPD may develop hypoxia without hypercarbia. (Dudley et al., 1980, p. 416)

Dudley et al. (1980) note in particular that during nonaction emotional states (e.g., apathy, depression, and deep relaxation), the COPD patient appears to decrease ventilation in excess of the change in metabolism that naturally accompanies such states. The result is relative ventilatory insufficiency—the pulmonary system simply does not supply enough oxygen or remove enough carbon dioxide, and resultant hypoxia and hypercarbia contribute to a vicious psychophysiological cycle. The dyspnea that results from such emotions increases the patient's psychological alarm, which, in turn, produces more physiologic changes. These physiologic responses increase the dyspnea, completing a vicious cycle which, according to Dudley and colleagues, "may completely incapacitate even (those) patients whose pulmonary function is relatively intact" (Dudley et al., 1980, p. 416).

As COPD progresses, the rigid avoidance of emotional conflict and emotional change that characterizes the emotional straight jacket phenomenon can increase the patient's frustration, anger, and despair. Misguided psychological coping strategies (e.g., denial, suppression, repression, displacement, and projection) can affect the patient's individual well-being as well as his or her relationships with health care providers and family members.

COPD Patients and Health Care Providers

It has often been observed that COPD patients seem to be particularly ambivalent about their relationships with their health care providers. The fear of alienating medical caregivers is a theme mentioned throughout the literature on the psychology of the COPD patient. Unfortunately, this fear often leads to passive-aggressive or passive-dependent behavior. We are wise to remember that patients with COPD are in a position of forced, typically uncomfortable dependence (Gilchrist, Phillips, Odgers, & Hoogendorp, 1985). They are forced to depend on the medical profession, and both medical professionals and the medical process can at once become targets and tools in their management of anger. Yellowlees (1987) theorized that such patients displace anger about their illness onto their physician, then punish the physician by requiring repeated hospital admissions or excessive or inappropriate medical treatment.

COPD Patients and Marital/Family Life

True understanding of the psychosocial experience of the COPD patient requires appreciation of the profound strains on the family and on individual caregivers that come with having a loved one suffering from this illness. As the patient's illness progresses, the family's social independence and quality of life diminishes. As the patient becomes progressively more homebound and dependent, the family loses its ability to function as a complete unit outside of the home. Both outside and in-home social activities then diminish. These patterns no doubt contribute to the fact that a predominant complaint of spouses of COPD patients is loneliness (Clough, Harnisch, Cebulski, & Ross, 1987; McSweeney, Grant, Heaton, Adams, & Timms, 1982). The interplay between individual patient and family-level coping patterns becomes ever more complex and important as COPD advances. As illness diminishes self-care abilities, family members typically become progressively more involved in the direct care of the patient. Loved ones also are progressively more affected by the patient's efforts to cope. The complexity of this interplay can become profoundly evident as the patient becomes dependent on home-based oxygen therapy.

Living With Home-Based Oxygen Therapy

Perhaps for the first time, the COPD patient who is faced with the need for home-based oxygen therapy is forced to deal with the chronic, deteriorating nature of his or her condition. Petty (1981) pointed out that the onset of home-based oxygen therapy represents the end of a useful and independent existence for the COPD patient and that both the patient's premorbid personality makeup and family situation will determine reactions to home oxygen use.

The COPD patient becomes dependent for his or her life on the oxygen concentrator, and the machine represents restricted activity, a reality that can diminish one's personal sense of worth. As the patient's physical state weakens, feelings of dependency deepen. This can lead to a generalized loss of any internal locus of control, as feelings of external locus of control grow. "Additional fears may become real issues—electricity failure can lead to death, the initial fear of being alone becomes exacerbated and his/her dependence on this environment is increased" (Sandhu, 1986, p. 79). This situation can only serve to increase already-existing fears and feelings of anger, helplessness, and dependency—feelings that are often projected onto the family.

The oxygen concentrator also "becomes a new entity in the family's interaction with the patient" (Sandhu, 1986, p. 78). In the later stages of COPD, the patient may use the oxygen concentrator for most parts of most days. Because the oxygen concentrator is controlled by the patient him- or herself, its use can become an integral part of the family's communication sequences. For example, resorting to use of the oxygen concentrator during conflict with a loved one can convey the communication-squelching metamessage, "This discussion is upsetting me. Be quiet!" Clinical experience suggests that it is fairly commonplace for family members to harbor tremendous ambivalence in reacting to the in-home oxygen machine. On the one hand, loved ones of COPD patients are often reassured by the presence of the machine. Their own fears and helplessness in responding to the patient's breathlessness are soothed by the fact that the machine can ease any respiratory crises.

But the oxygen machine can also become an object of loathing for family members; it can create distance between the patient and loved ones as the patient becomes ever more intimately attached to it. The wife of a COPD patient once commented, "I feel as if I am living with my husband and another woman. My husband spends more time interacting with that machine than with me. He gets more relief and soothing from that machine than he does from me. Whenever he is away from it, he is anxious to return to the 'loving presence' of that machine. And the next thing that always happens—no matter what the first thing was (us having an argument, us trying to make love, even a phone call from one of our children)—is him touching base with that machine. I know he needs the thing, but I'm sick and tired of it."

Of course, few spouses of COPD patients uniformly feel such frustrations. More typical is the pattern of mounting feelings of contempt followed by feelings of guilt over being angry in the first place. This guilt can then fuel overprotective behaviors on the part of the distressed family member (Sandhu, 1986).

HELPING COPD PATIENTS COPE

Many intervention strategies for promoting psychosocial adjustments in recovering cardiac and pulmonary patients have been outlined in preceding pages. However, special mention must be made of two additional factors as they relate specifically to the treatment of COPD patients.

The COPD Patient's Response to Formal Rehabilitation

As mentioned earlier, the use of multifaceted rehabilitation intervention in treating COPD patients has been recommended in the research literature. The extent to which such intervention leads to actual changes in pulmonary function remains a topic of debate and exploration. However, strong evidence exists that, independent of actual changes in physiologic measures of functional capacity, COPD patients who participate in some form of organized, multifaceted rehabilitation program do evidence marked enhancement of overall psychosocial functioning and activities of daily living (Hodgkin, 1988; Hodgkin et al., 1993).

For example, Baum and colleagues demonstrated the effectiveness of a treatment that combined standard medical management, breathing retraining, intensive graduated exercise, twice-weekly group therapy sessions, and voluntary vocational and social counseling. Patients met monthly and were followed for 1 year. At 1-year follow-up, the researchers noted improved ability to perform activities of daily living, even though many patients did not show corresponding demonstrable improvement in physiologic measures. These researchers hypothesized that by gradually increasing exercise in the reassuring presence of medical personnel, the intervention functioned as a form of desensitization of anxiety about physical exertion. This increased comfort with exertion evidently became generalized, thereby bolstering the patient's self-efficacy for solo physical activity outside of the rehabilitation setting (Agle, Baum, Chester, & Wendt, 1973; Baum, Agle, Chester, & Wendt, 1973).

Operationalizing the COPD Patient's Psychosocial Functioning

Perhaps more than most illnesses, in its early and intermediate stages, COPD tends to subtly shape the patient's daily style of living. As pulmonary debilitation silently and gradually progresses, patients often make subtle adjustments in their activity patterns without attributing these adjustments to the untreated illness. Often, the reasons attributed to such changes are far more pejorative than is warranted: Gradual withdrawal from hobbies that require physical exertion may be attributed to laziness; avoidance of intense emotional experiences may be attributed to disinterest; settling into a relatively even pace of life may be attributed to apathy or lack of ambition or boredom.

Explaining to patients and loved ones that such behavior patterns may have been fostered by the physical consequences of COPD, not by some negative psychological or relational factor, can be of tremendous value in helping the patient and his or her family use the crisis of the illness as an opportunity for psychosocial growth and healing. Exactly how the psychophysiological phenomena of living with COPD may be shaping the patient's daily patterns of living should be elucidated by obtaining a detailed account of the patient's daily activities. Such assessment can provide information to help in developing targets for change and markers of progress as the patient's rehabilitation program is designed.

 The following questions should be incorporated into routine assessment of the COPD patient:

- Under what circumstances do you feel best and worst?
- How have your daily activities changed over the past 5 years? What do you not do now that you used to enjoy doing?
- Do your symptoms fluctuate from day to day?
- Are your symptoms worse in the morning or evening?
- How does eating, sleeping, or exercising affect your symptoms?
- How does sexual excitement affect your symptoms?
- How does actual sexual activity affect your symptoms?
- What forms of work affect your symptoms?
- Are any of your symptoms likely to get worse when you feel certain emotions? Which emotions?
- How do you typically cope with those specific emotions?

- What brings relief from your symptoms?
- How has your family responded to [specify various areas mentioned above, one at a time]?
- How do you feel about their reactions?
- How have other health care providers responded to your concerns? In general, how would you describe your day-to-day mood?

Modified from Dudley et al. (1980)

In answering such questions, the patient's coping strategies are forced into conscious awareness. For some patients, simply enhancing insight in this way can lead to positive coping changes. For others, the information that surfaces can be processed and reflected back to the patient as a way of educating him or her about the associations that may exist between seemingly disparate aspects of his or her daily lifestyle. Finally, needed areas of coaching regarding alternative coping strategies can also surface from such questioning. An example of the usefulness of this operationalizing strategy is presented in the following case.

Luke Milano, a 68-year-old COPD patient, and his wife Julia were referred for help in dealing with stress reactions that were complicating his frequent bouts of dyspnea. According to his referring physician, a major stressor in this gentleman's life was unresolved marital tensions. This couple's responses during interview were telling of a misguided coping pattern in reacting to various aspects of Mr. Milano's illness and the marital dynamics involved in coping with the same.

WMS: "So, I understand that you are having quite a few bouts of dyspnea."

Luke: "Yes, far too many."

WMS: "Can you describe what happens during these episodes, Mr. Milano?"

Luke: "I just have trouble breathing . . . and the more it happens, the worse it gets."

WMS: "Sounds scary."

Luke: "It is. And aggravating."

WMS: "What do you do to cope at times like that?"

Luke: "Thank God for my oxygen machine. . . . I don't know what I would do if I didn't have it . . . it helps me breathe."

WMS: "Can you give me a picture of how your dyspnea comes and goes during a typical day?"

Luke: "What do you mean?"

WMS: "Are your symptoms predictably better at certain times of the day?"

Luke: [to his wife] "Well, I don't know. What do you think?"

Julia: "The mornings are the worst; the early mornings."

Luke: "You think so?"

Julia: "Yes. At least you don't use the oxygen machine as much in the late morning as you do in the early morning."

WMS: "So, early mornings are pretty tough times for you?"

Luke: "Yes."

Julia: "Yes."

WMS: "How so? What happens in the early mornings."

[uncomfortable silence]

Luke: "Well, when I sleep, I 'drain' a lot. So when I wake up I always have to cough a lot; I cough up a lot of mucus."

WMS: "That's a hard way to start the day, isn't it?"

Luke: "Well, I guess so. I know it's hard for her [his wife] to hear me hacking away, spitting up. I know that my wife doesn't like that."

WMS: "Is that right?"

Luke: [irritated] "Well, what am I supposed to do? I can't help it. I don't want this any more than she does."

WMS: "So is this a bone of contention between you? Your coughing?"

Julia: "No!"

Luke: "I think it totally disgusts her. But I can't help it. I go into the bathroom and close the door. But I know she hears me."

Julia: "Is that why you come out of the bathroom angry every morning?"

Luke: "I'm not angry every morning."

Julia: "Most mornings, the first thing I see is you looking red in the face, on your way to your oxygen machine. And you act like I have done something to make you angry. Half the time, all I've been doing is sleeping!"

WMS: "Wait, let me make sure I'm understanding this. Mr. Milano, you wake up, go into the bathroom to clear your lungs, and while you are doing so, you assume that Mrs. Milano is 'totally disgusted' by your coughing?"

Luke: "That's right."

Julia: "That's wrong."

WMS: "What happens next? What do you feel by the time you finish clearing your lungs?"

Luke: "Tired. And like I said, I can't help it that I have to cough. And then I have trouble breathing."

WMS: "It sounds like you end up feeling sort of angry and misunderstood about this."

Luke: "I guess so; sometimes. But not all the time."

WMS: "A lot of coughing can certainly make you have dyspnea. Also, a lot of folks find that if they get emotionally upset, it makes dyspnea worse. Does this happen to you?"

Luke: "I guess so."

Julia: "Definitely so."

WMS: "How so?"

Julia: "If he gets excited, he can't breathe."

WMS: "Is that so?"

Luke: "Yeah, I guess that's true."

WMS: "Excited how?"

Julia: "Like . . . angry."

WMS: "Is that right?"

Luke: "Yeah."

WMS: "So, what happens then; when you get angry?"

Luke: "Like I said: Thank goodness for my oxygen machine."

Julia: "That's right. He goes to the machine."

Luke: "Of course, that's not the only time I use the machine."

Julia: "No, of course not."

WMS: "So your dyspnea is especially likely to happen when you are excited, feeling something like anger."

Luke: "That's right."

WMS: "And you are especially likely to have dyspnea in the early mornings."

Luke: "Yes."

WMS: "Let's go back to a point that you made earlier, Mr. Milano. You were saying that you assume that Mrs. Milano is 'totally disgusted' by hearing you cough?"

Luke: "I would be if I were her."

Julia: "Luke, that's simply not true."

Luke: "Well you sure do act irritated with me when you finally get up each morning."

Julia: "I've told you before what that is about. I get tired of you 'disappearing' into that machine every morning. I feel like I can't even talk to you when I get up, because you are already upset!"

This form of questioning was useful in getting the Milanos to consciously examine several factors that were significantly affecting their overall well-being. First, Mr. Milano was angry and saddened by his deteriorating condition; he dreaded awakening in the mornings, for fear of the expectorating ordeal. He actually had no data upon which to base his assumption that his wife was "disgusted" by his expectoration; he had never asked, and she had never offered any information about her reactions in this regard. However, Mrs. Milano did clearly indicate that she resented her husband's daily "disappearing act"; she had repeatedly complained that she wished he did not need to use his home oxygen machine as frequently as he did.

Discussion of these points led to Mr. Milano's willingness to experiment with several new coping skills: (a) a direct yet noninflammatory method of expressing anger; (b) a direct style of communicating fears and anxieties about the impact of his illness on his marriage; and (c) relaxation procedures to help him cope with the distress and tension that he personally associated with the early-morning expectoration ordeal. With slight improvements in these areas, Mrs. Milano was able to renew her patience in enduring her husband's periodic need to use his oxygen machine, but she continued to complain that he sometimes used the machine as a way of manipulating her into silence.

CONCLUSIONS

The chronicity and diminishment of functioning that characterize COPD bring special challenges for such patients and require special awareness on the part of their health care providers. The official guidelines for pulmonary rehabilitation published by the AACVPR (Connors & Hilling, 1993) reemphasized that COPD patients need special help in attending to activities of daily living. The importance of providing help in managing anxiety, sexual concerns, and vocational adjustments has been discussed in preceding pages. But the AACVPR emphasizes that the COPD patient may even need help with fundamental aspects of daily living such as: ways to conserve time and energy; choosing leisure-time activities; ways to orchestrate travel; and identification and use of community resources.

Reasonable levels of daily activity are essential to overall psychosocial adjustment for COPD patients. The importance of promoting such adjustment is underscored by a caution that applies to any cardiopulmonary patient: "Unless the patient can learn techniques to handle emotional changes, the chance of long-term productive survival will be significantly diminished" (Dudley et al., 1980, p. 417).

SPECIAL NEEDS OF AGED PATIENTS

Medical advances over the past 50 years have extended the expected life cycle dramatically. The population of individuals over the age of 65 has increased 8-fold since the turn of the century, while the number of people over age 75 has grown 10-fold. In the United States, the over-65 segment of society represents the fastest growing population group. For most individuals, the later stages of the life cycle account for almost half of the entire life span (Wolinsky, 1990). Far too little attention has been paid in the professional literature to the differential psychosocial needs of adult patients of various ages. As mentioned in prior discussion, the adaptive challenges, available resources, and goals of intervention for the aged patient will typically be quite different from those of a younger patient. Medical intervention needs to be designed and delivered with sensitivity to the unique psychosocial and psychological processes that come with aging (Paine & Make, 1986).

THE DEVELOPMENTAL PROGRESSION FROM MIDLIFE TO OLD AGE: PSYCHOLOGICAL PERSPECTIVES

The decade of the 50s is considered the youth of the aging process. Contrary to popular mythology regarding the proverbial "midlife crisis," midlife tends to be a time of maximal capability, resourcefulness, and power for most people; a time when developmental tasks turn to clarifying, deepening, and finding use for what one has already learned in a lifetime of adapting (Gallagher, 1993).

Gerontology experts point out that the average member of the "young old" category of individuals aged 65-75 is personally attractive and physically active (Wolinsky, 1990). The span of life that begins with the climacteric and typically lasts for 30 to 40 years is a time of paradox. On the one hand, this stage of life is characterized by gradual waning of physical capacities and a gradual disengagement from the activities that have heretofore structured one's life. On the other hand, despite slowing of reaction time, there is a striking increment in the growth of wisdom and judgment in most aging individuals. In fact, IQ scores at age 56 are significantly higher than at age 22, especially if the variable of reaction time is controlled for (Gallagher, 1993; Levinson, 1978).

As clarified by renowned Duke University Medical Center gerontologist Dan Blazer in his timely essay on spirituality and aging well, wisdom has to do with knowledge of the larger system in which one lives and acceptance of the limits to which one can influence factors that are unchangeable (Blazer, 1991). As an example of this shift in perspective that often accompanies aging, he cites a poignant quote of Dame Edith Evans: "When you fall down at my age, the great secret is not to try to get up too quickly. Just lie there. Have a look at the world from a different perspective" (Dame Edith Evans, as quoted by Brian Forbes, 1977, p. 14).

Indeed, many aged cardiopulmonary patients who come into our care have already undergone this form of perspective shifting; others need our help in accomplishing this developmental task. The work of Pruyser (1975), also cited by Blazer, points to the adaptive directions that aged patients are developmentally compelled to take in reacting to both their aging and their illness:

Hypervigilance promoted by the rat race image of life can calm down to normal alertness. . . . Sexual attitudes and activities can become more relaxed—often with the effect of greater enjoyment and purer pleasure. Neuroticism tends to diminish with aging . . . and every diminution of a defense yields a quantum of energy that can now be put to freer use. (Pruyser, 1975, p. 114)

The psychosocial consequences of illness can either promote or deteriorate the developmental process that is ongoing with any aged person. Perhaps for the first time in the course of his or her life, the aged cardiopulmonary patient is psychologically capable of pursuing and enjoying a varied set of major activities and roles that provide a sense of self-worth, enjoyment, and meaning in life. Even if physical limitations prohibit varied activities of daily living, the aged patient may experience enhanced psychologic integration. Developmental psychologist Erik Erikson (1968) theorized that, starting around the age of 70, the individual is compelled to achieve psychological integrity. The developmental tasks that characterize this stage of growth include reviewing one's life decisions, accepting one's life as it was and is, and the development of pride in oneself and one's accomplishments in life. If all goes well, the aged person can bless his or her own life and, through that blessing, be able to accept the inevitability of death. This integration can enable the aged patient to engage in a direct, active, emotionally gratifying manner with the people and events that fill daily life. If this form of integrity does not occur, despair and the resort to more primitive psychological coping mechanisms results. For the despairing patient, aging and the losses associated with illness can reactivate narcissistic preoccupation with self, resulting in exaggerations of premorbid personality tendencies that make medical management very difficult (Erikson, 1968; Vaillant, 1977).

As they age, men and women tend to become more similar than dissimilar: Men become more receptive to affiliative and nurturant promptings, and women more responsive to and less guilty about aggressive and egocentric impulses. As they age, both "move toward more egocentric, self-preoccupied positions and attend increasingly to the control and satisfaction of personal needs" (Wolinsky, 1990, p. 36). Such attitudes can serve the recovering cardiopulmonary patient well, if channeled into an "I deserve to take better care of myself" perspective.

PSYCHOSOCIAL PERSPECTIVES ON AGING

It is only when physical and/or mental health fail that we see the changes more commonly associated with old age. Many individuals who live to an advanced age end up living in complex family systems. It has been estimated that by the year 2020, the typical family will consist of at least four generations, and that by 2040, nearly a quarter of the American population will be 65 and older. One out of three persons over the age of 65 has a living parent, and approximately 94% of people age 65 and over have family members (American Association of Retired Persons & the U.S. Department of Health and Human Resources, 1986; Hooyman & Lusbader, 1986).

Of those people aged 65 and over who have children, approximately 80% live less than an hour away from at least one child. It well may be the case that middle-generation women will spend more years with parents over 65 than with their children under 18, and that a far higher percentage of these aging adults will need hands-on and financial aid from their middle-aged children as they face a mix of rising health care and living costs and increased financial vulnerability. Currently, one out of three individuals over the age of 65 has a living parent, and one-third of adult child caregivers are aged themselves (Goldberg, 1992; Shanas, 1979; Simmons & Tiley, 1990).

IMPLICATIONS FOR TREATING AGED PATIENTS

These observations set the backdrop for a number of considerations that should be kept in mind in treating aged cardiopulmonary patients. First, note that the developmental action that characterizes the aging process creates special psychological needs for aging patients that can prove to be quite conducive to promoting a positive response to illness. The aged are developmentally predisposed to slow down, integrate the meaning of their experiences, reach out to others in new ways, and adjust their lifestyle to promote more biopsychosocial healthiness. They are also in need of an audience to whom they can tell their story and, in this telling, develop an integration of their life experiences. In short, these people are prime candidates for formal participation in cardiopulmonary rehabilitation, rich with its biopsychosocial emphasis (Hodgkin et al., 1993; Paine & Make, 1986).

Packa et al. (1989) called attention to the fact that, in addition to enhancing cardiopulmonary fitness, participation in a formal rehabilitation program may offer the elderly patient a significant degree of much-needed personal and social benefit that differs from that noted in younger populations. These authors presented data indicating that such participation leads to clear psychological and physiological benefits for most aged cardiac patients.

Unfortunately, relatively few elderly cardiopulmonary patients are referred for participation in formal cardiopulmonary rehabilitation programs. When they are referred, the aged cardiopulmonary population fares quite well; they generally show high levels of adherence to exercise training and to instructions in risk reduction. Most importantly, elderly men and women (over age 70) have been found to demonstrate responses to exercise training comparable to those of their youthful (below age 70) counterparts (Ades & Grunvald, 1990; Lavie et al., 1993; Williams, 1994).

Second, it is important to bear in mind the reference group to which your patient may be comparing him- or herself. Sensitivity to this issue tends to occur reflexively when treating young patients; it is assumed that part of the psychosocial distress being experienced by a young patient is questioning "Why me? My peers do not have these kinds of health problems." When an aged patient presents, we tend to erroneously assume that he or she is immune to this form of peer comparison. The data cited above suggest that most aged people know other aged people who are quite vibrant and reasonably healthy. The fact that many cardiac and most COPD patients have begun experiencing serious impairments in functioning at a relatively early age may blatantly and painfully distinguish them from their peers.

Finally, the longevity statistics cited above also raise an important psychosocial concern regarding the family systems of our patients. It is highly probable that the primary source of social support for any aged cardiopulmonary patient will be his or her grown offspring. Many of these grown children will be facing their own aging and health-related issues, a fact that can complicate reactions to cardiopulmonary illness for all members of the family system. An aged parent's physical deterioration may stir irrational fears or unresolved, painful dynamics within the aged, adult-child caregiver. For example, adult-child caregivers often report fears of their own mortality, of their own dependency needs, or of their own aging process (Wolinsky, 1990). Such fears may lead the distressed grown child to reject the role of caretaker for the elder. This is a bona fide problem in the contemporary health care system, given that the family system continues to supply approximately 80% of the hands-on care for the elderly frail (Lebowitz, 1978).

Even if they manage to escape the complexity of depending upon their children for physical or financial care, aged cardiopulmonary patients are likely to have their well-being affected by the developmental dramas that typify family relationships in the later stages of the family life cycle. Basically, aged parents and their offspring experience a renewal of the need to resolve issues of closeness/distance and individuation/separation. As old age is approached, even the most historically uninvolved parent tends to gravitate toward connection with family as a way of making amends, of connecting with his or her history, or simply out of loneliness and fear (Erikson, 1968; Levinson, 1978).

This can create a tremendous conflict for a middle-aged adult who has settled into a comfortable closeness or distance from his or her aged parent. Discomfort can come from changing this closeness/distance balance in either direction. Moving closer to a parent who is leaving as they age is likely to create a life crisis, either of a complex psychological sort (i.e., grieving) or a complex logistical sort (i.e., providing tangible assistance). On the other hand, moving away from aging parents as they experience illness or approach death is at least stressful and is sometimes heartbreaking.

At minimum, we should be sensitive to the complexities that come with aging while delivering care to our cardiopulmonary patients. Whether the patient is 45 or 75 years old, he or she is likely to be impacted, either personally or on a family level, by the factors outlined above. A number of specific strategies helpful in treating the aged follow, borrowing largely from the work of Anderson (1988).

- With aged patients, ask about their physical proximity to their children and grandchildren, bearing in mind the family developmental dramas outlined above, and the discussion of family issues in chapter 8. Ask young to middle-aged patients whether their parents are still living. If so, assume that caring for or concern about their parents is a major stressor in their lives. Useful references for such patients are *Parentcare Survival Guide: Helping Your Folks Through the Not-So-Golden Years* (Pritikin & Reece, 1993) and *Helping Your Aging Parents: A Practical Guide for Adult Children* (Halpern, 1987).

- Where appropriate, actively solicit the cooperation of grown children of aged patients. At minimum, a brief contact with another person who is a grown child actively involved in caring for an aged parent can encourage your patient's children to help in implementing your medical recommendations for their father or mother.

- When first getting to know an aged patient, take extra time gathering historical information. Remember, the aged make contact by reminiscing and by disclosing often painful information about themselves. A little bit of extra time spent in the initial phase of assessment can pay dividends in establishing rapport.

- Be respectful of elders. Taking a "one-down" position while gathering information conveys respect of the fact that your patient draws on a lifetime of experiences when deciding how to react to current challenges, including the challenges of illness and of dealing with you. Validate and confirm the coping patterns your patients have developed over the years, and avoid patented interventions that challenge and provoke. When it comes to making sense of their lives, the aged develop their own versions of "protective grooves," and these are to be respected, not stripped, as we try to help them change.

- Offer softer, more philosophical messages. Appealing to the "wisdom of the elders" is a positive and powerful frame of reference in validating what is important to the aged: protection, caring and nurturance. This strategy can also motivate an aging patient to implement rehabilitation recommendations. Examples of how this might be done follow:

    "We both know that a lot of what you are facing simply comes with age. But I want you to know that a lot can be done to help you cope with some of the 'givens' about aging. For example, by practicing these flexibility exercises, you can learn to protect yourself from the dangers of falling and breaking bones—a fear that you mentioned in your self-assessment questionnaire."

    "I appreciate that you have lived long enough to know what is and is not so important in life, and that one of the things that truly matters to you is staying healthy enough to be able to keep living independently. I also know that you worry about what will happen to your spouse if your own health fails. By following the recommendations we will give you about exercise and diet, I think you will find that you will bolster your ability to take care of your self and your spouse."

- Where possible, treat the aged on their own turf. The aged appreciate the familiar, and learning new coping skills within their most familiar contexts is a way of improving self-efficacy for activities of daily living. Home-based care for recovering cardiopulmonary patients will become progressively more important and timely as the aged population grows.

- Speak openly about the wisdom of growing beyond the ethic of individualism that pervades earlier stages of life. Older patients are soothed by normalizing their need for help and support. Emphasize that it is a sign of healthy aging to accept one's need for social support of the sort that comes from formal rehabilitation; family support from spouse, grown children, extended family, and surrogate family; and church or community involvements.

- Touch them. My clinical experiences have poignantly underscored a frequent pain in the lives of many aged individuals: As they age, they gradually stop receiving physical affection. My interviews with aged cardiac patients over the past seventeen years have consistently documented that one of the most appreciated and motivating aspects of participation in our cardiac rehabilitation program is the appropriate, friendly physical affection given to our patients by staff. This most often takes the form of a simple pat on the back, handshake, affectionate hug, or reassuring touch. For many patients, these are the only caring touches they receive in the course of a typical day or week. It is noteworthy that of the thousands of patients who have received such care in our program, sexually inappropriate responses from patients have been extremely rare.

- Help the aged accept the inevitable. Effective cardiopulmonary care of the aged most often entails helping them accept the inevitability of the progression of their illnesses, and always involves helping them accept the inevitability of diminished functioning (at least to some degree) as they age. Unlike younger populations, the aged might be motivated not so much by hope for change as by the hope of being able to more fully enjoy each remaining day of life.

- Remember that the aged remain quite capable of learning. The onus is on the health care provider to present relevant information in a manner appropriate to the aged person's learning style. Here, note that research has shown that most aged patients learn better from material that is presented auditorially, not visually (Yesavage & Karasu, 1982).

- Beware of ageism in delivering medical care. In a recent thought-provoking article, Rowe and Kahn (1987) reviewed a wealth of literature suggesting that age does not necessarily account for many of the physical and emotional struggles that we stereotypically associate with aging. The authors urge recognition of the fact that "successful aging" is mediated by factors such as support, enhancement of the patient's sense of control, exercise, management of health behaviors, and interventions that promote adaptive attitudes and coping skills in facing the challenges that come with aging. A burgeoning literature has documented that human beings remain capable of adaptive coping throughout their lives.

Unfortunately, many health care providers do not realize that the aged can change adaptively. Many assume that problems like depression, substance abuse, memory loss, and extended grieving are inevitable correlates of aging. Failure to accurately diagnose or treat such conditions can lead to increased morbidity and mortality in the aged. For example, it has been estimated that while one third of visits to physicians by the elderly include presentation of clear symptoms of depression that are accurately diagnosed by the consulting physician, only 10% of such patients are treated or referred for treatment of depression. This unchecked depression accounts for many of the supposed givens about aging, such as withdrawal, diminished cognitive abilities, increased anxieties, and somatic preoccupations (MacDonald, 1986). Furthermore, while substance abuse (defined as habitual substance use to the point of interfering with memory, sleep, emotional functioning, or cognitive abilities) occurs in 21-25% of medically ill older patients, it is accurately diagnosed only 37% of the time (compared to accurate diagnosis in 60% of younger patients) (Kemp, 1993).

It is also clear that the aged are quite responsive to psychosocial interventions when they are offered. Many supposedly demented aged patients with documented memory loss are able to significantly improve memory functions with appropriate cognitive and memory training (Schaie & Willis, 1986). In addition, when compared to non-treated controls, recently widowed patients have shown significant diminishment in mortality rates following participation in relatively brief, supportive grief counseling groups (Raphael, 1977).

Clearly, discounting the coping capabilities of the aged when delivering cardiopulmonary care is unwise, unnecessary, and inhumane.

CONCLUSIONS

Age is one of the few universals that face the patients we treat. Bearing in mind the individual and family-level dramas and opportunities that come with aging can enhance your ability to match interventions to relevant concerns and challenges that fill your patients' lives.

SUMMARY

For many, the adjustments faced when living with COPD and when aging obviously overlap. Both processes involve progressive diminishment in functioning and escalating tensions in family relationships. When treating both COPD and aged patients, special care should be taken to inquire regarding the patient's unique reactions to the challenges that come with his or her condition or age. Respectfully acknowledging awareness of the complexity of such issues—even if you do not personally struggle with the same—can go a long way in establishing and maintaining rapport with aged or COPD patients, an essential ingredient in formulating and implementing effective psychosocial interventions. An integrative discussion of both general and specific strategies for devising psychosocial interventions for these and other cardiopulmonary patients will close this book.

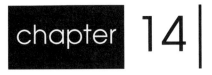

chapter 14

IMPROVING ADHERENCE
AND STRUCTURING INTERVENTIONS

The importance of getting patients to participate responsibly in their rehabilitation is becoming ever more urgent as the health care system increases its focus on outcomes. Unfortunately, nonadherence is a major problem in several areas that are crucial in the management of heart and lung illnesses.

Item 1: As time progresses throughout the first year of intervention, participants in formal rehabilitation programs drop out in steadily increasing numbers. Approximately 20% to 25% of patients drop out of formal participation in cardiac rehabilitation within the first 3 months, and 40% to 50% drop out between 6 and 12 months. Dropout rates then remain relatively flat for the next 3 or 4 years (Oldridge, 1988), but by some estimates, approximately 80% of patients drop out of formal rehabilitation within 48 months (Oldridge, 1982, 1984). In addition, dropout rates for lifestyle adjustment programs other than exercise also average 50% (Comoss, 1988).

Item 2: Despite the well-publicized fact that tobacco consumption is the single most preventable cause of death in the United States today, as recently as 1990, 46.3 million Americans identified themselves as smokers (American Lung Association, 1994; Guba & McDonald, 1993).

Item 3: Convincing evidence exists that dietary and medication interventions for controlling risk factors such as hypertension, obesity, and diabetes can decrease morbidity and mortality from CHD (Canner et al., 1986; Hjerman, Holme, Velve, Byer, & Leren, 1981). Yet it has been estimated that, on average, 50% of patients treated for chronic conditions such as obesity, hypertension, and diabetes do not follow treatment recommendations (Haynes, 1976a, 1979). The National Heart, Lung, and Blood Institute (1982) has specifically cautioned that the majority of patients do not take hypertensive medications as prescribed.

Item 4: It has been reported that only one-fourth to one-third of medical patients fully adhere to treatment recommendations (Sackett & Haynes, 1976). Approximately the same percentages of cardiac and pulmonary patients do not do so, and the remainder follow recommendations to varying degrees, depending upon the patient's—not the health care provider's—beliefs about what constitutes appropriate and necessary treatment.

THE CONSEQUENCES OF NONADHERENCE

The costs of nonadherence are formidable. For example, Psaty, Koepsell, Wagner, LoGerfo, & Inui (1990) reported that hypertensive patients who comply with beta-blocker treatment 100% of the time decrease the odds of having a cardiac event by one-half compared to those who take their medication between 80% and 99% of the time. Patients who comply less than 80% of the time have four times the risk of a cardiac event compared to those who take their medicines 100% of the time as prescribed. Similarly, the Beta-Blocker Heart Attack Trial Research Group (1982) found that a little bit of difference in compliance goes a long way in diminishing mortality: Patients who took more than 75% of prescribed medications (propranolol or placebo) evidenced a 2.2% mortality rate compared to a mortality rate of 5.4% for those taking 75% or less of prescribed medications (Horwitz et al., 1990).

Obviously, the stakes in this area of health care are quite high. Much of the published data regarding adherence might lead one to conclude that considerable amounts of the energy spent educating and caring for cardiopulmonary patients is being wasted. Fortunately, there is a brighter side to this picture. Some evidence suggests that even brief participation in formal rehabilitation programs seems to promote lasting changes in health behaviors such as exercise. In a noteworthy study, Daltroy (1985) investigated patients in a cardiac rehabilitation setting and found that, although less than 10% of patients were attending supervised sessions at 11 months, 78% reported exercising on their own. It may be that many so-called dropouts from supervised health-enhancement programs are implementing behavior changes in other locations more convenient or preferable to the patient (Oldridge & Spencer, 1985). Although many such patients may not be exercising at rates or intensities that would occur if participation in formal rehabilitation had continued, it is interesting to consider their plight in light of recent evidence of the efficacy of lower intensity exercise in improving aerobic capacity and safeguarding cardiovascular health (Blumenthal et al., 1988; Goble et al., 1991; Rechnitzer, Pickard, Paivio, Yuhasz, & Cunningham, 1972).

Also noteworthy is the fact that most professionals working in rehabilitation settings can readily identify a subset of patients who could be labeled "super adherers"—patients who have served as the social backbone for the rehabilitation program. For example, at the Wake Forest Cardiac Rehabilitation Program, we have a subset of patients who have been religious attenders and stalwart adherers since the outset of the program in 1976. An intriguing question for future researchers: If upwards of 80% of patients drop out of supervised rehabilitation programs within 12 months, shouldn't these be considered the normal patients? On the other hand, what motivates the

statistically "abnormal" patient who continues formal participation in rehabilitation beyond 1 year? What characterizes these "chronic attenders"? What
are the pros and cons of this orientation?

THE COMPLEXITY OF THE PROBLEM

I hope that the point of these last statements is obvious: In treating cardiopulmonary patients, it seems inappropriate to define *success* or *adherence* in
narrow terms. Harkaway and Madsen (1989) pointed out that the very
language of the compliance literature makes such a mistake. This literature
is filled with terms such as "noncompliers," "defaulters," "unmotivated,"
"lacking in willpower," "self-destructive," and the like in describing patients
who do not respond to the health care provider's notions regarding effective
treatment. Applying such negative and personalized connotations to noncompliance ignores several crucial facts.

First, despite the historical bent to blame difficulties in treatment on the
patient's "uncooperative personality," research in this area has consistently
failed to identify any demographic or personality characteristics per se that
definitively relate to compliance (Haynes, 1976a, 1979). Second, blaming
patients for treatment difficulties ignores the shared responsibility of the
family/treatment system in promoting treatment outcomes, a notion that
will be more fully discussed in the following pages.

Finally, Oldridge and Pashkow (1993) reminded us that, although some
compliance problems have to do with the patient not achieving reasonably
specified goals or not following reasonably explained procedures, not all
noncompliance problems have to do with an uncooperative patient resisting
our well-designed advice. For example, some patients evidence high degrees
of adherence but fail to attain desired goals. Others evidence low behavioral
adherence but manage to achieve rehabilitation goals due to underestimation
of their beginning functional status.

Based on these facts, observations, and speculations, I propose a lenient
frame of reference in assessing adherence in cardiopulmonary rehabilitation
settings. We need to structure our programs to educate and, to the extent
possible, shape our patients to ensure maximal generalization of the positive
effects of our treatments. Also, from the outset of rehabilitation we should
perhaps normalize that the patient is likely to participate for only 3 to 6
months. Doing so would prophylactically soothe any feelings of failure that
the patient might harbor when he or she does discontinue formal rehabilitation. In this way, the patient is more likely to leave our direct tutelage with
enhanced self-esteem, a crucial factor in promoting the self-efficacy that is
an indisputable key in maintaining lasting modification of health behaviors.
This point is demonstrated in the following excerpt from one of my counseling sessions with a cardiac patient who consulted me in my private practice
14 months after dropping out of participation in our cardiac rehabilitation
program at Wake Forest University.

WMS: "Hey, John. I remember you from the WFU program. How are you?"

John: "Well, if I was great I wouldn't be coming to see a 'shrink' like you, would I?" [laughing]

WMS: "I guess not; I know that I sure wouldn't come to see me unless I had to." [more laughter] "What can I do for you?"

John: "Well, I just thought I needed a stress management 'tune-up.' Nothing major is wrong, but I remember you talking about something you called 'stress-related depression' in one of the lectures out at WFU when I was in the program. I think that might be happening with me."

WMS: "You've got a good memory. I'm glad you paid attention to the lecture."

John: "Hell, yeah, I paid attention! I was scared half to death when I started that program. You guys really did help me—even if I did become another B-D-D-O."

WMS: "A what? A 'B-D-D-O?'"

John: [laughing] "Yeah. That's what we used to joke about—we patients; who's going to be the next B-D-D-O—Big Damn Drop-Out. We all knew that you guys seemed to take it personally when someone stopped coming to the program. The joke was if you became a B-D-D-O, you'd better not go to any of Wake Forest's ball games, because half of the rehab staff would be there and they'd look at you with that hurt look in their eyes."

WMS: "John, I've been working in that program for 17 years and I had no idea about this."

John: "That's because we didn't want to hurt your feelings. We all knew what a 'sensitive type' you are." [laughing]

WMS: "Now that's true. You're crushing my feelings right now, and after all I've done for you, John. . . . all the worrying, and advising, and encouraging. . . . this is my reward?" [laughing]

John: "No joke, I did get a lot out of the program. But after about 5 months, I don't know, I just decided it was time to test my wings on my own."

WMS: "Well, that's understandable. How have you done on your own?"

John: "Not bad, actually. Not perfectly, but pretty well. I exercise at least twice a week, usually more. And I monitor my heart rate the way the guys at the program taught me to when I do exercise. I do a lot of things I learned out there. Hell, I can't even smell a baked dessert without picturing that little woman nutritionist

> from WFU, Julie, looking at me with those schoolteacher eyes of hers. I'm not in the rehab program anymore, but I carry all of you guys around in my head. My head is filled with pictures of you all—Dr. Miller, Don, Dr. Ribisl, Dr. Brubaker, Dr. Rejeski, Julie, and that nice nurse, JoAnn—even you."

WMS: "Whew! That's a pretty ugly crew to have floating around in your head. No wonder you came to see a 'shrink.' " [laughter]

OVERVIEW OF
MODELS AND THEORIES OF ADHERENCE

Of course, many adherence problems are more serious than the circumstance described above. Nonadherence can lead to life-threatening consequences. What is to be done, then? In cases where blatant nonadherence is occurring, such as when patients are not taking medications as prescribed, the difficulty can be viewed from a variety of perspectives, four of which are elaborated below. Over 200 variables have already been identified in the literature as relating to adherence (or compliance) (Dracup & Meleis, 1982). Depending upon the theoretical model used, recommendations for ways to improve adherence vary.

THE MEDICAL MODEL

In the medical model, the provider has an active role and the patient or recipient has a passive role. Here noncompliance is assumed to be due to characteristics of the patient alone. Research has shown that, indeed, physicians tend to think of adherence from the medical model perspective: They are highly likely to focus on the patient in their explanations of nonadherence (Ross & Phipps, 1986). As a result, the medical model negates the importance of relationships—between the patient and his or her support system and between the patient and the health care provider—in affecting adherence (Dracup & Meleis, 1982).

THE HEALTH BELIEF MODEL

The Health Belief Model (Becker, 1979) introduced earlier emphasizes that interactions between the patient's and the provider's beliefs are especially important in determining adherence. This model is supported by research with cardiac patients which has demonstrated that communication between providers and patients that facilitated the patient's involvement in clinical decision making also led to improved patient satisfaction, patient adherence, and outcomes of treatment.

Sackett and Haynes (1976) pointed out that this model may be flawed by the lack of clarity about a crucial factor: Does change in adherence behavior precede or follow change in the patient's health beliefs? It may be that adherence is a cause, not an effect, of health beliefs, as suggested by the model. In addition, the Health Belief Model ignores the importance of the beliefs of the patient's family and social system in interaction with the factors specified above (Dracup & Meleis, 1982).

CONTROL THEORY

Control theory rests upon Rotter's seminal work regarding the concept of internal-external locus of control (Rotter, 1972). This theory poses that an individual falls somewhere along a continuum from believing that he or she is directly in control of his or her own life (internal locus) to believing that he or she has little or no control (external locus).

The effect of locus of control on motivation to take charge of health behaviors has been the focus of considerable research. It is generally suggested that internally oriented people are more likely to engage in behaviors that promote physical well-being and adhere to therapeutic regimens than those who are externally oriented (Dracup & Meleis, 1982).

SOCIAL LEARNING THEORY

Social learning theory focuses on two questions: how new behaviors are acquired, and once acquired, how their expression is affected by the interplay of internal and external forces (Bandura, 1977b; Jenkins, 1987). Bandura (1977b) theorized that new behaviors can be acquired through modeling. Furthermore, health behavior is said to be maintained through two processes: (a) through associative learning, a certain action becomes associated with cues or triggers that maintain that behavior; and (b) through operant learning, rewards and reinforcements associated with the behavior serve to perpetuate the behavior. Social learning theory has led to a focus on patients' self-efficacy (discussed earlier) in efforts to change health behaviors (Bandura, 1984).

Despite the fact that social learning theory emphasizes that modeling is important in determining health outcomes, approaches to enhancing adherence behavior based upon this theory have been criticized as "placing little emphasis on the quality of the interaction in which communication takes place, the characteristics of the health professional involved, or the social settings where information is communicated or where the prescription is (or is not) followed" (Dracup & Meleis, 1982, p. 32). In this manner, social learning theory essentially ignores the effect of the environment and the patient's significant others on adherence behaviors.

SYSTEMIC APPROACHES

Systemic approaches to adherence have attempted to overcome the objection that, to varying degrees, each of the previously discussed models overly focuses on the internal operations of the individual patient (i.e., the medical model, control theory) or on too limited a social field (i.e., social learning theory). The systemic approach has been elucidated by a number of authors who have posed that patients, their families, and health care providers need to be seen as sharing responsibility for responses to medical input (e.g., Dracup & Meleis, 1982; Harkaway & Madsen, 1989; McDaniel, Hepworth, & Doherty, 1992; Stein & Pontious, 1985). Accordingly, the focus of the systemic approach is on relationships: between patient and health care providers; between patient and his or her family; and between the family and health care providers. Doherty and Baird (1983) introduced the concept of "the health-care triad" that is formed between patient, family, and physician and emphasized the importance of focusing on the family system as the unit of intervention.

HARKAWAY AND MADSEN'S SYSTEMIC APPROACH

Harkaway and Madsen (1989) recommended a broadening of systemic thinking by presenting a model that incorporates many of the tenets from the various schools of thought outlined above. Here nonadherence is examined in the context of the family/treatment system. Within this model, the health care professional is viewed as a participant rather than as an observer (or victim), or as someone who must simply intervene to influence the patient or family. Harkaway and Madsen recommended use of the term *problematic treatment* in place of such terms as *nonadherence* or *noncompliance*. The implication of this switch in terminology is that "treatment difficulties occur in the context of interactions rather than existing as characteristics of the individual patient or family or, for that matter, of the health-care professional" (p. 44).

Harkaway and Madsen proposed that a true understanding of adherence requires a close examination of beliefs that drive the attitudes and behaviors of each member of the family/treatment system. Specifically, these authors emphasized four areas of beliefs that interplay in affecting adherence: (a) beliefs about the problem, (b) beliefs about the treatment of the problem, (c) beliefs about the role of the professional, and (d) beliefs about the role of the family.

Beliefs About the Problem

When a patient is not following a rehabilitation recommendation, several questions regarding beliefs about the problem of concern should be considered. First, it is important to clarify the definition of the targeted concern: Is the symptom of concern being defined as a problem? If not, how is the symptom being defined? Further, for whom and in what ways do these definitions apply. Harkaway and Madsen caution that it may be a mistake to assume that a patient's presence in the office represents a request for change. This assumption frequently conflicts with the assumptions of the patient or of the family system.

It is also important to clarify the various definitions of etiology within the family/treatment system. These definitions will influence how and if attempts are made to manage the problem. For example, some research has suggested that patients who view their health problems as being due to genetics may be less likely to commit to making behavioral changes than those who believe that the problem is due to poor health habits (Harkaway & Madsen, 1989).

Beliefs about volition also affect reactions to illness or to treatment interventions. These beliefs shape factors such as willpower and personal control of behavior. Of importance here is whether members of the family/treatment system believe that management of the problem is within or not within the patient's control. As pointed out by Harkaway and Madsen, differences within the family/treatment system in this area of belief can lead to escalating conflicts: "If part of the system insists that the problem is volitional and the patient insists it is not, the two can escalate their positions, each trying to prove a point to the other" (p. 47).

Idiosyncratic and special meanings within the family/treatment system can have profound effects on adherence. To demonstrate this point, Harkaway and Madsen presented the case study of a 380-pound 16-year-old boy whose family was concerned about his elevated blood pressure but proud of his weight. The pride in obesity was a family emotional legacy: A family "star" was a cousin who was renowned for being listed in a book of records as being the fattest man in the world.

Also crucial are the idiosyncratic meanings that the health care professional holds, either about the illness being treated or the intervention itself. These beliefs can directly affect interaction with the patient. It may be that the professional has had negative personal experiences with the problem at hand that affect his or her reactions to the patient's struggle with a similar problem. For example, the provider's response to an alcoholic, obese patient might be affected by his or her personal pains over having had an alcoholic parent or an overweight spouse, or a personal failure to control his or her own alcohol use or dietary behaviors. The professional might also be harboring frustrations from previous attempts to treat such patients with similar problems. Such personal experiences can lead either to blame or to conflict with the patient, or to a stirring of compassion to such a degree that the professional fails to assess the patient's and family's unique reactions. In this latter instance, the provider's lack of appropriate therapeutic distance and perspective on the patient may lead to the attitude, "I have struggled with this before myself, so I know how you feel without having to ask about your unique experience."

Beliefs About the Treatment

As has been demonstrated, any member of the family/treatment system can harbor beliefs about treatment that affect adherence. These can take several forms. First are beliefs about the effectiveness of treatment. Based upon past experiences or simply upon information, the patient, significant others, and/ or the professional will have either an enhanced or a diminished faith in the likelihood that treatment will help alleviate the targeted concern. Such experiences and biases will also color beliefs about what constitutes appropriate treatment. Harkaway and Madsen (1989) observed that "different members of the patient/treatment system may hold divergent beliefs about what should be done, and the conflict about appropriate therapy may block effective treatment" (p. 48).

Beliefs About the Role of the Health Care Professional

How is the relationship between the health care provider and the patient and his or her family to be structured? Will the provider be authoritarian—in control and directing—while the patient and family assume a passive stance? Will the provider offer guidance and the patient and family respond with grateful cooperation? Or will their be mutual participation in decision making and shared assumption of responsibility for decisions that affect the course of treatment and for the outcomes of these decisions?

Harkaway and Madsen (1989) again point out that personal experiences and biases on the part of any member of the family/treatment system will shape assumptions about the nature of the relationship among the provider, the patient, and the family, and these assumptions may simply be incorrect. For example, a patient (and/or his or her loved ones) may simultaneously manifest attitudes of respect and mistrust of a health care provider, resulting in pseudocompliance by the patient: Although they behave with respect and deference to the professional, their distrust may lead to failure to implement the recommendations that are so respectfully being accepted.

Beliefs About the Role of the Family

Finally, Harkaway and Madsen (1989) emphasize the importance of beliefs about the role of the family in determining the family/treatment system's effect on adherence. Here beliefs can vary from the notion that the family had nothing to do with the illness etiology and will have nothing to do with its treatment to the notion that the family was integrally involved in "causing" the illness and must be integrally involved in its treatment. Some families view heath care providers as outsiders who are to be resisted as they care for their own. Other families abdicate their own power and responsibility when faced with the challenges that come with having an ill member, turning to the health care provider to cure their sick loved one. A professional who pushes a certain style of treatment without first ascertaining the family's beliefs on the issue runs the risk of getting into unnecessary struggles with the family.

Harkaway and Madsen (1989) caution that in applying their systemic approach, the crucial factor is the ways in which the beliefs of different members of the family/treatment system interact. It is more likely that difficulties in treatment stemming from divergent beliefs (whether intra-familial or between the family and the treatment systems) will occur when these differences are ignored, minimized, or denied.

Support of the Notion That Beliefs Affect Adherence

Although the Harkaway and Madsen (1989) paper was a purely theoretical discussion of adherence, their notion that beliefs affect adherence is strongly supported in the cardiopulmonary literature. For example, Miller and Wikoff (1989) found that, for first-MI males, disagreement between couple members regarding their shared and respective responsibilities in rehabilitation tasks significantly interfered with adherence. In other studies, the patient's perception of what others believe about their need to comply have been found to be predictors of compliance in a variety of areas relevant to cardiac rehabilitation (Miller, Wikoff, McMahon, Garrett, & Ringel, 1985, 1988). In addition, data exist to support the notion that the spouse's attitude toward exercise may be a more important determiner of the cardiac patient's own physical activity and participation in supervised exercise programs than the patient's attitude (Dishman, Sallis, & Orenstein, 1985).

Unfortunately, as stated earlier, researchers in this area have essentially ignored the effects of the interplay between beliefs of the health care provider and those of the patient and his or her family (Sotile, Sotile, Sotile, & Ewen, 1993). A noteworthy exception is the investigation of Bar-On and Cristal (1987), which examined 89 male MI patients, 60 of their spouses, and 45 of the patients' physicians to determine the effects on rehabilitation of differences in beliefs about what caused the MI and what needed to be done to cope with it. Patients and their spouses tended to agree on the assumed causes of the MI, regardless of the content of these assumptions (e.g., some couples assumed that the MI was caused by fate, others that the MI was caused by risk factors). However, the physicians consistently tended to assume that the illness was caused by risk factors. Unfortunately, the authors did not extensively investigate the interactive sequences between patient, family, and physician as they were affected by differences in beliefs (when such occurred) or the effects of such interactions on adherence.

IMPROVING ADHERENCE

What can be done to increase adherence with medical or rehabilitation recommendations? Several researchers have offered specific guidelines in this regard. The current approach to enhancing adherence revolves around four factors: (a) managing the partnership that exists between patient, family, and health care provider; (b) helping the patient develop a clear understanding of what is expected of him or her; (c) using a combination of adherence-enhancing strategies; and (d) facilitating overall psychosocial adjustment to rehabilitation for the patient and his or her loved ones.

Clearly, the communication process between patient and health care professional is the overriding factor affecting each of these four keys to enhancing adherence. But unfortunately the compliance literature (e.g., Oldridge & Pashkow, 1993) is filled with suggestions that provider-patient communication problems abound in clinical practice. These observations set the stage for the first category of recommendations regarding ways to bolster adherence.

FIRST, EVALUATE YOURSELF

Before focusing on the patient, evaluate yourself and your program. Ask:

Have your interventions matched the patient's reading or cognitive levels, learning styles, and current concerns? Most of these issues have been discussed in prior pages. Here it is reiterated that information may be presented prematurely or at inappropriate times, or in ways that mismatch the patient's learning styles and preferences. Bear in mind that some patients respond better to written material, others to material that is verbally presented; some prefer group interaction, others require individualized attention; some respond best to brief interventions, others to lengthy interventions. Effective programs tend to provide a menu of interventions. More keys to structuring interventions will be presented later in this chapter.

Also bear in mind the importance of matching interventions to the patient's goals. As Oldridge and Pashkow (1993) noted: "We frequently cannot motivate our patients to walk 1 mile to save their lives, but they will walk a hundred miles for a T-shirt" (p. 343).

Is the prescription appropriate in pursuing the stated goals? Does the issue of concern really need to change to promote health and well-being for this patient? Will the potential benefits of changing be worth the patient's efforts to change? Avoid the mistake that many health care providers make: We grow insensitive to the fact that most people find it difficult to change health behaviors. Compassionately help the patient choose which battles of this sort are worth facing at this time.

Does the patient understand what is being asked of him or her? Although you may be clear about what you are trying to convey, the patient's interpretations may lead to behavior quite different from your intention. Ask the patient and his or her loved ones to reflect back their understanding of your input, and keep communicating until their response is the one you intend.

Is your interaction with the patient rewarding desired change? Busy health care providers often skip a crucial step in effective communication:

They fail to give appropriate feedback or rewards for progress. Notice the patient, and comment on what is being done right, not solely on what he or she needs to change.

IDENTIFY PATIENTS AT RISK OF NONADHERENCE

A number of guidelines have been published (e.g., Rose & Robbins, 1993) for flagging cardiopulmonary patients who may be at high risk of having psychosocial factors interfere with adherence to rehabilitation prescriptions. What follows is a summary of these recommendations. It is important to underscore that adherence is a complex, multidetermined process. Family systems researcher Thomas Campbell has pointed out that "it is difficult to determine which factors correlated with compliance actually play a causal role" (Campbell, 1986, p. 164). With this caveat in mind, it is recommended that any patient who evidences a combination of the following characteristics be given special consideration for adherence-enhancing interventions:

- Patients who live alone
- The recently divorced or widowed
- The socially isolated
- Patients from multiproblem families
- Young, impoverished women
- Smokers
- Obese patients
- Patients who have multiple chronic illnesses
- Active substance abusers
- Patients who have cultural or religious values that work against the philosophy of self-reliance and optimism
- Patients who have impaired cognitive functioning
- Patients working in nonprofessional occupations
- Those with chronically low levels of activity
- Depressed or anxious patients
- Hypochondriacal patients
- Patients with chronic cough
- Patients with persistent chest pain
- Patients who evidence poor left ventricular function
- Patients with low ego strength
- The socially introverted

In a previously mentioned investigation of the causal attributions made by MI patients, their mates, and their physicians regarding their illness and rehabilitation, Bar-On and Cristal (1987) found that patients at high risk of struggling with the adaptive tasks of living with heart illness can be flagged with two questions: "Why did it happen to you?" and "What will help you cope with it?" Positive copers recognized the limitations and the need for help from the medical profession and family and were therefore more likely to be responsive to input. They also tended to assume that something they have done, not fate, caused the MI. On the other hand, patients and spouses who attributed their MI to external, uncontrollable causes evidenced poorer psychosocial adjustment.

Family members (especially spouses) at high risk of posthospital adjustment struggles should also be flagged and provided extra support. Shanfield (1990) suggested that wives of recovering male MI patients who are especially likely to have difficulty adjusting during the course of rehabilitation are those who are depressed, have preexisting psychiatric and marital problems, are younger in age (under age 65) and blue-collar in socioeconomic status, are psychologically dependent, and have diminished capacity to express feelings.

USE STRATEGIES FOR IMPROVING ADHERENCE

It should now be apparent that adherence is an outcome in a dynamic process. The rehabilitation tasks for individuals and their family members can differ drastically, as can those for inpatients, outpatients who have only recently been discharged from the hospital, and long-term outpatients. For this reason, enhancing adherence with medical treatments is an individualistic, sometimes idiosyncratic, matter (Miller et al., 1985). At different points in the course of rehabilitation, a given patient may need more or less structure, guidance, directive advice, monitoring, emotional support, tangible support, and so on (Rogers, 1987).

Below is a menu of options regarding adherence-enhancing strategies that have been suggested by research:

1. Structural programmatic changes, such as staggered start times (in formal programs) that allow for increased personal contact between staff and patients (Comoss, 1988).

2. Contingency management, such as pairing a reward with a desired health behavior (Stalonas, Johnson, & Christ, 1978).

3. Cueing strategies, such as leaving exercise apparel or equipment in sight (Rejeski & Kenney, 1988).

4. Cognitive strategies, such as distraction or reframing (Leventhal, Zimmerman, & Gutman, 1984).

5. Patient education (Mullen, Green, & Persinger, 1985).

6. Written behavioral contracts/goal setting (Martin & Dubbert, 1984; Oldridge & Jones, 1983).

7. Increasing the patient's sense of control.

8. Increasing encouragement and support from peers (Beneke & Paulsen, 1979).

9. Emphasizing the importance of and the expectation that the patient will receive family support in the form of:

   a. physical assistance, material aid, or resources;

   b. cooperation and participation in behavioral modification efforts;

   c. shared participation in an exercise program (Oldridge & Jones, 1986);

   d. an expressed positive attitude toward the medical treatment or rehabilitation program (Andrew et al., 1981).

10. Coaching the patient's family in how to provide verbal and emotional support (Doherty, Schrott, Metcalf, & Iasiello-Vailas, 1983; Sotile, Sotile, Ewen, & Sotile, 1993).

11. Use of diaries for self-monitoring (Rejeski & Kenney, 1988).

12. Use of telephone counseling (Daltroy, 1985).

13. Use of rewards (Thoresen & Coates, 1976).

14. Use of relapse prevention strategies (Marlatt, 1985).

15. Openly examining the beliefs held by the patient, by the patient's family, and by the rehabilitation specialist regarding the condition being treated, its etiology, and the respective roles of patient, provider, and family (Harkaway & Madsen, 1989).

16. Enhancing the patient's self-efficacy for making desired changes (O'Leary, 1985).

Regardless of the specific intervention used, the major goal of adherence-enhancing strategies is "to instill and strengthen patients' beliefs in both treatment effectiveness and their own abilities to effect positive changes in their health" (O'Leary, 1985, p. 448). As can be seen from this list, a wealth of options can facilitate this outcome. In clinical practice, multiple adherence-enhancing strategies should be used, usually consisting of some combination of cognitive/behavioral interventions or skill training and provision of tangible and emotional social support.

EXAMPLES OF MULTIPHASIC PROGRAMS TO ENHANCE ADHERENCE

Research in the areas of diet modification/weight reduction and behavioral control of hypertension provide pertinent examples of the importance of incorporating various adherence-enhancing strategies into intervention designs.

DIET MODIFICATION
AND WEIGHT-REDUCTION PROGRAMS

Considerable research has documented the effectiveness of multidisciplinary interventions geared toward lowering lipids, both with and without use of lipid-lowering drugs (e.g., DeBusk et al., 1994). In some instances, such interventions have also led to significant regression of coronary athero-sclerosis (i.e., Ornish et al., 1990; Schuler et al., 1992). Admittedly, several of the most publicized of these programs employed interventions that were far more intensive than is possible in many treatment settings (i.e., Karvetti & Hamalainen, 1993; Ornish et al., 1990; Schuler et al., 1992).

Well-controlled studies comparing various weight-reduction techniques with cardiopulmonary rehabilitation populations are lacking in the litera-ture—especially with reference to controlling such factors as pretreatment needs for weight loss and motivational levels for losing weight (Engblom et al., 1992). However, a wealth of potentially useful information in structuring dietary modifications and weight-reduction efforts with cardiopulmonary patients can be gleaned from this body of research. The most effective inter-ventions noted in the general literature on weight loss and dietary modifica-tions have typically combined some form of exercise training, behavioral counseling, and dietary instruction.

Carmody et al. (1982) pointed out that the principal factors shown to influence patient compliance both with medication and with behavioral prescriptions for lowering lipids have been the quality of the patient-doctor relationship; the amount of information the patient needs to learn about the disease and treatment; the complexity of the instructions or prescriptions offered to the patient; family support; social isolation; health beliefs that may conflict with treatment recommendations; and the cost/benefit ratio computed by the patient regarding the relative inconvenience versus benefits of adhering to treatment recommendations.

Carmody et al. (1982) further specified that primary prevention trials for modifying high-fat, high-cholesterol diets and promoting weight control have typically employed a combination of educational counseling, family-oriented interventions, and a wealth of individual and group behavioral modification strategies of the types listed above (e.g., reinforcement, model-ing, self-monitoring, stimulus control, contingency management), as well as educational counseling and family-oriented interventions. It has been shown that the most effective dietary modification programs employ variations of many of the strategies for enhancing overall adherence. With reference to dietary behavior, these include:

- self-monitoring of calories and eating patterns with an eye toward modest dieting,
- stimulus control,
- development of alternative behavioral responses to eating urges,
- changes in nutrition,
- involving the family of the patient in treatment,
- maintenance training and relapse prevention, and
- combining various of these strategies with regular physical exercise into a multicomponent program.

BEHAVIORAL CONTROL OF HYPERTENSION

Hypertension can be controlled if the patient will adhere to recommendations to take their medicines, control their body weight, and make needed changes in dietary choices and alcohol use (Hypertension Detection and Follow-up Program Cooperative Group, 1979, 1988). In addition, regular exercise has been shown to reduce blood pressure an average of 7 mmHg systolic and 4 mmHg diastolic (Hamalainen et al., 1989; Kallio et al., 1979). Given how controllable this illness typically is if treatment recommendations are followed, nonadherence by such patients can prove to be one of the more frustrating problems faced by cardiopulmonary specialists.

Self-management of hypertensives can be improved by interventions that target specific aspects of the biopsychosocial substratum that contributes to this problem. This can be accomplished through health education that simplifies the treatment regimen, and with interventions that enhance social support, self-monitoring, and stress management skills. Specific interventions described in the literature have included relaxation therapy (Johnston, 1985; McCaffrey & Blanchard, 1985) and interpersonal skill training geared to quieting the physiologic responses experienced during conflictual marital communication (Levenson & Gottman, 1983, 1985; Smith & Brown, 1991).

The importance of facilitating family support, and especially spouse support, in promoting adherence to antihypertensive regimens cannot be overemphasized (Sotile, Sotile, Ewen, & Sotile, 1993). Home visits that incorporate a conscientious effort by the home visitor to promote family support have been found to be profoundly effective in increasing adherence behaviors and decreasing incidences of morbidity and mortality in hypertensive patients. Storer et al. (1987) reported an amazing 90% hypertension control success rate in 2 years of follow-up of a family-based self-help group study conducted in rural Mississippi involving 1,700 subjects. The intervention involved educating a selected family member about blood pressure measurement and control strategies and having that family member conduct monthly family blood pressure monitoring and education sessions.

A landmark investigation of the effects of health education for hypertensive patients (Levine et al., 1979; Morisky et al., 1983) demonstrated the effectiveness of including a spouse in each home visit session given to a group of 400 hypertensive patients. Three educational interventions were compared. Educating a spouse led to an overall improvement in compliance and to a significant 65% increase in blood pressure control (versus a nonsignificant 22% increase in blood pressure control for patients who received standard care). Five-year follow-up also indicated a 57% reduction in mortality when various combinations of health education intervention were added to the usual care given to the hypertensive patient.

Such behavioral management strategies seem to be best suited to patients who are only mildly hypertensive, to those who are not on a pharmacological regimen, or as an adjunct to—not a replacement for—pharmacological and other nonpharmacological treatments (Hatch, Klatt, & Supik, 1985).

SUMMARY REGARDING ADHERENCE

In summary, it appears that many factors need to be considered in promoting adherence with our treatment and rehabilitation recommendations. We need to be clear about what we are selling, be certain that the patient understands what we are selling, and allow the patient to make an informed decision about the prescribed therapeutic regimen. In a nutshell: "Patients who are fully convinced both of the effects of the treatment and their abilities to carry out the regimen will be more likely to practice them faithfully" (O'Leary, 1985, p. 448).

Several decades of research have demonstrated that virtually all of the interventions discussed thus far in this chapter can, in some instances, be effective in promoting adherence; however, it is also true that research has failed to provide consistent evidence of the effectiveness of any single procedure in maintaining health behavior changes across various patient populations (Carmody et al., 1982). For example, studies of obese patients have shown that interventions that bolster perceptions of self-efficacy to manage food and body weight are particularly effective for individuals with an internal locus of control but not for those who view their behavior as externally controlled (Chambliss & Murray, 1979).

It remains for future researchers to discern the most effective intervention strategies for ensuring adherence by various personality types and various family constellations faced with various rehabilitation challenges. We also must be resigned to the fact that, because we are in the business of treating chronic illnesses that in some cases progress rapidly and diminish the quality of our patients' lives, patients will not always maintain motivation to make changes. Oldridge and Pashkow (1993) recommended that if no modifications can be made, we have two options: (a) Accept nonadherence and provide as much assistance as possible—change from a "curing" to a "caring" mode; or (b) withdraw our care.

Despite the aforementioned important point that the research has clearly shown that nonadherence with medical recommendations does not correlate with individual psychopathology, this literature does suggest a relationship between overall psychosocial adjustment and medical adherence. Recall, for example, that adherence has been shown to be affected by realistic acceptance and understanding of medical recommendations, marital and family support and involvement in treatment, and facility in using a range of psychosocial coping skills. It therefore seems logical that any effort to increase patient adherence should focus on the design, implementation, and assessment of creative approaches to enhancing patients' overall psychosocial adjustment. The remainder of this book presents a summary, integration, and expansion of the various guidelines for structuring such interventions.

STRUCTURING PSYCHOSOCIAL INTERVENTIONS: GENERAL GUIDELINES

The next two sections will offer a number of guidelines for structuring psychosocial interventions. Exploration of three broad concepts will set the backdrop against which eight specific recommendations for structuring interventions will be made. These recommendations are drawn from the integration of a broad research literature and my own clinical experiences (see Indexed Bibliography).

INCORPORATE PRACTICAL PSYCHOSOCIAL INTERVENTIONS FROM THE OUTSET OF CLINICAL CARE

It generally is agreed that intervention is best begun early, preferably before the patient enters the hospital or, in the case of emergency hospitalizations, before the patient leaves the CCU. In inpatient, outpatient, or rehabilitation settings, the stigma sometimes attached to seeking psychosocial help can be circumvented by framing psychosocial evaluation and services as natural, ongoing aspects of care.

Regarding this last issue, I recommend that you take an open, honest approach, exercising special care to show compassion, confidence, and forthrightness in underscoring the importance of attending to psychosocial concerns. Except in specialized treatment settings, psychosocial interventions with cardiopulmonary patients should incorporate supportive, concrete, didactic, nonexploratory approaches that do not resemble or bear the label of "psychotherapy." Gruen (1975) offered the very wise suggestion that in-hospital psychological consultation be framed as intervention from the "Department of Patient Care Improvement." Remember: Psychosocial care should always be framed in nonthreatening terminology.

Effective intervention can be provided in either group or individualized formats. In my opinion, no definitive data exist regarding any overall differential effectiveness of group versus individual treatments. Regardless of the treatment format, the tenets of behavior modification and behavior therapy have generally been used to structure psychosocial interventions with recovering cardiopulmonary patients. Even when dealing with personality-based coping patterns and family systems factors (two of the distinguishing features of the Effective Emotional Management model), actual advice and intervention with cardiopulmonary patients tends to follow these tenets.

BEHAVIOR MODIFICATION

As has been demonstrated throughout this book, behavior modification with cardiopulmonary patients is aimed at promoting self-control through such strategies as pairing reinforcement with desired behaviors, disrupting chains of maladaptive behaviors, and contracting. A typical behavior modification intervention might include a period of self-observation by the patient plus questions that help the patient identify circumstances and rewards that are positively reinforcing. The patient is then instructed in ways to contract with him- or herself to provide those rewards contingent upon the performance of a desired rehabilitation behavior such as exercising. Instructions in self-rewards often accompany this method of intervention (Atkins et al., 1984).

BEHAVIOR THERAPY

Preceding discussions have also demonstrated how behavior therapy approaches focus on skill-building, pattern disruption, and the establishment of new stimulus-response connections. Here patients are taught methods of behavior change such as contracting, cueing, eliciting social support, contingency management techniques for self-administration of reinforcers, and behavioral rehearsal of new, desired behavior patterns. The various smoking cessation interventions detailed in chapter 12 exemplify a number of behavior therapy techniques such as disrupting stimulus-response chains that lead to cigarette smoking by placing cigarettes in hard-to-find places; rehearsal of ways to manage the urge to smoke in certain high-risk situations by displacing smoking behavior with other, less costly behaviors; and so on. As will be shown in the following pages, such techniques can be effectively incorporated into brief interventions throughout various stages of recovery and rehabilitation and in treating various target behaviors.

STRUCTURING
PSYCHOSOCIAL INTERVENTIONS: SPECIFICS

A number of specific guidelines can also be followed in structuring psychosocial interventions. Of course, these should be modified to shape interventions that fit the patient's particular needs and the treatment setting.

PROVIDE MULTIPLE, BRIEF SESSIONS

Clinicians who work extensively with medical patients tend to agree that lengthy psychosocial interventions are often perceived as being burdensome and sometimes irrelevant to a patient who is in crisis. More effective is a treatment strategy that employs repeated, brief contacts with the patient during the crisis at hand. For example, Kendall et al. (1979) demonstrated the powerful effectiveness of repeated therapeutic contacts (three times in 2 days) in helping patients anticipating cardiac catheterization manage the stress of the procedure. These contacts should ideally be brief, supportive, and relevant to one of the patient's targeted, imminent concerns. Beyond the crisis point, repetition of psychosocial interventions remains important, given that salient issues shift as the course of rehabilitation unfolds.

TAILOR INTERVENTIONS
TO MEET THE PATIENT'S LEARNING STYLE

Interventions should not only match the patient's needs, they should also be tailored to the individual's learning style and reading level, bearing in mind that the reading level of the average American adult is between grades 6 and 8 (Connors & Hilling, 1993). Hoop and Maddox (1984) advised that retention of educational material can be significantly enhanced by employing audiovisual aids and multisensory stimuli that allow the patient to hear, see, feel, and do something related to what is being taught. In orienting the patient and his or her loved ones to events that will accompany upcoming medical or rehabilitation interventions and their sequence of occurrence, it is especially important to emphasize the anticipated sensory components of the intervention and immediate postintervention experience (Pimm & Feist, 1984). At their best, such interventions teach commonsense implications for better understanding and managing the physiological and emotional consequences of stress and do so in a manner that motivates the patient to change his or her style of managing (or mismanaging) stress. Both standard and slide-sound educational programs have been found to be effective in lessening anxiety and promoting health-enhancing behavior in hospitalized cardiopulmonary patients (Barbarowicz, Nelson, DeBusk, & Haskell, 1980) and in their spouses (Thompson & Meddis, 1990).

COMBINE STRATEGIES

As pointed out earlier when discussing adherence-enhancing strategies, it appears that the most powerful way to promote positive psychosocial adjustment is to use a combination of interventions. For example, research with heart patients has documented that combining relaxation training with coaching regarding effective coping strategies (Anderson, 1987) or with the provision of emotionally supportive counseling (Mumford et al., 1982) is a more effective intervention than simply providing presurgical education about surgery and the postoperative period. Leserman, Stuart, Mamish, and Benson (1989) demonstrated that a combined intervention consisting of a brief presurgical education session, written handouts, brief relaxation training, a taped recording of a relaxation procedure, and very brief daily encouragement from a nurse was successful in lowering the incidence of postoperative supraventricular tachycardia in cardiac patients.

Similar findings were reported by Pimm and Feist (1984), who found that supportive counseling paired with relaxation training led to a lower incidence of postoperative tachycardia following CABG and to reduced levels of depressed mood in the weeks following surgery. Combinations of relaxation induction, coping skills rehearsal, and presurgical teaching have been found to reduce complaints of pain, the need for analgesics, the incidence of postoperative complications, the length of hospital stays, levels of emotional distress, and the incidence of postoperative delirium for patients undergoing open heart surgery (Kendall & Watson, 1981; Mumford et al., 1982). In treating children undergoing cardiac catheterization, intervention combinations that included the use of puppet therapy, support, and education were found to enhance postprocedure behavioral, emotional, and medical adjustments (Cassell, 1965; Cassell & Paul, 1967). In addition, children exposed to these interventions were more willing to return to the hospital for postdischarge medical follow-up.

Combination interventions have also been used effectively in treating COPD patients. A home care program that included reconditioning, relaxation, and breathing exercises increased exercise tolerance and decreased symptom ratings of perceived dyspnea and muscle fatigue in a group of COPD patients (Strijbos, Koeter, & Meinesz, 1990). Ambrosino et al. (1981) demonstrated that combination approaches can have surprising effects with COPD patients. This study compared 23 patients who were treated with rehabilitation and medical therapy to a group of 28 control patients treated with medical therapy alone for 1 month. Intervention consisted simply of combined relaxation training with the teaching of slow breathing, diaphragmatic breathing, and pursed-lip breathing. No vital changes were noted in the control group, but the rehabilitation intervention significantly improved maximal exercise tolerance on cycle ergometer testing, enhanced efficiency of ventilatory patterns, and decreased respiratory rates and increased tidal volume. The most interesting aspect of the Ambrosino et al. study is that experimental subjects improved maximal exercise tolerance even though no specific exercise training was given as part of the treatment intervention.

Treatment programs with strong combined approaches to modifying psychosocial functioning of recovering cardiac patients have also been found to reduce 1- to 3-year mortality rates (Frasure-Smith & Prince, 1989; Friedman & Ulmer, 1984; Friedman et al., 1986) and to promote changes in CHD risk-factor status over a 12-month period (Lovibond et al., 1985). Such treatments typically employ realistic, short-term goal setting, education, detailed feedback regarding changes in specific coronary risk, follow-up, training in behavioral self-management procedures, and detailed self-monitoring of target behaviors. Such combination approaches have specifically proved effective in promoting smoking cessation, resumption of sexual activity, and return to work (Sallis, Flora, & Fortmann, 1981; Sivarajan et al., 1981).

IDENTIFY OBVIOUS AND SUBTLE STRESSORS

In addition to providing information, psychosocial interventions should help the targeted individuals to begin analyzing what thoughts, behaviors, and interpersonal or environmental factors might be important to control in facing their current stressors. As has been emphasized throughout this book, I believe that the major causes of stress are often obvious in our patients' lives and should never be overlooked for the sake of exploring esoteric psychological issues. A patient facing the terror of major surgery is not in need of psychoanalysis; he or she is in need of help in coping with the terror at hand.

However, in more extended treatment settings, patients often want help in understanding why they are distressed, given their perceptions that their life circumstances may no longer warrant crisis reactions. Here it is helpful to remember that we often overlook the "subtle" stressors that tend to fill contemporary life. Three strategies can be particularly helpful in identifying subtle stressors.

First, help the patient to quantify the number of major life transitions being dealt with. Brief, self-administered scales such as the Holmes-Rahe Social Readjustment Scale (Holmes & Rahe, 1967) can be used to underscore a variety of commonsense stress management points such as: life is a constant series of adaptations; stress is an inevitable correlate to adapting; and both positive and negative changes promote stress. If the patient reports a high level of transition-related stress, underscore this fact to motivate the patient to implement the stress management strategies being recommended.

Another method for specifying a subtle factor that serves as both a stress stimulus and a stress response is to have a patient keep a thought diary. This technique was explicitly demonstrated in chapter 9. The point of such a diary is to help the patient learn to recognize how certain thinking habits occur reflexively during stressful times and how these same thought patterns then stir further stress reaction.

Finally, patients often benefit from examining whether a subtle form of stress is coming from their living out of "position" with reference to this question: "When it comes to your personal values, are you living such that your behavior is aligned (more than less) with what you really think, feel, need, and want?" In the wake of illness, such existential questioning is often stirred on subtle levels and can be made explicit by having the patient complete a simple values inventory of the sort presented in Form 14.1.

Form 14.1 A Values Inventory

Instructions:

Read through the list of words that follows.

Next reread the list and check the three or four words that describe values that are important to you. Use as a guideline the notion: "If I could have only four of these factors in my life, and no more, I would choose these."

My values

Security	Acceptance
Status	Power
Being liked	Achievement
Approval	Service
Affection	Glamour
Belongingness	Wealth
Spirituality	Meaningful friendships
Family unity	Romance
Sex	Fortune
Fame	Protecting the environment
Contributing to humanity	

The point of this exercise comes in the clinical processing. Once the patient has responded, encourage him or her to examine exactly how he or she is living. Often, patients report that doing this exercise helps them pinpoint ways they are stressing themselves by not living in harmony with their values. This information can be quite potent in motivating patients to take advantage of the crisis of illness by redoubling their efforts to live in healthier, more balanced ways.

OPERATIONALIZE COPING STRATEGIES

Successful psychoeducational interventions ultimately help patients do two things, each of which contains two parts: (a) identify and stop maladaptive coping patterns; and (b) learn about and begin to use better coping strategies.

Maladaptive coping strategies can be gleaned from clinical interview data or from formal questionnaires. Simply inquiring "What tends to happen next?" while interviewing a patient regarding coping sequences can shed light on this issue. The following excerpt from a counseling session demonstrates this point.

WMS: "So, your concern is the fact that, as the week wears on, you get progressively more fatigued, and then you start to worry about your health?"

Patient (Pt.): "That's right."

WMS: "I'm interested in how this happens. When do you typically start to feel tired in the course of a week?"

Pt.: "I don't know. It varies. But I guess I'm pretty tired by the time most Wednesdays roll around."

WMS: "That's interesting. I wonder what usually happens in your life on Mondays and Tuesdays?"

Pt.: "Well, I do hit the ground running at the start of every week. That's for sure. In my business, new stock arrives every Monday at 4:30 a.m., so I get an early start on my week."

WMS: "That's a tough way to get going each week. What happens then?"

Pt.: "It depends on how much I get done on Monday. I usually have to work late into Monday evening to get the stock recorded and shelved."

WMS: "Is that so? How do you manage to get through those long days?"

Pt.: "I don't know, I just do it. Of course, that 'never-ending cup of coffee' helps."

WMS: "What happens after such a long day of work and coffee?"

Pt.: "I go home and don't sleep very well, that's what."

WMS: "So Monday is also a day that you typically skip your exercising."

Pt.: "Well, yeah. When would I have time to exercise?"

WMS: "So you work all day, drink coffee by the pot-load, go home, and don't sleep. Then what?"

Pt.: "Then Tuesday comes. That's usually a better day, except that I'm always sleepy."

WMS: "Coffee?"

Pt.: "What?"

WMS: "So you drink more coffee?"

Pt.: "Well, I guess I do. [laughs] At least a pot."

WMS: "So, does this mean another sleepless night?"

Pt.: "No, usually not. My wife and I go Western dancing every Tuesday evening. I dance until my feet hurt, and then I sleep like a baby. Of course, those 'few' beers I drink at the dance probably help. But I still wake up tired as a dog on most Wednesday mornings."

Such informal conversation was used to teach this patient about his coping sequences and the cause-and-effect relationships between these and the symptoms of concern. Pointing out the links between stress, lack of exercise, sleeplessness, excessive caffeine consumption, and eventual sedation with alcohol helped put the "mysterious" Wednesday-morning bouts of fatigue into more manageable perspective.

This is an example of the "disrupt the coping dominoes" principle that underlies the EEM model. This sort of pinpointing of coping sequences should lead to commonsense recommendations for ways to disrupt a maladaptive coping pattern.

In orchestrating such assessments, special care should be taken to flag maladaptive coping strategies such as substance abuse or pseudosoothing of anxieties with unhealthy escapism or engagement in compulsive behaviors such as overeating or overworking. Of course, in long-term rehabilitation settings, much more elaborate operationalization of the change process and coaching regarding needed behavioral changes is sometimes necessary.

PREPARE THE PATIENT AND FAMILY
FOR UPCOMING ADJUSTMENT CHALLENGES

As mentioned in chapter 1, the psychosocial needs of patients and family are fairly often attended to in hospital settings, but these tend to be ignored by health care providers once discharge occurs (Dracup, 1994). This is most unfortunate, given the high incidence of depression and anxiety seen in both recovering patients and their loved ones for up to several years posthospitalization. At minimum, the patient and family should be cautioned regarding what they are likely to encounter during the immediate next stage of rehabilitation.

Advise those who are being discharged from the hospital that their immediate coping challenges will involve at least two predictable hurdles: (a) adjusting to the relative lack of hands-on support and guidance from medical providers (compared to the degree received in the hospital); and (b) the homecoming depression and anxiety that often result from a combination of lessened support, posttraumatic stress syndrome, grief over anticipated or actual losses, and the frightening reality that this rehabilitation will last a lifetime.

In outpatient medical or rehabilitation settings, too, patients and their families can greatly benefit from brief discussions of what is likely to come. Here intervention can be structured by referring to the prior discussions regarding the adjustment course often seen in outpatient rehabilitation: Exaggerated versions of typical personality-based coping patterns may strain family relationships for a while, and elation over initial rehabilitation strides may only lead to overreacting depressively to setbacks encountered post-hospitalization (Dudley et al., 1980; Ell & Dunkel-Schetter, 1994).

During early convalescence, patients particularly need help in anticipating and warding off marital conflicts about respective spousal roles in the patient's resumption of activities (Gillis, 1984; Sotile, 1992). Warn patients and their loved ones of the costs of disagreeing about the patient's medical status (Finlayson & McEwen, 1977) or interpretations of medical advice (Sotile, 1992). Including the spouse, significant caretakers, or adult children of the patient in discharge planning and in outpatient visits soon after hospitalization can help avoid such tensions (Mayou, Williamson, & Foster, 1976; Ries, 1990).

REFER TO SELF-HELP OR SUPPORT GROUPS

Referral to self-help groups can provide much-needed support for the recovering patient and his or her family. Support groups can be structured in a variety of ways. Separate groups can be offered to patients, to their mates, or to couples. Issues that are often addressed in patient groups include concerns regarding illness, medication, discharge, sex, and attitudes of family (with special emphasis on aggravation about being treated in an overprotective manner) (Bilodeau & Hackett, 1971). Group themes in support programs for spouses of recovering patients might include catharsis, discussion of depression and anger management, dealing with loss, communication within marriage and family, fear of death of spouse, concerns regarding work return and other activities (especially sexual fears) (Harding & Morefield, 1976).

Support groups designed specifically for couples can directly explore various of the important marital themes mentioned in chapter 8: differences in interpretations of medical advice; clarification of respective rehabilitation roles; relationship patterns that help versus hurt each other's ability to cope with rehabilitation; concerns regarding children and grandchildren; communication issues; and so on.

Two observations from my own clinical and consultation experiences with many rehabilitation specialists throughout the country are worth discussing. First, it is important to know that we all periodically struggle in reacting to the challenges of running support programs. Don't expect that you will design the perfect program. No matter how you structure it, no single program will satisfy the needs of everyone you would like to help. Be prepared for complaints. If you offer a program for patients only, some will comment that they wish their significant others had been included. If your program targets couples, some will lament that certain issues may have been more comfortably explored in sessions attended only by patients or by significant others. Brief, time-limited programs will be criticized by some for "ending too soon"; open-ended groups as "lasting too long."

It is also important to realize that spotty attendance patterns at your support programs may be rather disheartening. You must learn not to discontinue your programs out of the pain of taking low attendance personally.

Noteworthy colleagues of mine have jokingly shared their versions of a frequent occurrence in my own practice: "Monday, I traveled across the country and had the privilege of presenting my ideas to an audience of hundreds of cardiopulmonary patients and their loved ones. It was a heart-warming experience. I came home on Tuesday, made the same ideas available in a support group open to any of our patients, and three of them showed up!"

Don't take it personally; and don't stop offering the programs. I have repeatedly had versions of the experience conveyed in the previously discussed case of John: Often, years after the fact, a patient indicates that even brief participation in a support/educational program was helpful to him or her. For some, simply noticing that a group probing a certain theme is being offered serves to validate that, indeed, that issue must be a legitimate topic of concern in rehabilitation. This awareness alone has spurred some patients I have known to discuss relevant matters more openly with their loved ones and health care providers.

In my opinion, the support program format that proves to be most helpful to the most people combines the following elements:

- Offer time-limited programs, such as a four- to six-session group.
- Specify a group theme. For example, offer a four-session stress management group or a six-session diet-change group.
- Make the sessions revolve around brief presentations of relevant material followed by "ticklers" that stir group discussion. Video- or audiotaped presentations of relevant material can be quite helpful in this regard. Excellent resources here include the *Healthy Heart* video series from the American Heart Association, 7320 Greenville Avenue, Dallas, TX 75232 (214-750-5300) and the *Portrait of a Heartmate* video series, available from Heartmates, Inc., P.O. Box 16202, Minneapolis, MN 55416 (800-946-3331).

My own video-educational series, *Coping With Heart Illness* (Sotile, 1995), is specifically designed to facilitate the teaching format under discussion (available from Human Kinetics, P.O. Box 5076, Champaign, IL 61825-5076 or call 800-747-4457). Brief vignettes of clinical interviews with patients, couples, spouses, and children of patients are presented. Each vignette is followed by a short educational segment related to the theme of the vignette. Themes include a range of topics addressed in this book: Tape 1 covers individual patients issues (how to identify and cope with depression, coping patterns, how to manage stress and emotions); tape 2 covers family issues (the importance of family teamwork in making lifestyle changes, how to talk about heart illness with children and grandchildren, and the importance of support); and tape 3 covers spouse issues (the experiences of heart patient spouses, sexual fears and concerns after heart illness, sex and aging). Each segment closes with a series of questions relevant to the issue under discussion, at which point the viewer is encouraged to stop the tape and discuss the topic. This format has proven to be quite valuable in stirring even the most reticent of patients and family members to discuss their concerns and experiences.

Various support programs delivered in-hospital have been described in the literature. Mended Hearts, a program that involves recovered patients visiting preoperative and postoperative patients, has been employed with CABG, MI, and percutaneous transluminal coronary angioplasty (PTCA) patients (Ell & Dunkel-Schetter, 1994). In addition, many educational and emotion-focused group programs have been described (Ibrahim et al., 1974; Rahe, Ward, & Hayes, 1979), and such educational and counseling interventions have consistently been found to improve measures of psychological well-being and lessen indicators of morbidity, at least throughout the first year of recovery (Oldenburg et al., 1985).

The effectiveness of group interventions for recovering cardiopulmonary populations has been discussed extensively (e.g., Ibrahim et al., 1974; Rahe et al., 1979). The usefulness of such group support for spouses of recovering patients has also been explored (Harding & Morefield, 1976; Levin, 1987).

Dracup et al. (1984) summarized efforts to meet the special needs of family members during the crisis of hospitalization. These have included such interventions as specialized "spouse care plans" in intensive care units (Dracup & Breu, 1978), rehabilitation care plans that included provision of brief supportive interactions with the loved ones of hospitalized patients (Dracup & Bryan-Brown, 1992; Janis, 1958), educational classes during post-intensive care stays (Scalzi et al., 1980), and formal support groups in waiting-room areas (McGrath & Robinson, 1973).

Information regarding formal support group programs can be gotten from the Support Group Clearing House, the American Lung Association, and the American Heart Association, as well as from formal cardiac or pulmonary programs that may be identified by contacting the American Association of Cardiovascular and Pulmonary Rehabilitation (see Appendix A for addresses and telephone numbers).

REFER TO FORMAL CARDIAC OR PULMONARY REHABILITATION PROGRAMS

A worldwide literature has documented that participation in a formal rehabilitation program can promote both physical and emotional recovery for a wide range of heart and lung patients. A few of the countries from which convincing data in this regard have been published are: the United States, Finland, the Netherlands, Sweden, and Australia (see Indexed Bibliography).

It remains for future researchers to differentiate the necessary versus the optimal components of these multifaceted programs in promoting given physical and emotional outcomes. However, few experts in cardiopulmonary rehabilitation would argue with the statement that a profoundly powerful factor inherent in the formal rehabilitation process is the psychosocial component. Dracup (1994) pointed out that formal participation in a cardiac rehabilitation program provides four dimensions of social support that were described by House (1981) as being crucial to wellness:

1. Emotional support is provided by both staff and fellow participants, especially if the program establishes an emotional climate in which individuals feel free to express their feelings and fears.

2. Instrumental support is provided by programs that help patients obtain appropriate community and government services.

3. Informational support is provided through educational sessions that augment the exercise component of the program.

4. Sense of self-worth is bolstered by the patient's affiliation with others who have had similar experiences or reaction to the recovery process. Here normalization and affirmation come from group processes inherent in ongoing participation in a formal rehabilitation program.

In my opinion, the inherent benefits of a formal cardiopulmonary rehabilitation program transcend the provision of social support. As was mentioned earlier, well-run rehabilitation programs epitomize the implementation of the Effective Emotional Management model. Such programs literally help patients to see their rehabilitation as a challenge, promote a lifelong commitment to healthy living, and teach biopsychosocial methods for establishing and maintaining control of adaptive coping processes. In so doing, the program itself becomes part of the nurturing "fencing" that forms the patient's life territory.

If my speculation is accurate, then participation in formal rehabilitation should lead to benefits that transcend improvements in physical functioning. Is this the case? The research literature answers this question with a resounding yes. Descriptions of but a few studies from this literature follow.

Lustig et al. (1972) reported that participation in a formal pulmonary rehabilitation program consisting of 15 to 20 treatments that included graded exercises, postural drainage, relaxation, and breathing retraining resulted in greater psychological improvement for pulmonary patients than did psychotherapy. Other researchers (e.g., Agle et al., 1973; Baum et al. 1973) reported that participation in a brief rehabilitation program that combined such interventions as intensive graduated exercises, breathing retraining, and group therapy led to sustained improvement in the ability to perform activities of daily living despite the lack of corresponding improvement in physiologic measures. Similar psychological benefits have been noted from comprehensive rehabilitation programs for chronic bronchitis and emphysema (Fishman & Petty, 1971).

These later claims match anecdotal reports from a variety of pulmonary ehabilitation specialists who note the frequency with which patients who participate in a formal rehabilitation program evidence marked improvements in self-confidence, mood, and daily functioning long before any actual changes in pulmonary function or in overall functional capacity have been noted. Clinical experience with such patients has repeatedly indicated that the various forms of EEM intervention inherent in the routine cardiopulmonary rehabilitation program are key mechanisms of change underlying this observed improvement of subjectively determined well-being.

McPherson et al. (1967) found that patients with heart disease who participated in a 24-week program of graduated exercise reported an enhanced sense of well-being and reduced anxiety and mood disturbances compared to subjects in a control group. Similar findings have been reported more recently from Roviaro, Holmes, & Holsten (1984).

Research in this area has also pinpointed many psychosocial interventions that have led to improvements in mood, lessening of distress, increased knowledge of risk factors, and increased social support—all important variables when measuring overall quality of life for the cardiopulmonary patient (Miller et al., 1990). These include health education and counseling, individual and group psychotherapy, stress management, relaxation training, and education regarding the effects of exercise on mood. Obviously, such treatments can be incorporated into rehabilitation programs for cardiac and pulmonary patients seen in either formal rehabilitation, office-based consultation, or hospital settings (Emery, 1991; Houston-Miller et al., 1990).

A number of specific strategies can be used to bolster the treatment milieu's psychosocial support factor. Following is a list of strategies that have been anecdotally reported to me by rehabilitation specialists throughout the country regarding effective ways to bolster the supportive component in office or rehabilitation settings, coupled with my own observations in this regard.

- Frequently touch patients in friendly, nonsexual ways.
- Exercise with patients.
- Regularly take the time, however brief, to chat with patients in a caring manner. Inquire about their families, church, work, or community activities. Let them know that you recognize them as people who have full and important lives, not simply as a bearer of the illness that you are treating.
- Note anniversaries, birthdays, and special occasions through monthly or weekly newsletters.
- Acknowledge illnesses or deaths as having effects on the group, and take program time to memorialize a participant who has died.
- Pair social gatherings with educational sessions. For example, serve refreshments before and after a monthly lecture.
- Hold yearly holiday celebrations for participants and their loved ones.

- Stage reunions that unite current and former participants and their loved ones.

- Conduct awards banquets, acknowledging progress. Here it is perhaps more important to acknowledge every participant for something (e.g., "the patient with the brightest-colored workout clothes") than to promote competition regarding weight loss, MET capacity, and so on.

- Provide buddy systems that pair certain individuals as identified supports for each other.

- Structure exercise sessions so that the same people exercise together each week—a variant of the buddy system.

- Include spouses in adjunctive exercise/wellness programs. As discussed in the preceding chapter, a number of authors (e.g., Shanfield, 1990; Sotile, 1993) have recommended that spouses should be included in formal rehabilitation programs with patients.

- Use the telephone to contact patients who have missed scheduled sessions or simply to inquire about the patient's overall well-being.

Specific suggestions have also been offered for ways to provide support and psychosocial follow-up for cardiopulmonary patients being seen in outpatient treatment settings, as listed below.

- Take advantage of routine follow-up visits to physicians to inquire about relevant psychosocial issues.

- Encourage participation in maintenance exercise groups.

- Encourage involvement with organizations such as the American Lung Association or the American Heart Association.

- Train all office personnel in ways to provide support and encouragement to visiting patients.

- Offer office-based psychosocial educational or treatment sessions as special aspects of care.

- Make educational materials regarding relevant psychosocial issues readily available to visiting patients.

- Conduct periodic, brief phone follow-ups.

- Send newsletters with articles on relevant issues.

- Administer questionnaires that solicit input from patients regarding their concerns.

- Provide home-health referrals.

- Conduct home visits.

OFFICE MANAGEMENT
OF PSYCHOSOCIAL CONCERNS

The challenges of promoting positive psychosocial adjustment in recovering cardiac and pulmonary patients are especially obvious to practitioners working in outpatient medical and rehabilitation settings. The long-term relationships that develop between providers and patients and their family members in these settings can be a great boon to adaptive psychosocial functioning.

By choice or by default, most treatment for psychosocial concerns and mental health disorders is provided in primary care medical settings, not in the offices of specialists in mental health. Research in this area suggests that approximately three-fifths of mental health concerns of patients are treated in the general medical sector (Doherty, 1986), particularly in the offices of specialists in family medicine (Reiger, Goldberg, & Taube, 1978). Cassata and Kirkman-Liff (1981) randomly surveyed 207 general practitioners and residency-trained family physicians in North Carolina and Ohio and found that fully one-third of their diagnoses were "behavioral-psychological" in nature, with the four most common problems being depression, anxiety, obesity, and marital discord. Despite this apparent onslaught of patients in need of psychosocial intervention, the Cassata and Kirkman-Liff survey also noted that only 2% to 4% of the physician-patient encounters were reported as counseling or referral-making sessions.

Unfortunately, most primary care practitioners have limited time, energy, and expertise to devote to treating the psychosocial concerns of their patients (Reiger et al., 1978). In an effort to remedy this situation, models for the role of medical practitioners in psychosocial treatment have been published (Christie-Seely, 1984; Doherty & Baird, 1983). Doherty and Baird (1983) developed a model for understanding the interplay of marital or family treatment in family medicine settings that can be modified to apply to the delivery of psychosocial care in the treatment of cardiopulmonary patients in outpatient settings. Such care should center on education, prevention, support, and challenge.

The educational component might focus on coaching patients and their loved ones regarding stress management, the coping tasks that come with rehabilitation, anticipated family problems, and communication issues, especially as they relate to the illness and to the rehabilitation process.

Prevention efforts can entail providing anticipatory help before psychosocial problems arise. This might take the form of forewarning the patient and family of certain predictable, unavoidable coping hurdles in the path of rehabilitation, such as the inevitable demoralization and fear that accompany less than linear progression in indicators of recovery.

The importance of recovering patients receiving support from medical personnel has already been discussed extensively. Many elderly patients rate emotional and informational support received from their physician as being more important to their well-being than family support. Times of transition are especially likely to stir high needs for support. Transitions such as retirement, progression of illness to the point of the need for specialized interventions (e.g., home ventilation), or death of a loved one should be acknowledged with bolstered supportive efforts on the part of medical staff.

Finally, Doherty and Baird recommend that office-based psychosocial interventions challenge the patient and his or her loved ones to attend to psychosocial concerns. Psychosocial issues should be presented as a normal and integral part of overall rehabilitation, and the patient and family should be caringly confronted to mobilize themselves to make changes or to accept referral for specialized help.

Each of these areas of office-based psychosocial intervention can be enhanced by use of videotaped and multimedia educational resources of the types already mentioned (Hollis et al., 1993). In addition, the benefits of nurse-delivered counseling can be immeasurable. In the reality of a busy outpatient medical practice, it is most often the nurse, not the physician, who assumes responsibility for patient education and counseling. However, the importance of physician-delivered sanctioning and encouragement of participation in psychosocial counseling cannot be overemphasized. As mentioned in prior discussion of office-based smoking cessation counseling, brief, unequivocal endorsement of the importance of attending to psychosocial concerns, followed by a combination of educational and nurse-delivered counseling interventions, can be tremendously effective in promoting positive psychosocial changes.

Medical offices have an unlimited range of options for designing effective psychosocial interventions. If health care personnel follow the basic principles described in this book, they can tailor their programs to suit their unique situations. A few examples of structures that might be used follow.

Blake et al. (1990) described a practical, office-based program for enhancing psychosocial adjustments of recovering COPD patients. The intervention consisted of two to three nurse-delivered counseling sessions that focused primarily on appraisal of coping strategies, teaching new coping skills, and reinforcing the use of adaptive coping tools. Skill building included brief education regarding stress management, relaxation exercises, systematic breathing exercises, and visual imagery. The importance of social support was emphasized, and cognitive restructuring and reframing were also taught. For example, the patient was instructed to depersonalize during episodes of dyspnea, quieting the emotional reactions to the episode by attributing the symptoms to the underlying disease process instead of to a personal weakness or defect. Audiotaped and reading materials were also provided to each patient. Following a single 60- to 90-min session during which the above interventions were delivered, each patient was contacted by telephone at least once to review progress and reinforce or modify their coping plan. One or two face-to-face follow-up sessions at intervals of 2 to

4 weeks were then provided. When possible, the spouse or some significant other of the patient was included.

The results of this study by Blake and colleagues suggested that relatively brief office-based psychosocial interventions can be effective in helping COPD patients cope. Compared to controls, the 37 treatment patients evidenced immediate, significant improvements in physical functioning and in overall psychosocial functioning. Modest delayed beneficial effects on overall functional status were also noted.

Gift et al. (1992) demonstrated the effectiveness of brief relaxation training in improving pulmonary function indicators in a small group of COPD patients. Intervention subjects received a taped relaxation message teaching progressive muscular relaxation. The patients first listened to the tape in a quiet room in an outpatient medical office setting. They then took the tape home, with instructions to practice and to record practice times. They returned at weekly intervals for three more sessions to present practice diaries to a nurse and to demonstrate ability to achieve relaxation. Compared to controls who received a similar degree of medical attention but no relaxation training, the experimental subjects evidenced significantly greater reductions in levels of anxiety and dyspnea and significantly improved pulmonary function. Specifically, their peak expiratory flow rates (PEFR) improved from 173 to 184 L/min, whereas the control group subjects' PEFR decreased from 208 to 193 L/min.

Effective office-based interventions have also been described with cardiac patients. Kallio et al. (1979) demonstrated the effectiveness of a multidisciplinary approach to office-based rehabilitation of acute MI patients. Intervention with 150 male and 37 female MI patients began 2 weeks postdischarge. Treatment consisted of medical examinations performed monthly for the first 6 months after MI, then when necessary, or at least at 3-month intervals. In addition, a treatment team consisting of a social worker, psychologist, dietitian, and physiotherapist provided patients with health education consisting of antismoking and dietary advice, discussions of psychosocial problems, and physical exercise recommendations. This counseling, too, was delivered intensively during the first 3 months of rehabilitation and then tapered thereafter.

Compared to 151 male and 37 female patients who received routine cardiac care, the intervention group evidenced significant improvements in blood pressures at 1-, 2-, and 3-year follow-ups. Compared to controls, the intervention group also evidenced significantly lowered serum cholesterol levels, serum triglyceride levels, and body weight. Most noteworthy was that the cumulative reduction in the percentage of sudden deaths for the intervention group (5.8%) was significantly lower than for controls (14.4%), as were the number of CHD-related deaths in the intervention group (n = 35) compared to controls (n = 55).

Office-based interventions hold tremendous promise in promoting enhanced overall psychosocial adjustment for cardiopulmonary patients. Of course, not all psychosocial concerns of patients can be dealt with effectively by nonspecialists. Whether or not a primary care provider can intervene effectively will depend on several factors: problem severity and chronicity; provider skill; provider time and resources; and the patient's adaptability (Doherty & Baird, 1983). The three kinds of problems identified by Doherty (1986) as possible candidates for primary care counseling are (a) illness-related events; (b) life-cycle transitions; and (c) recent-onset problems that do not reflect long-standing dysfunction.

Guidelines published by the National Cancer Institute (NCI) for office management of smoking cessation (Glynn & Manley, 1992) can be broadened to apply to treatment of any of these circumstances outlined by Doherty (1986). At minimum, the outpatient milieu should be structured to provide psychosocial interventions that follow the "four As" approach recommended by the NCI: ask, advise, assist, and arrange.

Ask about the patient's psychosocial functioning.

Advise about the importance of attending to psychosocial concerns.

Assist psychosocial adjustments by presenting age-appropriate educational, self-help, or counseling interventions.

Arrange for follow-up regarding the effects of interventions or for further specialized consultation.

COLLABORATING WITH MENTAL HEALTH PROFESSIONALS

Adjustment problems that persist despite initial efforts to educate and support, or those of long-standing duration, indicate the need for referral for specialized care. Even in the routine delivery of medical or rehabilitation care, the patient's biopsychosocial functioning can be enhanced by sensible input from a mental health professional. The Kallio et al. (1979) study cited above highlighted the importance of interdisciplinary collaboration in caring for recovering cardiopulmonary patients.

Other research has demonstrated the effectiveness of even limited involvement of a mental health professional in treating medical patients, especially those prone to somatization. Single-session psychiatric consultation has been shown to lead to a 50% reduction in health care charges over a 3-month period compared to the health care charges of a group of highly somaticizing patients who did not receive such psychiatric consultation (Smith, Monson, & Ray, 1986). In treating this same population, case studies have documented the effectiveness of a variety of behavioral strategies, including reinforcement for systematic increases in physical activities, exercise, and independent self-care; and relaxation therapies (Levenkron, Goldstein, Adamides, & Greenland, 1985).

When available, affordable, and necessary, formal evaluation and treatment by a mental health specialist should be considered. It is worthwhile for any cardiopulmonary rehabilitation program, hospital, or outpatient medical provider to foster relationships with mental health specialists who are either knowledgeable about cardiopulmonary rehabilitation or, minimally, are willing to learn about the unique adaptive challenges faced by recovering patients in the population being served. Once identified, such specialists can be used to provide interventions along the continuum of complexity proposed in this book, but especially at levels V and VI, where specialized assessment, feedback, and follow-up regarding specified psychosocial concerns is indicated. Such assessments typically incorporate data from extended clinical interviews with the patient and his or her loved ones and the results of a battery of standardized personality, neuropsychological, and family systems inventories (Rose & Robbins, 1993; Wright & Leahey, 1984). In addition, extended cognitive/behavioral therapy, marital/family therapy, and individual or group psychotherapy can enhance overall psychosocial adjustment and adherence to medical recommendations (Dudley & Pattison, 1969; Kolman, 1983). It has also been recommended that many COPD patients could benefit from formal psychotherapy geared to working through losses that are entailed in living with their illness (Greenberg, Ryan, & Bourlier, 1985; Lusting, Haas, & Castillo, 1972; Rabinowitz & Florian, 1992). Similarly, as discussed earlier, the fear of death experienced by many recovering cardiac and pulmonary patients can have profound effects on the patient's functioning and create timely opportunities for helping the patient to examine and resolve long-standing psychodynamic conflicts.

Also as mentioned earlier, it is wise to frame referral for specialized psychological or psychiatric help in terms that bolster the patient and the family and allow them to save face. Here the use of frames of reference that compliment, rather than humiliate, is essential. In making referrals, avoid frames such as the following:

"I just don't believe that you are going to be able to cope with this. You need to be seen by a mental health professional."

"You people just don't know how to get along. Let me refer you to a family therapist."

"If you don't get a better handle on this, your stress is going to kill you. I'm going to refer you to a psychiatrist."

Do use frames such as the following:

"I know that you are coping with a lot right now. Would you be open to talking with someone who is a specialist in this area—a 'coping coach'?"

> "Families go through hard struggles when coping with this. Let me suggest a friend of mine who can help you figure out how to organize your efforts to help each other. She specializes in teaching family stress management."
>
> "A key part of your rehabilitation will be to learn effective stress management techniques. This is just as important as the other medical recommendations that you are hearing. I would like for you to get at least a brief consult regarding the latest stress management strategies that have proven to be effective for recovering cardiopulmonary patients and their families. Would you be willing to talk with one of my friends who specializes in this area?"

Doherty and Baird (1983) called attention to the fact that, once referral is made, a new therapeutic triangle of influence exists consisting of the primary medical provider, the family, and the mental health specialist. It is important that the primary care provider and the mental health specialist share responsibility for communicating directly with each other and not undermine each other's efforts to care for the patient. Family therapist Mara Selvini-Palazzoli and colleagues (Selvini-Palazzoli, Cecchin, Prata, & Boscolo, 1978) discuss the problems faced by therapists when treating families referred by physicians who have inadvertently become codependent caretakers. As long as the patient or family has problems, the "intimacy" of the caretaking arrangement persists; if the patient or family rehabilitate, the pain of lost caretaking is suffered. In such circumstances, both the family and the doctor may be unconsciously relieved when the therapy fails (Doherty & Baird, 1983). These observations underscore the need for ongoing, open dialog between health care providers, patients, and patients' families. Discussion of this issue will conclude this book. But first, an overview of specialized psychosocial interventions will be presented.

THE EFFECTIVENESS OF SPECIALIZED PSYCHOSOCIAL INTERVENTIONS WITH CARDIOPULMONARY PATIENTS

Throughout this book, the benefits of brief, simple psychosocial interventions with cardiopulmonary patients have been emphasized. It is also true that more extensive interventions are sometimes called for. An overview of the effectiveness of various types of specialized psychosocial interventions with recovering cardiopulmonary patients can be best gleaned from the literature on the treatment of cardiac patients. In addition to relaxation therapy (described above), three types of specialized interventions have been incorporated into overall cardiac care: intensive multifaceted treatment programs; psychotherapy; and supportive counseling delivered in a series of very brief contacts, often by phone. As will be seen in the following, research has shown that each of these types of treatment can be effective in promoting a variety of important physical, behavioral, and psychological outcomes for recovering patients.

Extensive Treatment Programs

Several extensive treatment interventions have been described in the literature. Gruen (1975) demonstrated the effectiveness of what the author termed *brief psychotherapy* delivered to MI patients during hospitalization. As will be seen below, the intervention provided in this study actually incorporated a number of psychotherapeutic techniques and was delivered throughout the course of hospitalizations that were quite lengthy by today's standards of stringently managed care.

In contrast to many publications in this literature, the Gruen study is noteworthy for the author's specification of the psychological intervention employed. Seventy first-MI patients were randomly assigned to treatment or control groups. As mentioned earlier, the 38 treatment subjects received an intervention framed as help from "The Department of Patient Care Improvement"—not as psychotherapy. Intervention was begun during either the first or second day of hospitalization and continued "for an average of 1/2 hour initially for 6 days a week and, later, 5 days a week until . . . release from the hospital" (p. 225). Unfortunately, the author did not specify the average length of stay for treated patients nor the average number of treatment sessions delivered. However, the indication that psychological testing was administered to each patient "on about the eleventh day of hospitalization" (p. 226) suggests that considerable lengths of stay afforded the opportunity to provide fairly extensive psychological intervention with each patient.

Psychotherapy was geared toward exploration, feedback, and positive reinforcement of effective coping. The goal of intervention was to provide support and gentle reframing to help each patient become aware of positive aspects of his or her coping style that could serve well in coping with hospitalization and illness. Ten therapeutic components were integrated into the intervention:

1. The therapist attempted to develop genuine interest in the patient and to convey regard for the patient's positive qualities.

2. Reassurance and normalization regarding fears, anxieties, or feelings of depression were offered.

3. The patient's positive coping mechanisms, strengths, and positive personality resources were highlighted.

4. During discussions, the therapist listened supportively, reflecting back the patient's feelings and tentative conclusions.

5. The therapist also reflected back to the patient his or her catastrophizing or erroneous perceptions. This was not done in a confrontational

style; reflection was offered along with the invitation and advice that there might be other ways to look at the issue of concern.

6. Intervention was done with sensitivity to the patient's capacity for absorbing input. Confrontation was not used; only feedback about the patient and his or her social environment that he or she could and was willing to assimilate was offered. If the patient evidenced denial, this denial was not challenged.

7. The patient was encouraged to get medical advice through being appropriately assertive, rather than passively waiting for information.

8. Throughout intervention, the patient was offered constant reassurance of the therapist's faith in his or her capacity to cope. Any signs of strength such as humor, extension of interests, concern for others, religious faith, or planning for the future were reinforced by the therapist.

9. The patient was encouraged to resolve conflicts and unsolved dilemmas in his or her life.

10. In general, intervention provided constant reinforcement of adaptive coping strategies and of use of existing or formerly hidden resources by the patient.

An impressive use of medical data in assessing outcomes was reported by Gruen. Compared to controls, intervention patients were discharged from the hospital 2.5 days sooner, from ICU 1 day sooner, and were taken off cardiac monitoring 1.8 days sooner. Analysis of nursing notes and of results of psychological testing (again, administered on about the 11th day of hospitalization) indicated that intervention patients also evidenced significantly fewer congestive heart failure days; less weakness, depression, anxiety, and sadness; and greater degrees of positive feelings. Blind ratings of at-home follow-up interview data gathered between 4 and 4-1/2 months posthospitalization indicated that, compared to controls, intervention patients evidenced significantly less anxiety and significantly greater return to normal activities.

The landmark work of Dean Ornish and colleagues (Ornish et al., 1983, 1990) also deserves mention as an example of a multifaceted treatment program that employed providers with specialized training in the delivery of psychosocial interventions. The Ornish treatment program is both extensive and intensive. Here intervention combined stringent dietary reductions in fat and caloric intake, minimal exercise, and extensive stress management training. The stress management intervention consisted of group support, group exploration of psychosocial issues, and training in relaxation and meditation procedures, particularly emphasizing the use of yoga. Intervention was delivered in an intensive, 24-day format. Compared to non-randomized controls, intervention subjects evidenced statistically significant increases in duration of exercise and total work performed, lowered levels of plasma cholesterol and triglycerides, improved left ventricle performance, lessened chest pain, and lessened severity of CHD as assessed by angiography.

Psychotherapy

An example of a psychotherapy-type stress management intervention with recovering MI patients was provided by Rahe et al., (1979). In a controlled comparison study, these researchers assessed the effects of six group psychotherapy sessions aimed at reducing stress, providing emotional and social support, offering advice on modifying coronary-prone behavior—but not on altering risk factors such as smoking or excess body weight. Compared to controls who received no special intervention, treated subjects experienced significantly reduced rates of reinfarction, and there were significantly fewer CHD deaths during 3 years of follow-up posthospitalization. Similar positive results from psychotherapy with COPD patients have also been reported (Greenberg et al., 1985; Lustig et al., 1972).

Clearly, effective psychosocial interventions can be structured in various ways. Treatment settings, staff time, and patient needs obviously shape inclusion of such interventions into the delivery of care. However, the range of interventions that have led to positive outcomes in this area suggests that doing something to help patients cope with stress is always more advisable than doing nothing.

THE IMPORTANCE OF FOLLOW-UP

Finally, the need for follow-up in promoting psychological adjustment to cardiac and pulmonary patients is crucial. Unfortunately, this aspect of the psychosocial component of cardiopulmonary rehabilitation is far too often overlooked. To assess and educate patients upon entry into our care and then never again makes no more sense within the psychosocial realm than within any other realm of rehabilitation.

Both clinical experience and empirical research supports this call for bolstered follow-up in the delivery of cardiopulmonary care. Data from the Recovery from Heart Surgery: Bio-Behavioral Factors research project at the Boston University School of Medicine and the Harvard Medical School (Stanton et al., 1984) underscored this need. This project followed 249 heart patients for 6 months postsurgery, evaluating the adequacy of the education offered in facilitating their psychosocial adjustment posthospitalization. More than half the patients reported that they had not been adequately prepared for the emotional and relationship stresses faced during rehabilitation. Both patients who rated their postsurgery preparation as adequate and those who thought it inadequate agreed that they were faced with more fears and more adjustments following surgery than they had anticipated. Furthermore, the researchers found a direct association between the patients' incidence and degree of angina and their subjective ratings of fears and adjustment struggles following surgery.

Follow-up should take two forms. First, use of the telephone to provide monitoring and brief counseling is recommended. Second, all medical and rehabilitation specialists should remember that because psychosocial adjustment is an ever-evolving process, periodically repeating psychosocial assessment is an important part of delivering comprehensive cardiac and pulmonary care.

EXCHANGE TELEPHONE NUMBERS

Cardiac rehabilitation specialist Nancy Houston-Miller has been quoted as saying that the telephone is the most underused health behavior change tool available to contemporary medical professionals (Houston-Miller, 1990). This claim has been supported by research documenting that interventions that incorporate brief telephone consultation into multifaceted rehabilitation efforts for cardiac illness can help promote a range of positive posthospitalization outcomes, including:

- maintenance of smoking cessation (DeBusk et al., 1994; Taylor, Houston-Miller, Kilen, & DeBusk, 1990);
- enhanced patient and family confidence in their ability to manage rehabilitation and corresponding diminishment in levels of posthospital depression and a more rapid return to work during the 9 months following discharge (Follick et al., 1988);
- improved patient adherence to exercise regimens (Daltroy, 1985);
- improved functional capacity and diminished plasma LDL concentrations at 1-year follow-up (DeBusk et al., 1994);
- enhanced overall psychosocial adjustment and subsequently decreased mortality (Frasure-Smith & Prince, 1985, 1989);
- diminished anxiety and reduced incidence of rehospitalization for CABG patients (Beckie, 1989); and
- enhanced patient satisfaction with the quality of their medical care (DeBusk et al., 1994).

Lewin et al. (1992) demonstrated the effectiveness of a simple, cost-effective home-based self-help program in rehabilitating MI patients that made use of telephone follow-up. A sample of 176 patients were treated with a 10-min in-hospital consult, followed by 10-min telephone contacts at 1, 3, and 6 weeks posthospitalization. During the telephone contacts, the patient's use of a self-instructive manual describing home-based exercise and stress management concepts was reviewed. The intervention also included a tape-based relaxation and stress management program. The telephone contacts were primarily supportive in nature and were purposely kept brief, in line with research suggesting that minimal contact from a treatment facilitator can potentiate self-help treatments (Glasgow & Rosen, 1987). Controls received an equal amount of the facilitator's attention and a packet of leaflets covering various issues relevant to rehabilitation rather than the heart manual and taped relaxation and stress management program.

Follow-up conducted at 6 weeks, 6 months, and 1 year indicated that, compared to controls, treated subjects showed strikingly less general emotional disturbance as measured by a standardized measure of emotional symptomatology (the General Health Questionnaire). Specifically, the controls were significantly more anxious and depressed at all follow-up periods. Even more striking was the fact that the treatment group evidenced fewer consultations with their general practitioners at 6 months and at 1 year. Patients in the control group made a mean of 1.8 more visits to their physicians than did the treatment group in the first 6 months, and a mean of 0.9 more visits than treatment patients in the subsequent 6 months. Also, significantly more control patients than treatment patients were readmitted to the hospital in the first 6 months posthospitalization (8% of the treatment patients were readmitted versus 24% of the control patients).

Such data suggest that telephone follow-up may be one of the most cost-effective ways to enhance outcomes of medical interventions. If telephone follow-up is not possible, postcard reminders of key points covered in the discharge plan should be sent.

DO IT AGAIN!

Information presented as part of the delivery of medical care often seems to fall on deaf ears. This may be due to the disruptions in attention, concentration, and memory that often accompany the crisis of hospitalization or entry into rehabilitation. This fact, considered in conjunction with the work of Prochaska and DiClemente on the stages of change, underscores the importance of periodically repeating psychosocial assessment and feedback throughout the course of outpatient rehabilitation.

The need for follow-up regarding patients' psychosocial issues has been underscored by both researchers and clinicians. Follow-up studies are needed to determine the effects of interventions and to discern what interventions are needed in promoting long-term changes (Hill et al., 1992). The original position paper on pulmonary rehabilitation published by AACVPR (Ries, 1990) lamented the general lack of extended follow-up with pulmonary patients beyond 3 months.

From a clinical standpoint, the importance of providing regular follow-up evaluation and input regarding relevant psychosocial issues should be obvious but is often ignored in actual practice. The relationships between rehabilitating cardiopulmonary patients and their health care providers often span years, and as life progresses, the psychosocial issues impacting patients change. To initially evaluate, educate, and advise a patient who entrusts you to be his or her medical caretaker, and then to never again inquire regarding psychosocial issues that are known to be important in the patient's life, is not only poor clinical practice; it is uncaring. Follow-up should be sensitive to the implications of the patient's current physical status, age, occupational status, and family developmental process.

FUTURE DIRECTIONS

It remains for future researchers to clarify the specific causes and effects of overall psychosocial adjustment in recovering cardiopulmonary populations (Dracup, 1994). This area of research is complex and challenging. Even the measurement of important variables relevant to psychosocial adjustment is difficult, and available instruments have all been found to have various limitations (Sarason & Sarason, 1994). As has been noted, this fact seriously clouds comparative interpretation of research in this area. For example, Heitzmann and Kaplan (1988) pointed out that the lack of consensual definition of social support makes it impossible to compare studies that link social support to stress, health outcomes, and general psychological and physical well-being. These authors further caution that "a caring, supportive spouse or confidant may be treated (in measurement) just as a spouse with whom there is frequent stressful conflict" (Heitzmann & Kaplan, 1988, p. 77).

With these cautions duly noted, I offer several thoughts about needed research in this area. First, the strong indication that a supportive milieu is crucial to both physical and psychosocial well-being, coupled with the research evidence that the family may be the most crucial and important aspect of social support for heart patients (Sotile, Sotile, Sotile, & Ewen, 1993), suggests that future research exploring the intimacy factor within cardiopulmonary populations would be especially timely. In this realm, the differential social support needs and overall psychosocial adjustment patterns of men and women cardiopulmonary patients and of their spouses need to be clarified. Some researchers have suggested that no differences exist between men's and women's psychosocial responses to heart illness (Foley, Sivarajan, & Woods, 1983; Rankin, 1990). Other researchers have long held that significant sex differences do exist, both in response to one's own illness (e.g., Stern, Pascale, & McLoone, 1976) and to illness in a spouse (Shanfield, 1990).

In my opinion, this is an area that proves the point that incorporation of information beyond our targeted area of study can greatly clarify that which we are viewing. As discussed in chapter 8, a broad-based literature has documented male/female differences in such rehabilitation-relevant areas as caretaking activities in families, stress management tendencies, and the definition of the role of work in one's life (Sivarajan & Newton, 1984). Male and female CHD patients have even been shown to evidence differential reactions to physical touch by attending nurses. In the aforementioned study by Weiss (1990), women showed a preference for less frequent, gentle, brief touching of only a few select body parts, whereas men preferred firm touching of long duration and over a greater extent of the body.

Preliminary data from our laboratory at Wake Forest University suggest that male and female cardiac patients have different social networks and differ significantly in the extent to which they receive out-of-program social support. In a pilot study reported by Ribisl et al. (1994) that used the social support inventory from the Medical Outcomes Study (Tarlov et al., 1989), 58 male heart patients were found to have significantly more family members living in their household, whereas 25 female patients tended to live alone and to have significantly more potential out-of-home members of their social network. In addition, female patients reported lower levels of tangible support (e.g., help with activities such as driving, meal preparation, and chores), affection support (love, hugs, feeling wanted), positive support (good times, relaxation, enjoyment), and emotional support (someone to listen, offer advice, confide in, or offer understanding) than their male counterparts.

My clinical experiences in counseling thousands of women and men regarding various individual and relational concerns strongly suggests that even in this age of supposed enlightenment regarding gender roles, most women continue to struggle with conflicting feelings about whether or not they "dare to claim entitlement" when it comes to inconveniencing their loved ones for the sake of their own rehabilitation. I continue to regularly encounter tremendous disparity in male and female medical patients as they grapple with the home-life implications of their rehabilitation. Classic examples of this discrepancy came from two of my cardiac patients during last year's holiday season.

WMS: "So, Becca, how was your Thanksgiving?"

Becca: "Great. It was great. This was the first time since my bypass surgery that I cooked a holiday meal—and the first time since surgery that I got a chance to visit with my husband's brother and his family."

WMS: "Well, how did it go?"

Becca: "It was okay. I sorta missed eating all that yummy, high-fat food, though. I love that stuff! But I was happy to prepare it for everyone else, and I enjoyed watching them enjoy eating it. It was a good day."

WMS: "Well, what did you eat?"

Becca: "Oh, I took care of myself. I cooked myself a few low-fat side dishes and had a little of the turkey white meat."

WMS: "Hey, A.J. How are you?"

A.J.: "I'm great. Still stuffed from Thanksgiving, though."

WMS: "Did you and your family have a nice holiday?"

A.J.: "We had a great holiday. My mother, one of my sisters, and one of my favorite cousins and his family all came to our house for dinner on Thursday, and then my family and I went and had another feast on Saturday at my other sister's."

WMS: "Sounds like fun."

A.J.: "It was. Since I had this heart attack last year, I realize more and more how important my family is to me."

WMS: "That's good stuff, A.J. It sounds like you have a close family. I'm happy for you."

A.J.: "Yeah. They're great. I just wish I could get them to stop all that whining about having to eat low-fat meals when they're around me. [laughs] My mother said, 'This seems un-American—or at least un-North Carolinian: Thanksgiving dinner with no fatty casseroles or pecan pies!'

"But, hey, they'll get used to it. They understand—this heart illness is serious business. If I can stop eating all that food that I love, they can, too. They'll catch on, eventually."

Of course, these cases represent rather extreme reactions of selflessness and self-focusedness, and neither of these roles is confined to either gender. I have worked with selfless males and self-focused females. But my point—and that made by the clinical experiences of many of my colleagues—is that, predominantly, one problem faced in rehabilitation of women patients is their paltry sense of self-entitlement and cooperation in creating in-home environments that are supportive of their rehabilitation changes. In my opinion, it is naive to believe that the psychosocial adjustment challenges faced by men and women during the course of rehabilitation do not diverge in marked ways. This issue is yet to be definitively researched with recovering cardiopulmonary patients.

This observation dovetails with those of many researchers of overall psychosocial adjustment patterns in rehabilitation. In summarizing the state of information on the issue of quality of life post-cardiovascular disease, Richard Mayou (1990) cautioned that, in various ways, we have unfortunately neglected attending to the design and evaluation of treatment interventions that take the individual needs of patients and their families into consideration. Among others, he offers these criticisms of exiting research in this area: It overemphasizes general concepts and neglects individual meaning of well-being (he uses the term *quality of life*); it neglects the range of individual responses; it overly relies on use of measures that are often insensitive to clinically important issues and underuses the more clinically rich method of structured interviewing for data gathering; and it overemphasizes research on the consequences of specific illnesses (i.e., MI) while underresearching the different quality-of-life issues faced by patients suffering various forms of illness or patients who undergo various forms of surgery.

CONCLUDING COMMENTS

The information presented in this book documents that even brief psychosocial interventions that are caringly and strategically implemented can significantly enhance the biopsychosocial functioning of both cardiac and pulmonary patients. At any level of psychosocial intervention, patients can be helped to become more effective emotional managers. In structuring psychosocial interventions, several points should always be kept in mind.

By choice or by default, health care providers are profoundly important agents of psychosocial adjustment for patients. In this age of medical specialization, all patients are faced with input from various, often conflicting, sources. This is an evident fact when dealing with maladies that require multidisciplinary care, such as cardiopulmonary illness. This fact underscores the importance of health care providers taking responsibility for actively collaborating about the needs and treatments of individual patients (Delbanco, 1992; Friedman, 1990; Gorlin, 1992). Interdisciplinary or interspecialty communication is particularly crucial at times of important transition in the patient's care or physical condition. Specifically, taking time to contact and communicate with other professionals is key to providing ongoing psychosocial adjustment during transfer from hospital to outpatient care; upon diagnosis of new levels of illness; or upon recommending new levels of care (e.g., referral to formal rehabilitation or prescription of home-based procedures such as supplemental oxygen therapy). The days of remaining narrowly confined to the cubbyhole of one's own specialty—and simply diagnosing and referring patients with no intention of initiating and continuing an active collaboration with other professionals treating the patient and his or her family—should be put to rest.

Just as every patient and every family holds certain unique perspectives on illness and rehabilitation, every health care specialist develops his or her unique perspectives on a given patient. We need to communicate these to each other. Our collective perspectives can paint a more full and accurate picture of the patient. Comprehensive cardiopulmonary care requires collaboration among patients, their families, and health care providers. To truly collaborate in delivering comprehensive cardiopulmonary care, we need to share these perspectives with each other. Disjointed, compartmentalized care only serves to stress, not support, the recovering patient.

The necessity and advisability of open and active interdisciplinary collaboration in providing care for cardiopulmonary patients is being magnified by the call for efficient delivery of treatment from the managed care movement predominating our emerging health care system. As health care reform unfolds over the next decade, it is likely that collaborative family health care will become the standard in treating all medical patients. This will certainly prove to be the case in treating heart and lung patients, given the biopsychosocial nature of recovery from these illnesses.

Regardless of the level of psychosocial intervention offered, several points should be kept in mind:

First, each of the factors in the model presented in this book should be legitimized as a bona fide area of concern in the treatment of cardiac and pulmonary patients. Patients' personal needs are important to them, even when these needs do not fit conveniently into our own professional agendas.

Second, it is important to be clear about (a) your expectations that patients and their loved ones will address these psychosocial concerns as part of their overall rehabilitation process; (b) your availability for consultation in these areas; and (c) the limits of your expertise and comfort in addressing these issues.

Third, the patient and his or her loved ones should be surrounded with information and interaction that can facilitate adjustment. Combinations of handouts, newsletters, audiovisual aids, and—most importantly—caring conversations should be offered throughout the course of treatment.

In general, it is our job to create success experiences for our patients. No matter what the patient's physical or emotional status at the time of consultation, it is important to remember that he or she is seeking more than mere mechanical input. Patients seek our help in healing their bodies, their emotional wounds, their spirits, their families, and their worries. In addition to our concerns and admonitions, patients need to hear about what they are doing well—where progress is occurring or where stability is being maintained. In delivering medical or rehabilitation care, it is wise to follow a simple credo: Find something to reward, and reward it!

In closing, I propose that it is not farfetched to conceptualize health care providers who work with recovering cardiac and pulmonary patients as agents of hope and of faith. We must remember to offer the people we serve not only our assistance in caring for their bodies, but also our help in mustering hope—hope that the adjustments they face can be managed, and hope that in adjusting to illness, they can find renewed meaning in their lives. We must also treat our patients in ways that promote their faith—not in our ability to deliver them eternal life, but in our willingness to ensure that our care will always be delivered with respect for the psychosocial realities that fill their lives.

■ INDEXED BIBLIOGRAPHY ■

Preface

For a discussion of reengineering, see:
Hammer, M., & Champy, J. (1993). *Reengineering the corporation.* New York: Harper Business.
Methodological problems with the cardiac psychosocial literature:
Blumenthal, J.A., & Emery, C.F. (1988). Rehabilitation of patients following myocardial infarction. *Journal of Consulting and Clinical Psychology, 56*(3), 374-381.
Razin, A.M. (1982). Psychosocial intervention in coronary artery disease: A review. *Psychosomatic Medicine, 44*(4), 363-381.
Methodological problems with the pulmonary psychosocial literature:
Fishman, D.B., & Petty, T.L. (1971). Physical, symptomatic and psychological improvement in patients receiving comprehensive care for chronic airway obstruction. *Journal of Chronic Diseases, 24,* 775-785.
Lustig, F.M., Haas, A., & Castillo, R. (1972). Clinical and rehabilitation regime in patients with chronic obstructive pulmonary disease. *Archives of Physical Medicine and Rehabilitation, 53,* 315-322.
Pattison, E.M., Rhodes, R.J., & Dudley, D.L. (1971). Response to group treatment in patients with severe chronic lung disease. *International Journal of Group Psychotherapy, 21,* 214-225.
Williams, R. (1989). *The trusting heart: Great news about Type A behavior and your heart.* New York: Time Books.

PART I INTRODUCTION

CHAPTER 1 The Importance of Psychosocial Interventions in the Treatment of Cardiopulmonary Patients

For statistics regarding COPD in America, see:
American Lung Association (1994). *Lung disease data: 1994.* New York: Author.
Williams, S.J., & Bury, M.R. (1989). "Breathtaking": The consequences of chronic respiratory disorder. *International Disability Studies, 11,* 114-120.
Call for bolstering psychosocial care in cardiac rehabilitation:
Hill, D.R., Kelleher, K., & Shumaker, S.A. (1992). Psychosocial interventions in adult patients with coronary heart disease and cancer. *General Hospital Psychiatry, 14,* 28-42.
World Health Organization Expert Committee. (1992). *Rehabilitation after diseases, with special emphasis on developing countries: Report of a WHO expert committee.* Geneva, Switzerland: World Health Organization.
Early studies of the psychological effects of medical procedures:
Henrichs, T.J., MacKenzie, J.W., & Almond, C.H. (1971). Psychological adjustment and psychiatric complications following open-heart surgery. *Journal of Nervous and Mental Disease, 152,* 332-345.
Weiss, S.M. (1966). Psychological adjustment following open heart surgery. *Journal of Nervous and Mental Disease, 143,* 363-368.

Stresses of cardiac and pulmonary illness for patients and family:
Houston-Miller, N., Taylor, C.B., Davidson, D.M., Hill, M.N., & Krantz, D.S. (1990). The efficacy of risk factor intervention and psychosocial aspects of cardiac rehabilitation. *Journal of Cardiac Rehabilitation, 10*, 198-209.

Rejeski, W.J., Morley, D., & Sotile, W. (1985). Cardiac rehabilitation: A conceptual framework for psychologic assessment. *Journal of Cardiopulmonary Rehabilitation, 4*, 172-180.

Sotile, W.M., Sotile, M.O., Ewen, G.S., & Sotile, L.J. (1993). Marriage and family factors relevant to effective cardiac rehabilitation: A review of risk factor literature. *Sports Medicine, Training and Rehabilitation, 4*, 115-128.

Sotile, W.M., Sotile, M.O., Sotile, L.J., & Ewen, G.S. (1993). Marital and family factors relevant to cardiac rehabilitation: An integrative review of the psychosocial literature. *Sports Medicine, Training and Rehabilitation, 4*, 217-236.

Wise, T.N., Schiavone, A.A., & Sitts, T.M. (1988). The depressed patient with chronic obstructive pulmonary disease. *General Hospital Psychiatry, 10*, 142-147.

Psychosocial factors predict morbidity for CHD patients:
Maeland, J.G., & Havik, O.E. (1989). Use of health services after a myocardial infarction. *Scandinavian Journal of Social Medicine, 17*, 93-102.

Shaw, R.E., Cohen, F., Fishman-Rosen, J., Murphy, M.C., Stertzer, S.H., Clark, D.A., & Myler, R.K. (1986). Psychologic predictors of psychosocial and medical outcomes in patients undergoing coronary angioplasty. *Psychosomatic Medicine, 48*, 582-597.

Williams, R.B., Jr., Haney, T.L., McKinnis, R.A., Harrell, F.E., Jr., Lee, K.L., Pryor, D.B., Califf, R., Kong, Y., Rosati, R.A., & Blumenthal, J.A. (1986). Psychosocial and physical predictors of anginal pain relief with medical management. *Psychosomatic Medicine, 48*, 200-210.

Mental stress and sudden cardiac death:
Willich, S.N., Maclure, M., Mittleman, M., Arntz, C., & Muller, J.E. (1993). Sudden cardiac death, support for a role of triggering in causation. *Circulation, 87*, 1442-1450.

Emotional factors and the course of COPD:
Agle, D.F., Baum, G.L., Chester, E.H., & Wendt, M. (1973). Multidiscipline treatment of chronic pulmonary insufficiency. 1. Psychological aspects of rehabilitation. *Psychosomatic Medicine, 35*(1), 41-49.

Beck, G., Scott, S., Teague, R., Perez, F., & Brown, A. (1988). Correlates of daily impairment in chronic obstructive pulmonary disease. *Rehabilitation Psychology, 33*(2), 77-84.

Jones, P.W., Baveystock, C.M., & Littlejohns, P. (1989). Relationships between general health measured with the sickness impact profile and respiratory symptoms, physiological measures, and mood in patients with chronic airflow limitation. *American Review of Respiratory Diseases, 140*, 1538-1543.

Ries, A.L. (1987). The role of exercise testing in pulmonary diagnosis. *Clinics of Chest Medicine, 8*, 81-89.

Traver, G.A. (1988). Measures of symptoms and life quality to predict emergent use of institutional health care resources in chronic obstructive airways disease. *Heart and Lung, 17*, 689-697.

The importance of attending to psychosocial factors in outpatient rehabilitation of COPD patients:
Atkins, C.J., Kaplan, R.M., Timms, R.M., Reinsch, S., & Loftback, K. (1984). Behavioral exercise programs in the management of chronic obstructive pulmonary disease. *Journal of Consulting and Clinical Psychology, 52*(4), 591-603.

Bebout, D.E., Hodgkin, J.E., Zorn, E.G., Yee, A.R., & Sammer, E.A. (1983). Clinical and physiological outcomes of a university-hospital pulmonary rehabilitation program. *Respiratory Care, 28*, 1468-1473.

Lertzman, M.M., & Cherniack, R.M. (1976). Rehabilitation of patients with chronic obstructive pulmonary disease. *American Review of Respiratory Diseases, 114*, 1145-1165.

The incidence and costs of cardiac surgeries:
Nair, C., Colburn, H., McLean, D., & Petrasovits, A. (1989). Cardiovascular disease in Canada. In D.F. Bray (Ed.), *Health reports* (pp. 1-22). Ottawa, ON: Statistics Canada—Canadian Centre for Health Information.

Polister, P., & Cunico, E. (1988). *Social-economic factbook for surgery.* New York: American College of Surgeons, Socioeconomic Affairs Department.

Hospitalization statistics for COPD patients:

Yellowlees, P.M., Alpers, J.H., Bowden, J.J., Bryant, G.D., & Ruffin, R.E. (1987). Psychiatric morbidity in patients with chronic airflow obstruction. *The Medical Journal of Australia, 146,* 305-307.

Incidence of positive psychosocial adjustment following cardiac illness:

Havik, O.E., & Maeland, J.G. (1990). Patterns of emotional reactions after a myocardial infarction. *Journal of Psychosomatic Research, 4*(3), 271-285.

Mayou, R., Foster, A., & Williamson, B. (1978a). The psychological and social effects of myocardial infarction on wives. *British Medical Journal, 1,* 699-701.

Prince, R., Frasure-Smith, N., & Rolicz-Woloszyk, E. (1982). Life stress denial and outcome in ischemic heart disease patients. *Journal of Psychosomatic Research, 26,* 23-31.

Stern, M.J., Pascale, L., & McLoone, J.B. (1976). Psychological adaptation following an acute myocardial infarction. *Journal of Chronic Diseases, 29,* 513-526.

The psychosocial struggles of recovering cardiac patients and their families:

Gundle, M.D., Reeves, B.R., & Tate, S. (1980). Psychosocial outcome after coronary artery surgery. *American Journal of Psychiatry, 137,* 1591-1594.

Haywood, J., & Obier, K. (1971). Psychosocial problems of coronary care unit patients. *Journal of the National Medical Association, 63,* 425-428.

Hill, D.R., Kelleher, K., & Shumaker, S.A. (1992). Psychosocial interventions in adult patients with coronary heart disease and cancer. *General Hospital Psychiatry, 14,* 28-42.

Houston-Miller, N., Taylor, C.B., Davidson, D.M., Hill, M.N., & Krantz, D.S. (1990). The efficacy of risk factor intervention and psychosocial aspects of cardiac rehabilitation. *Journal of Cardiac Rehabilitation, 10,* 198-209.

Pimm, J.B., & Feist, J.R. (1984). *Psychological risks of coronary artery bypass surgery.* New York: Plenum Press.

Sotile, W.M., Sotile, M.O., Ewen, G.S., & Sotile, L.J. (1993). Marriage and family factors relevant to effective cardiac rehabilitation: A review of risk factor literature. *Sports Medicine, Training and Rehabilitation, 4,* 115-128.

Sotile, W.M., Sotile, M.O., Sotile, L.J., & Ewen, G.S. (1993). Marital and family factors relevant to cardiac rehabilitation: An integrative review of the psychosocial literature. *Sports Medicine, Training and Rehabilitation, 4,* 217-236.

Wishnie, H., Hackett, T., & Cassem, N. (1971). Psychological hazards of convalescence following myocardial infarction. *Journal of the American Medical Association, 215,* 1292-1296.

Affective distress of COPD patients:

Gift, A.G., & Cahill, C. (1990). Psychophysiologic aspects of dyspnea in chronic obstructive pulmonary disease: A pilot study. *Heart and Lung, 19,* 252-257.

Gift, A.G., Palut, S.M., & Jacox, A. (1986). Psychologic and physiologic factors related to dyspnea in subjects with chronic obstructive pulmonary disease. *Heart and Lung, 15*(4), 595-601.

Long-range adjustment struggles of cardiac patients and family:

Gundle, M.D., Reeves, B.R., & Tate, S. (1980). Psychosocial outcome after coronary artery surgery. *American Journal of Psychiatry, 137,* 1591-1594.

Pimm, J.B., & Feist, J.R. (1984). *Psychological risks of coronary artery bypass surgery.* New York: Plenum Press.

Wishnie, H., Hackett, T., & Cassem, N. (1971). Psychological hazards of convalescence following myocardial infarction. *Journal of the American Medical Association, 215,* 1292-1296.

Razin, A.M. (1982). Psychosocial intervention in coronary artery disease: A review. *Psychosomatic Medicine, 44*(4), 363-381.

Attitudes of COPD patients toward rehabilitation:

Gift, A.G., & McCrone, S.H. (1993). Depression in patients with COPD. *Heart and Lung, 22*(4), 289-297.

Light, R.W., Merrill, E.J., Despers, J.A., Gordon, G.H., & Mutalipassi, L.R. (1985). Prevalence of depression and anxiety in patients with COPD: Relationship to functional capacity. *Chest 87*, 35-43.

Morbidity for CHD and MI patients:

Gruen, W. (1975). Effects of brief psychotherapy during the hospitalization period on the recovery process in heart attacks. *Journal of Consulting Clinical Psychology, 43*, 252-270.

Ibrahim, M., Feldman, J., Sultz, H.A., Staiman, M., Young, L., & Dean, D. (1974). Management after myocardial infarction: A controlled trial of the effect of group psychotherapy. *International Journal of Psychiatry Medicine, 5*(3), 253.

Medalie, J., Snyder, M., & Groen, J. (1973). Angina pectoris among 10,000 men: 5-year incidence and univariate analysis. *American Journal of Medicine, 55*, 583-594.

Psychosocial factors and morbidity for CABG patients:

Aiken, L.H., & Henricks, T.F. (1971). Systematic relaxation as a nursing intervention technique with open heart surgery patients. *Nursing Research, 20*(3), 212-216.

Psychosocial factors and mortality from CHD:

Berkman, L., & Syme, S.L. (1979). Social networks, host resistance, and mortality: A nine-year follow-up study of Alameda County residents. *American Journal of Epidemiology, 109*, 186-204.

Garrity, T.F., & Klein, R.F. (1975). Emotional response and clinical severity as early determinants of six-month mortality after myocardial infarction. *Heart and Lung, 4*, 730-737.

Positive results from specific brief interventions:

• **Relaxation training**

Oldenburg, B., Perkins, R.J., & Andrews, G. (1985). Controlled trial of psychological intervention in myocardial infarction. *Journal of Consulting and Clinical Psychology, 53*, 852-859.

• **Brief counseling in-hospital**

Gruen, W. (1975). Effects of brief psychotherapy during the hospitalization period on the recovery process in heart attacks. *Journal of Consulting Clinical Psychology, 43*, 252-270.

Langosch, W., Seer, P., Brodner, G., Kallinke, D., Kulich, B., & Heim, F. (1982). Behavior therapy with coronary heart disease patients: Results of a comparative study. *Journal of Psychosomatic Research, 26*(5), 475-484.

• **Long-range adjustment from brief counseling**

Gruen, W. (1975). Effects of brief psychotherapy during the hospitalization period on the recovery process in heart attacks. *Journal of Consulting Clinical Psychology, 43*, 252-270.

Langosch, W., Seer, P., Brodner, G., Kallinke, D., Kulich, B., & Heim, F. (1982). Behavior therapy with coronary heart disease patients: Results of a comparative study. *Journal of Psychosomatic Research, 26*(5), 475-484.

CHAPTER 2   Assessment

Cardiopulmonary illness as a crisis:

Havik, O.E., & Maeland, J.G. (1990). Patterns of emotional reactions after a myocardial infarction. *Journal of Psychosomatic Research, 4*(3), 271-285.

Moos, R.H. (1982). Coping with acute health crisis. In T. Millon, C. Green, & R. Maegher (Eds.), *Handbook of clinical health psychology* (pp. 76-90). New York: Plenum Press.

For seminal discussions of psychosomatic invalidism, see:

White, K.L., Grant, J.L., & Chambis, W.N. (1955). Angina pectoris and angina innocens. *Psychosomatic Medicine, 17*, 128-135.

Specific approaches to treating psychosomatic invalidism:

• **Systematic desensitization of anxiety**

Rifkin, B.G. (1968). The treatment of cardiac neurosis using systematic desensitization. *Behavioral Research Therapy, 6*, 239-241.

• **Behavior therapy**

Baile, W.F., & Engel, B.T. (1978). A behavioral strategy for promoting treatment compliance following myocardial infarction. *Psychosomatic Medicine, 40*, 413-419.

- **Biofeedback**
  Wickramasekera, I. (1974). Heart rate feedback and the management of cardiac neurosis. *Journal of Abnormal Psychology, 83,* 578-580.
- **Supportive psychotherapy**
  Stein, E.H., Murdaugh, J., & MacLeod, J.A. (1969). Brief psychotherapy of psychiatric reactions to physical illness. *American Journal of Psychiatry, 8,* 1040-1047.
- **Coaching regarding hyperventilation control**
  Razin, A.M. (1982). Psychosocial intervention in coronary artery disease: A review. *Psychosomatic Medicine, 44*(4), 363-381.
- **Family interventions**
  Doherty, W.J. (1986). Marital therapy and family medicine. In N. Jacobson & A Gurman (Eds.), *A clinical handbook of marital therapy* (pp. 185-198). New York: Guilford Press.

Prevalence and course of depression and anxiety in cardiac patients:

Carney, R.M., Rich, M.W., Tevelde, A., Saini, J., Clark, T., & Jaffe, A.S. (1987). Major depressive disorder in coronary artery disease. *American Journal of Cardiology, 60,* 1273-1275.

Hackett, T.P. (1985). Depression following myocardial infarction. *Psychosomatics, 26*(Suppl.), 23-28.

Hackett, T.P., Cassem, N.H., & Wishnie, H.A. (1968). The coronary care unit: An appraisal of its psychological hazards. *New England Journal of Medicine, 279,* 1365-1370.

Kornfeld, D.S., Heller, S.S., Frank, K.A., Wilson, S.N., & Malm, J.R. (1982). Psychological and behavioral responses after coronary artery bypass surgery. *Circulation, 66*(Suppl. III), 24-28.

Kornfeld, D.S., Zimberg, S., & Malm, J.R. (1965). Psychiatric complications of open heart surgery. *New England Journal of Medicine, 273,* 287-292.

Schleifer, S.J., Macari-Hinson, M.M., Coyle, D.A., Slater, W.R., Kahn, M., Gorlin, R., & Zucker, H.A. (1989). The nature and course of depression following myocardial infarction. *Archives of Internal Medicine, 149,* 1785-1789.

Schockern, D.D., Green, A.F., Worder, T.J., Harrison, E.E., & Spielberger, D.C. (1987). Effects of age on the relationship between anxiety and coronary artery disease. *Psychosomatic Medicine, 49,* 118-126.

Taylor, C.B., DeBusk, R.F., Davidson, D.M., Houston, N., & Burnett, K.F. (1981). Optimal methods for identifying depression following hospitalization for myocardial infarction. *Journal of Chronic Disease, 34,* 127-133.

Verwoerdt, A., & Dovenmuhle, R.H. (1964). Heart disease and depression. *Geriatrics, 19,* 856-863.

Wishnie, H., Hackett, T., & Cassem, N. (1971). Psychological hazards of convalescence following myocardial infarction. *Journal of the American Medical Association, 215,* 1292-1296.

The course of anxiety and depression in recovery from cardiopulmonary illness:

Cassem, N.H., & Hackett, T.P. (1979). "Ego infarction." Psychological reactions to a heart attack. *Journal of Practicing Nurses, 29,* 17-39.

Granger, J.W. (1974). Full recovery from myocardial infarction: Psychosocial factors. *Heart and Lung, 3,* 600-610.

Longitudinal studies of depression and MI:

Lebovitis, B.Z., Shekelle, R.B., Ostfeld, A.M., & Paul, O. (1967). Prospective and retrospective psychological studies of coronary heart disease. *Psychosomatic Medicine, 29*(3), 265-272.

Malan, S.S. (1992), Psychosocial adjustment following MI: Current views and nursing implications. *Journal of Cardiovascular Nursing, 6*(4), 57-70.

Ostfeld, A.M., Lebovitis, B.Z., Shekelle, R.B., & Paul, O. (1964). A prospective study of the relationship between personality and coronary heart disease. *Journal of Chronic Diseases, 17,* 265-276.

Schleifer, S.J., Macari-Hinson, M.M., Coyle, D.A., Slater, W.R., Kahn, M., Gorlin, R., & Zucker, H.A. (1989). The nature and course of depression following myocardial infarction. *Archives of Internal Medicine, 149,* 1785-1789.

Factors that affect adjustment to cardiac illness:

Croog, S.H. (1983). Recovery and rehabilitation of heart patients: Psychosocial aspects. In D.S. Krantz, A. Baum, & J.S. Singer (Eds.), *Handbook of psychology and health. Vol. 3: Cardiovascular disorders and behavior.* London: Erlbaum.

Prevalence of depression in COPD patients:

Beck, G., Scott, S., Teague, R., Perez, F., & Brown, A. (1988). Correlates of daily impairment in chronic obstructive pulmonary disease. *Rehabilitation Psychology, 33*(2), 77-84.

Further information regarding treatment strategies for postoperative delirium:

Kornfeld, D.S., Zimberg, S., & Malm, J.R. (1965). Psychiatric complications of open heart surgery. *New England Journal of Medicine, 273,* 287-292.

Leigh, H., Hofer, M.A., Cooper, J., & Reiser, M.F. (1972). A psychological comparison of patients in "open" and "closed": Coronary care units. *Journal of Psychosomatic Research, 16,* 449-458.

Prevalence of anxiety disorders in COPD patients:

Dudley, D.L., Glaser, E.M., Jorgenson, B.N., & Logan, D.L. (1980). Psychosocial concomitants to rehabilitation in chronic obstructive pulmonary disease: Part I. Psychosocial and psychological considerations. *Chest, 77*(3), 413-420.

Kinsman, R., Fernandez, E., Schocket, M., Dirks, J., & Covino, N. (1982). Multidimensional analysis of the symptoms of chronic bronchitis and emphysema. *Journal of Behavioral Medicine, 6*(4), 339-357.

Wise, T.N., Schiavone, A.A., & Sitts, T.M. (1988). The depressed patient with chronic obstructive pulmonary disease. *General Hospital Psychiatry, 10,* 142-147.

Critical comments regarding research on anxiety disorders in COPD:

Porzelius, J., Vest, M., & Nochomovitz, M. (1992). *Behaviour Research and Therapy, 30*(1), 75-77.

Prevalence of depressive disorders in COPD patients:

Kersten, L. (1990b). Changes in self-concept during pulmonary rehabilitation, part 2. *Heart and Lung, 19*(5), 463-470.

Light, R.W., Merrill, E.J., Despers, J.A., Gordon, G.H., & Mutalipassi, L.R. (1985). Prevalence of depression and anxiety in patients with COPD: Relationship to functional capacity. *Chest, 87,* 35-43.

McSweeney, A., Grant, I., Heaton, R., Adams, K., & Timms, R. (1982). Life quality of patients with chronic obstructive pulmonary disease. *Archives of Internal Medicine, 142,* 473-478.

Negative effects of depression on medical recovery in general:

Katon, W., & Sullivan, M.D. (1990). Depression and chronic medical illness. *Journal of Clinical Psychiatry, 51*(Suppl. 6), 3-11.

Ways that depression complicates recovery for CHD and post-MI patients:

- **Early mortality and higher morbidity with depressed patients**

  Frasure-Smith, N., Lesperance, F., & Talajic, M. (1993). Depression following myocardial infarction. *Journal of the American Medical Association, 270*(15), 1819-1825.

  Roose, S.P., Dalack, G.W., & Woodring, S. (1991). Death, depression and heart disease. *Journal of Clinical Psychiatry, 52*(Suppl. 6), 34-39.

- **Predisposes affected individuals to ventricular fibrillation and to decreased parasympathetic activity**

  Lown, B., & Verrier, R.L. (1976). Neural activity and ventricular fibrillation. *New England Journal of Medicine, 294,* 1165-1170.

  Lown, B., Verrier, R.L., & Rabinowitz, S.H. (1977). Neural and psychological mechanisms and the problem of sudden death. *American Journal of Cardiology, 39,* 890-902.

- **Responses to cardiac catheterization**

  Carney, R.M., Rich, M.W., Freedland, K.E., Saini, J., Tevelde, A., Simeone, C., & Clark, K. (1988). Major depressive disorder predicts cardiac events in patients with coronary artery disease. *Psychosomatic Medicine, 50,* 627-633.

- **Affects outcome in exercise tolerance for recovering CHD patients**

  Milani, R.V., Littman, A.B., & Lavie, C.J. (1993). Depressive symptoms predict functional improvement following cardiac rehabilitation and exercise program. *Journal of Cardiopulmonary Rehabilitation 13,* 406-411.

- **Lack of physical, vocational, and general psychosocial improvement for CHD patients**
  Hlatky, M.A., Haney, T., & Barefoot, J.C. (1986). Medical, psychological, and social correlates of work disability among men with coronary artery disease. *American Journal of Cardiology, 58,* 911-915.

  Pancheri, P., Bellaterra, M., Matteoli, S., Christofari, M., Polizzi, C., & Puletti, M. (1978). Infarct as a stress agent: Life history and personality characteristics in improved versus not-improved patients after severe heart attack. *Journal of Human Stress, 4,* 16-22.

  Stern, M.J., Pascale, L., & Ackerman, A. (1977). Life adjustment postmyocardial infarction. *Archives of Internal Medicine, 137,* 623-633.

- **Interferes with maintenance of behavioral changes**
  Finnegan, D.L., & Suler, J.R. (1985). Psychological factors associated with maintenance of improved health behaviors in post coronary patients. *Journal of Psychology, 119,* 87-94.

- **Poor compliance with medical recommendations**
  Blumenthal, J., Williams, R.S., Needels, T., & Wallace, A. (1982). Psychological changes accompany aerobic exercise in healthy middle-aged adults. *Psychosomatic Medicine, 44,* 529-536.

Other discussions of effects of depression on recovery from cardiac illnesses:
  Ahern, D.K., Gorkin, L., Anderson, J.L., Tierney, C., Hallstrom, A., & Ewart, C., for the Cardiac Arrhythmia Pilot Study (CAPS) Investigators. (1989, November). *Biohavioral variables and mortality or cardiac arrest in the CAPS.* Paper presented at the annual meeting of the American Heart Association, New Orleans.

  Bruhn, H., Wolf, S., & Philips B. (1971). Depression and death in myocardial infarction: A psychosocial study of screening male coronary patients over nine years. *Journal of Psychosomatic Research, 15,* 305-313.

  Garrity, T.F., & Klein, R.F. (1975). Emotional response and clinical severity as early determinants of six-months mortality after myocardial infarction. *Heart and Lung, 4,* 730-737.

  Stern, M.J., Pascale, L., & Ackerman, A. (1977). Life adjustment postmyocardial infarction. *Archives of Internal Medicine, 137,* 623-633.

  Swenson, J.R., & Abbey, S.E. (1993). Management of depression and anxiety disorders in the cardiac patient. In F.J. Pashkow & W.A. Dafoe (Eds.), *Clinical cardiac rehabilitation: A cardiologist's guide.* Baltimore: Williams & Wilkins.

Symptoms of anxiety disorders:
  Greist, J.H., Jefferson, J.W., & Marks, I.M. (1986). Anxiety and its treatment. New York: Warner Books.

  Marks, I.M. (1986). *Fears, phobias, and rituals: An interdisciplinary perspective.* Cambridge, MA: Oxford University Press.

  Swenson, J.R., & Abbey, S.E. (1993). Management of depression and anxiety disorders in the cardiac patient. In F.J. Pashkow & W.A. Dafoe (Eds.), *Clinical cardiac rehabilitation: A cardiologist's guide.* Baltimore: Williams & Wilkins.

  Taylor, C.B., & Arnow, B. (1985). *The nature and treatment of anxiety disorders* (pp. 313-314). New York: Free Press.

  Taylor, C.B., Sheikh, J., Argras, W.S., Roth, W.T., Margraf, J., Ehleys, A., Maddock, R.J., & Gossard, D. (1986). Ambulatory heart rate changes in patients with panic attacks. *American Journal of Psychiatry, 143,* 479-482.

Psychosocial stressors that cause anxiety and depression in recovering patients:
  O'Malley, P.A., & Menke, R. (1988). Relationship of hope and stress after myocardial infarction. *Heart and Lung, 17,* 184-190.

Exercise caution when interpreting data from standard assessments of depression and anxiety:
  Taylor, C.B., DeBusk, R.F., Davidson, D.M., Houston, N., & Burnett, K.F. (1981). Optimal methods for identifying depression following hospitalization for myocardial infarction. *Journal of Chronic Disease, 34,* 127-133.

Psychotropics with cardiac patients:
  Swenson, J.R., & Abbey, S.E. (1993). Management of depression and anxiety disorders in the cardiac patient. In F.J. Pashkow & W.A. Dafoe (Eds.), *Clinical cardiac rehabilitation: A cardiologist's guide.* Baltimore: Williams & Wilkins.

Veith, R.C., Raskind, M.A., Caldwell, J.H., Barnes, R.F., Gumbrecht, G., & Ritchie, J.L. (1982). Cardiovascular effects of tricyclic antidepressants in depressed patients with chronic heart disease. *New England Journal of Medicine, 306*, 954-959.

Psychotropics with COPD patients:

Gordon, G.H., Michiels, T.M., Mahutte, C.K., & Light, R.W. (1985). Effect of desipramine on control of ventilation and depression scores in patients with severe chronic obstructive pulmonary disease. *Psychiatry Research, 15*(1), 5-32.

CHAPTER 3 Approaching Cardiopulmonary Patients for Psychosocial Intervention

Seminal works on medical hypnosis:

Erickson, M. (1948). Hypnotic psychotherapy. *The Medical Clinics of North America.*

Erickson, M.H., Hershman, S., & Secter, I. (1961). *The practical application of medical and dental hypnosis.* New York: The Julian Press.

How health behaviors organize interpersonal relationships:

Stuart, R.B., & Davis, B. (1972). *Slim chance in a fat world: Behavioral control of obesity.* Chicago: Research Press.

Coppotelli, H.C., & Orleans, C.T. (1985). Partner support and other determinants of smoking cessation maintenance among women. *Journal of Consulting and Clinical Psychology, 53*, 455-460.

For further discussion of the stages of change theory, see:

DiClemente, C.C., Prochaska, J.O., Fairhurst, S., Velicer, W.F., Velasquez, M.M., & Rossi, J.S. (1991). The process of smoking cessation: An analysis of precontemplation, contemplation and preparation stages of change. *Journal of Consulting and Clinical Psychology, 59*, 295-304.

Prochaska, J.O., & DiClemente, C.C. (1983). Stages and processes of self-change of smoking: Toward an integrative model of change. *Journal of Clinical and Consulting Psychology, 51*, 390-395.

Prochaska, J.O., DiClemente, C.C., & Norcross, J.C. (1992). In search of how people change: Applications to addictive behaviors. *American Psychologist, 47*(9), 1102-1114.

Prochaska, J.O., Velicer, W.F., Rossi, J.S., Goldstein, M.G., Marcus, B.H., Rakowski, W., Fiore, C., Harlow, L., Redding, C.A., Rosenbloom, D., & Rossi, S.R. (1994). Stages of change and decisional balance for 12 problem behaviors. *Health Psychology, 13*(1), 39-46.

Methods for assessing an individual's stage of change:

- **A discrete categorical measure that assesses the stage of change from a series of mutually exclusive questions**

DiClemente, C.C., Prochaska, J.O., Fairhurst, S., Velicer, W.F., Velasquez, M.M., & Rossi, J.S. (1991). The process of smoking cessation: An analysis of precontemplation, contemplation and preparation stages of change. *Journal of Consulting and Clinical Psychology, 59*, 295-304.

- **A continuous measure that yields separate scales for precontemplation, contemplation, action, and maintenance**

McConnaughy, E.A., DiClemente, C.C., Prochaska, J.O., & Velicer, W.F. (1989). Stages of change in psychotherapy: A follow-up report. *Psychotherapy: Theory, Research and Practice, 4*, 494-503.

McConnaughy, E.A., Prochaska, J.O., & Velicer, W.F. (1983). Stages of change in psychotherapy: Measurement and sample profiles. *Psychotherapy: Theory, Research and Practice, 20*, 368-375.

Methods of assessing repression and sensitization:

Byrne, D., Barry, J., & Nelson, D. (1963). Relation of the revised repression-sensitization scale to measures of self-description. *Psychology Report, 13*, 323-334.

Weinberger, D.A., Schwartz, G.E., & Davidson, J.R. (1979). Low anxious and depressive coping styles: Psychometric patterns and behavioral physiological responses to stress. *Journal of Abnormal Psychology, 88*, 369-380.

Weinberger, Schwartz, and Davidson developed a method for assessing repression-sensitization that is a refinement of the original Byrne Repression-Sensitization Scale and that uses a combination of the Taylor Manifest Anxiety Scale from the Minnesota Multiphasic Personality Inventory and the Marlowe-Crowne Social Desirability Scale. However, the construct validity of this method has not yet been established.

For seminal discussion of denial in cardiac patients, see:

Hackett, T.P., Cassem, N.H., & Wishnie, H.A. (1968). The coronary care unit: An appraisal of its psychological hazards. *New England Journal of Medicine, 279,* 1365-1370.

Hackett, Cassem, & Wishnie, who differentiated between "major deniers" (those who report no fear at all at any time during their cardiac crisis), "partial deniers" (who at first deny but eventually admit some fear), and "minimal deniers" (who readily acknowledge fear).

For further discussion of the need for research regarding denial in cardiac populations:

Razin, A.M. (1982). Psychosocial intervention in coronary artery disease: A review. *Psychosomatic Medicine, 44*(4), 363-381.

How TYABP sometimes promotes positive adjustments during cardiac rehabilitation:

Rejeski, W.J. (1983). Rehabilitation and prevention of coronary heart disease: An overview of the Type A behavior pattern. *Quest, 33*(2), 154-165.Rejeski, 1983

Rejeski, W.J., Morley, D., & Miller, H.S. (1983). Coronary prone behavior as a moderator of GTX performance. *Journal of Cardiac Rehabilitation, 3,* 339-346.

Rejeski, W.J., Morley, D., & Miller, H.S. (1984). The Jenkins Activity Survey: Exploring its relationship with compliance to exercise prescription and MET gain within a cardiac rehabilitation setting. *Journal of Cardiac Rehabilitation, 4,* 90-94.

Data that strongly validate the efficacy of taking care to first point out what the patient and family are doing that is working, and then gently stretch their awareness as a means of promoting coping flexibility:

Kendall, P.C., Williams, L., Pechacek, T.F., Graham, L.E., Shisslak, C., & Herzoll, N. (1979). Cognitive-behavioral and patient education interventions in cardiac catheterization procedures: The Palo Alto Medical Psychology Project. *Journal of Consulting and Clinical Psychology, 47,* 49-58.

Sanctioning of use of goal setting in rehabilitation:

American Association of Cardiovascular and Pulmonary Rehabilitation. (1991). *Guidelines for cardiac rehabilitation programs.* Champaign, IL: Human Kinetics.

American Thoracic Society. (1981). Official ATS Statement—pulmonary rehabilitation by the American Lung Association. *American Review of Respiratory Disease, 124,* 663-666.

Connors, G., & Hilling, L. (1993). *Guidelines for pulmonary rehabilitation programs.* Champaign, IL: Human Kinetics.

Ries, A.L. (1990). Position paper of the American Association of Cardiovascular and Pulmonary Rehabilitation: Scientific basis of pulmonary rehabilitation. *Journal of Cardiopulmonary Rehabilitation, 10,* 418-441.

Houston-Miller, N., Taylor, C.B., Davidson, D.M., Hill, M.N., & Krantz, D.S. (1990). The efficacy of risk factor intervention and psychosocial aspects of cardiac rehabilitation. *Journal of Cardiac Rehabilitation, 10,* 198-209.

Use of goal setting in modifying risk factors:

Lovibond, S.H., Birrell, P.C., & Langeluddecke, P. (1985). Changing coronary heart disease risk-factor status: The effects of three behavioral programs. *Journal of Behavioral Medicine, 9*(5), 415-437.

Discussion of how the provider's goals for the patient might differ from the patient's own goals during rehabilitation:

Feinstein, A.R., Josephy, B.R., & Wells, C.K. (1986). Scientific and clinical problems in indexes of functional disability. *Annals of Internal Medicine, 105,* 413-420.

Using modeling to help patients overcome fears:

Kazdin, A.E. (1974). Covert modeling, model similarity, and reduction of avoidance behavior. *Behavior Therapy, 5,* 325-340.

Kendall, P.C., Williams, L., Pechacek, T.F., Graham, L.E., Shisslak, C., & Herzoll, N. (1979). Cognitive-behavioral and patient education interventions in cardiac catheterization procedures: The Palo Alto Medical Psychology Project. *Journal of Consulting and Clinical Psychology, 47,* 49-58.

The form of coping modeling in which the provider normalizes fears and subsequently discusses the methods for overcoming them has been shown to be more effective than interventions delivered by health care providers who act fearless throughout their interactions with patients (Kazdin). Patients facing cardiac catheterization have been shown to benefit from such modeling in the form of information from former patients (Kendall et al).

Further discussion of the social support factor in rehabilitation:

Thoits (1986) pointed out that social support should provide three forms of coping assistance—problem-focused coping (direct action that alters circumstances appraised as threatening); perception-focused coping (altering the meaning of the situation so that it is perceived as less threatening); and emotion-focused coping (controlling undesirable feelings through actions and thoughts).

Thoits, P.A. (1986). Social support as coping assistance. *Journal of Consulting and Clinical Psychology, 54,* 416-423.

Education in rehabilitation:

• **Teaching health management techniques**

Cowan, M.J. (1990). Cardiovascular nursing research. *Annual Review of Nursing, 8,* 333.

to inpatients

Scalzi, C., Burke, L., & Greenland, S. (1980). Evaluation of an inpatient education program for coronary patients and families. *Heart and Lung, 9,* 846-853

to outpatients

Lertzman, M.M., & Cherniack, R.M. (1976). Rehabilitation of patients with chronic obstructive pulmonary disease. *American Review of Respiratory Diseases, 114,* 1145-1165.

Ott, C.R., Sivarajan, E.S., Newton, K.M., Almes, M.J., Bruce, R.A., Bergren, M., & Gibson, B. (1983). A controlled randomized study of early cardiac rehabilitation: The Sickness Impact Profile as an assessment tool. *Heart and Lung, 12,* 162-170.

Sivarajan, E.S., Bruce, R.A., Almes, M.J., Green, B., Belanger, L., Lindskog, B.D., Newton, K.M., & Mansfield, L.W. (1981). In-hospital exercise after myocardial infarction does not improve treadmill performance. *New England Journal of Medicine, 305*(7), 357-362.

Sivarajan, E.S., & Newton, K.M. (1984). Exercise, education, and counseling for patients with coronary artery disease. *Clinics in Sports Medicine, 3,* 349-369.

Sivarajan, E.S. (1989). *Ten-year prognostic value of clinical and exercise test variables in patients after myocardial infarction.* Unpublished doctoral dissertation, University of California, Los Angeles.

Psychosocial benefits of education:

Cowan, M.J. (1990). Cardiovascular nursing research. *Annual Review of Nursing, 8,* 3-33.

Godin, G. (1989). The effectiveness of interventions in modifying behavioral risk factors of individuals with coronary heart disease. *Journal of Cardiopulmonary Rehabilitation, 9,* 223-236.

Limitations of education in promoting risk factor changes:

Farquhar, J.W., Macoby, N., Wood, P.D., Alexander, J.K., Breitrose, H., Brown, B.W., Haskell, W.L., McAlister, A.L., Meyer, A.J., Nash, J.D., & Stern, M.P. (1977). Community education for cardiovascular health. *Lancet, 1,* 1192-1195.

Hosay, P.M. (1977). The unfulfilled promise of health education. *New York University Education Quarterly, 2,* 16-22.

Rose, G., Heller, R.F., Pedoc, H.T., & Christie, D.G. (1980). Heart disease prevention project: A randomised controlled trial in industry. *British Medical Journal, 279,* 747-751.

PART II   THE EFFECTIVE EMOTIONAL MANAGEMENT MODEL

CHAPTER 4   Effective Emotional Management: A Model for Structuring Practical Psychosocial Interventions in Medical Settings

Stress management with cardiopulmonary patients:

Razin, A.M. (1982). Psychosocial intervention in coronary artery disease: A review. *Psychosomatic Medicine, 44*(4), 363-381.

Hill, D.R., Kelleher, K., & Shumaker, S.A. (1992). Psychosocial interventions in adult patients with coronary heart disease and cancer. *General Hospital Psychiatry, 14s,* 28-42.

Blake, R.L., Vandiver, T.A., Braun, S., Bertuso, D.D., & Straub, V. (1990). A randomized controlled evaluation of a psychosocial intervention in adults with chronic lung disease. *Family Medicine, 22*(5), 365-370.

Friedman, M., Thoresen, C.E., Gill, J.J., Ulmer, D., Powell, L.H., Price, V.A., Brown, B., Thompson, L., Robin, D., Breall, W.S., Bourg, E., Levy, R., & Dixon, T. (1986). Alteration of Type A behavior and its effect on cardiac recurrences in postmyocardial infarction patients: Summary results of the recurrent coronary prevention project. *American Heart Journal, 112,* 653-665.

Friedman, M., & Ulmer, D. (1984). *Treating Type A behavior and your heart.* New York: Knopf.

A problem with the "stress management" literature with cardiopulmonary patients is that a wide variety of psychosocial treatments have been encompassed under the rubric of "stress management training." Reviewers (e.g., Razin; Hill et al.) have noted that a shortcoming of literature that has examined psychosocial issues in cardiopulmonary patients is lack of specificity regarding treatment procedures. A close reading of stress management studies that have employed cardiopulmonary samples suggests that what is referred to as "stress management" actually encompasses a wealth of treatment interventions delivered in treatment formats ranging from a single session of psychoeducation (Blake et al.) to support groups meeting for up to 4-5 years (Friedman et al.; Friedman & Ulmer).

Stress hardiness:

Noted family researchers Holahan & Moos (1986) offered practical descriptions of stress-hardiness characteristics of their patient samples that should be kept in mind in counseling recovering cardiopulmonary patients. These researchers found that stress-hardy individuals manifest the following four characteristics: (1) When bothered or when faced with stress, they approach, and don't avoid; (2) they work to maintain an easy-going disposition; (3) they create and maintain positive family relationships (especially important for women); (4) they find ways to bolster their self-confidence.

Stress and cardiac reactions:

Emery, C.F., Pinder, S.L., & Blumenthal, J.A. (1989). Psychological effects of exercise among elderly cardiac patients. *Journal of Cardiopulmonary Rehabilitation, 9,* 46-53.

Krantz, D.S. (1993, October). *Stress and myocardial ischemia: New insights.* Presented to the Eighth Annual Meeting of the American Association of Cardiovascular and Pulmonary Rehabilitation, Orlando, FL.

Krantz, D.S., Contrada, R.J., Hill, D.R., & Friedler, E. (1988). Environmental stress and biobehavioral antecedents of coronary heart disease. *Journal of Consulting and Clinical Psychology, 56,* 333-341.

Research on the effects of positive emotions:

Waltz, M., & Bandura, B. (1988). Subjective health, intimacy and perceived self-efficacy after a heart attack: Predicting life quality five years afterwards. *Social Industrial Research, 20,* 303-332.

CHAPTER 6   Relaxation

Biofeedback with respiratory patients:

Tiep, B.L. (1993). Biofeedback and respiratory muscle training. In J.E. Hodgkin, G.L. Connors, & C.W. Bell (Eds.), *Pulmonary rehabilitation: Guidelines to success* (2nd ed.) (pp. 403-421). Philadelphia: Lippincott.

For a discussion of guided imagery:

Naparstek, B. (1995). *Staying Well with Guided Imagery.* New York: Warner Publications.

Effects of physical fitness level on cardiovascular reactivity:

When stressed, the physically fit have been shown to evidence

• **Smaller increases in systolic blood pressure**

Lake, B.W., Suarez, E.C., Schneiderman, N., & Tocci, N. (1985). The Type A behavior pattern, physical fitness, and psychophysiological reactivity. *Health Psychology, 4,* 169.

Light, K.C., Obrist, P.A., James, S.A., & Stogatz, D.S. (1987). Cardiovascular responses to stress: II. Relationships to aerobic exercise patterns. *Psychophysiology, 24,* 79-86.

Cantor, J.P., Zillman, D., & Day, K.D. (1978). Relationship between cardiovascular fitness and physiological responses to films. *Perceptive Motor Skills, 46,* 1123-1130.

• **Smaller increases in diastolic blood pressure**

Light, K.C., Obrist, P.A., James, S.A., & Stogatz, D.S. (1987). Cardiovascular responses to stress: II. Relationships to aerobic exercise patterns. *Psychophysiology, 24,* 79-86.

Hull, E.M., Young, S.H., & Ziegler, M.G. (1984). Aerobic fitness affects cardiovascular and catecholamine responses to stressors. *Psychophysiology, 21,* 353-360.

• **Less increase in heart rate**

Holmes, D., & Roth, D. (1985). Association of aerobic fitness with pulse rate and subjective responses to psychological stress. *Psychophysiology, 22,* 525-529.

• **Faster heart rate recovery**

Sinyor, D., Schwartz, S.G., Peronnet, F., Brisson, S., & Saraganian, P. (1983). Aerobic fitness level and reactivity to psychosocial stress: Physiological, biochemical and subjective measures. *Psychosomatic Medicine, 45,* 205-217.

Cox, J.P., Evans, J.F., & Jamieson, J.L. (1979). Aerobic power and tonic heart rate responses to psychosocial stressors. *Personal Social Psychology Bulletin, 5,* 160-163.

For a general discussion and overview of fitness and cardiac reactivity, see:

Emery, C.F., Pinder, S.L., & Blumenthal, J.A. (1989). Psychological effects of exercise among elderly cardiac patients. *Journal of Cardiopulmonary Rehabilitation, 9,* 46-53.

Seraganian, P., Roskies, E., Hanley, J.A., Oseasohn, R., & Collu, R. (1987). Failure to alter psychophysiological reactivity in Type A men with physical exercise or stress management programs. *Psychological Health, 1,* 195-213.

Psychological benefits of exercise in nonclinical populations:

Folkins, C.H., & Sime, W.E. (1981). Physical fitness training and mental health. *American Psychologist, 36,* 373-389.

Taylor, C.B., Bandura, A., Ewart, C.K., Miller, N.H., & DeBusk, F. (1985). Exercise testing to enhance wives' confidence in their husbands' cardiac capability soon after clinically uncomplicated acute myocardial infarction. *American Journal of Cardiology, 55,* 635-638.

Effects of regular exercises on reducing the cardiovascular impact of emotional stressors:

Perkins, K.A., Dubbert, P.M., Martin, J.E., Faulstich, M.E., & Harris, J.K. (1988). Cardiovascular reactivity to psychological stress in aerobically trained versus untrained mild hypertensives and normotensives. *Health Psychology, 7,* L329-340.

Positive emotional changes from exercise occur independent of actual changes in physical fitness:

Goff, D., & Dimsdale, J.K. (1985). The psychologic effects of exercise. *Journal of Cardiopulmonary Rehabilitation, 5,* 274-290.

Jasnoski, M., & Holmes, D. (1981). Influence of initial aerobic fitness, aerobic training and changes in aerobic fitness on personality functioning. *Journal of Psychosomatic Research, 25,* 553-556.

Jasnoski, M., Holmes, D., Soloman, S., & Aguiar, C. (1981). Exercise, changes in aerobic capacity and changes in self-perceptions: An experimental investigation. *Journal of Research in Personality, 15,* 460-466.

CHAPTER 7   Personality-Based Coping Patterns

For extensive discussion of the theory upon which the information regarding coping patterns and pitfalls is based, see:

Stewart, I., & Joines, V. (1987). *TA today: A new introduction to transactional analysis.* Nottingham, England: Lifespace.

Regarding the incidence of TYABP:

Moss, G.E., Dielman, T.E., Campanelli, P.C., Leech, S.L., Harian, W.R., VanHarrison, R., & Horvath, W.J. (1986). Demographic correlates of 51 assessments of Type A behavior. *Psychosomatic Medicine, 4,* 564-674.

Baker, L.J., Dearborn, M.J., Hastings, J., & Hamberger, K. (1984). Type A behavior in women: a review. *Health Psychology, 3,* 477-497.

Demographic characteristics of those who show TYABP:

Davidson, M.J., Cooper, C.L., & Chamberlain, D. (1980). Type A coronary-prone behavior and stress in senior female managers and administrators. *Journal of Occupational Medicine, 22,* 801-805.

Moss, G.E., Dielman, T.E., Campanelli, P.C., Leech, S.L., Harian, W.R., VanHarrison, R., & Horvath, W.J. (1986). Demographic correlates of 51 assessments of Type A behavior. *Psychosomatic Medicine, 4,* 564-674.

Waldron, I., Zyzanski, S.J., Shekelle, R., Jenkins, C.D., & Tannenbaum, S. (1977). The coronary prone behavior pattern in employed men and women. *Journal of Human Stress, 3,* 2-18.

Investigations that have questioned whether or not TYABP really relates to:
• **The development of CHD**

Shekelle, R.B., Gale, M., Ostfeld, A., & Paul, O. (1983). Hostility, risk of coronary heart disease and mortality. *Psychosomatic Medicine, 45,* 109-114.

Shekelle, R.B., Hulley, S.B., Neaton, J.D., Billings, J.H., Borhani, N.O., Gerace, T.A., Jacobs, D.R., Lasser, N.L., Mittlemark, M.B., & Stamler, J. (1985). Incidence of coronary heart disease. *American Journal of Epidemiology, 122*(4), 559-570.

• **The prognosis of CHD**

Ragland, D.R., & Brand, R.J. (1988). Type A behavior and mortality from coronary heart disease. *New England Journal of Medicine, 318,* 65-69.

• **Rehabilitation responses**

Matthews, K.A. (1982). Psychological perspectives on the Type A behavior pattern. *Psychological Bulletin, 91,* 293-323.

Seminal descriptions of various defining characteristics of TYABP:

Friedman, M., & Rosenman, R.H. (1974). *Type A behavior and your heart.* New York: Knopf.

Friedman, M., & Ulmer, D. (1984). *Treating Type A behavior and your heart.* New York: Knopf.

Jenkins, C.D. (1971). Psychologic and social precursors of coronary disease. *New England Journal of Medicine, 284,* 244-255.

Price, V.A. (1982). *Type A behavior patterns: A model for research and practice.* New York: Academic.

Williams, R. (1989). *The trusting heart: Great news about Type A behavior and your heart.* New York: Time Books.

Various perspectives on the mechanisms of action underlying TYABP:

Haaga, D.A. (1987). Treatment for the Type A behavior pattern. *Clinical Psychology Review, 7,* 557-574.

Nunes, E., Frank, K.A., & Kornfeld, D.S. (1987). Psychologic treatment for the Type A behavior pattern and for coronary heart disease: A metanalysis of the literature. *Psychosomatic Medicine, 48,* 159-173.

Price, V.A. (1988). Research and clinical issues in treating Type A behavior. In B.K. Houston & C.R. Snyder (Eds.), *Type A behavior pattern: Research, theory, and intervention* (pp. 275-311). New York: Wiley.

Seminal work on the biologic interaction model of TYABP:

Kahn, J.P., Kornfeld, D.S., Frank, K.A., Heller, S.C., & Hoar, P.F. (1980). Type A behavior and blood pressure during coronary artery bypass surgery. *Psychosomatic Medicine, 42,* 407-414.

Krantz, D.S., Arabian, J.M., Davia, J.E., & Parker, J.S. (1982). Type A behavior and coronary artery bypass surgery: Intraoperative blood pressure and perioperative complications. *Psychosomatic Medicine, 44,* 273-284.

Krantz, D.S., Arabian, J.M., Davia, J.E., & Parker, J.S. (1982). Type A behavior and coronary artery bypass surgery: Intraoperative blood pressure and perioperative complications. *Psychosomatic Medicine, 44,* 273-284.

Hostility as the key component of TYABP that relates to the etiology of CHD:

MacDougall, J.M., Dembroski, T.M., Dimsdale, J.E., & Hackett, T.P. (1985). Components of Type A, hostility, and anger. *Health Psychology, 4,* 137-152.

Matthews, K.A., Glass, D.C., Rosenman, R.H., & Bortner, R.W. (1977). Competitive drive, pattern A and coronary heart disease: A further analysis of some data from the Western Collaborative Group study. *Journal of Chronic Diseases, 31,* 489-498.

Hecker, M.H.L., Chesney, M.A., Black, G.W., & Frautschi, N. (1988). Coronary-prone behaviors in the Western Collaborative Group Study. *Psychosomatic Medicine, 2,* 153-164.

For example, investigations of the "potential for hostility"—a predisposition to respond to frustration with reactions of anger, irritation, contempt, etc.—have found a significant association between hostility and the future occurrence of CHD, even among sample groups who had not shown positive relationships between global measures of TYABP and coronary disease (MacDougall, Dembroski, Dimsdale, & Hackett). In addition, the very measures of TYABP employed in seminal research that led to declaring TYABP a major risk factor for CHD have been found to load on assessment of the hostility factor. For example, reanalysis of components of the Structured Interview method that is most often used to assess TYABP in research (Matthews et al.; Hecker et al.) clearly implicates hostility as a primary factor in elevating ratings of TYABP.

Effect of TYABP on one's spouse:

Burke, R.J., Weir, T., & DuWors, R.E., Jr. (1979). Type A behavior of administrators and wives' reports of marital satisfaction and well-being. *Journal of Applied Psychology, 63*(1), 57-65.

High levels of TYABP in males correlated with wives' feelings of: worthlessness, anxiety, tension, guilt, and marital dissatisfaction (Burke, Weir, & DuWors, 1979).

Discussion of literature regarding modifying TYABP:

Nunes, E., Frank, K.A., & Kornfeld, D.S. (1987). Psychologic treatment for the Type A behavior pattern and for coronary heart disease: A metanalysis of the literature. *Psychosomatic Medicine, 48,* 159-173.

Price, V.A. (1982). *Type A behavior patterns: A model for research and practice.* New York: Academic.

Razin, A.M. (1982). Psychosocial intervention in coronary artery disease: A review. *Psychosomatic Medicine, 44*(4), 363-381.

Razin, A.M., Swencionis, C., & Zohman, L.R. (1986). Reduction of physiological, behavioral, and self-report responses in Type A behavior: A preliminary report. *International Journal of Psychiatric Medicine, 16*(1), 32-47.

Smith, T.W., & Rhodewalt, F. (1986). On states, traits and processes: A transactional alternative to individual difference assumptions in Type A behavior and physiological reactivity. *Journal of Research in Personality, 20,* 229-251.

Sotile, W.M. (1992). *Heart illness and intimacy: How caring relationships aid recovery.* Baltimore: Johns Hopkins University Press.

Sotile, W.M., Sotile, M.O., Ewen, G.S., & Sotile, L.J. (1993). Marriage and family factors relevant to effective cardiac rehabilitation: A review of risk factor literature. *Sports Medicine, Training and Rehabilitation, 4,* 115-128.

Thoresen, C.E., Telch, M.J., & Eagleston, J.R. (1981). Approaches to altering the Type A behavior pattern. *Psychosomatics, 22,* 472-482.

Various perspectives on the most important target of treatment of Type As:

Gill, J.J., Price, V.A., Friedman, M., Thoresen, C.E., Powerll, L.H., Ulmer, D., Brown, B., & Drews, F.R. (1985). Reduction in Type A behavior in healthy middle-aged American military officers. *American Heart Journal, 110,* 503-501.

Jenni, M.A., & Wollersheim, J.P. (1979). Cognitive therapy, stress management training, and the Type A behavior pattern. *Cognitive Therapy and Research, 3,* 61-73.

Levenkron, J.C., Goldstein, J.G., Adamides, O., & Greenland, P. (1985). Chronic chest pain with normal coronary arteries: A behavioral approach to rehabilitation. *Journal of Cardiopulmonary Rehabilitation, 5,* 475-479.

Roskies, E., Seraganian, P., Oseasohn, R., Hanley, J.A., Collu, R., Martin, N., & Smilga, C. (1986). The Montreal Type A intervention project: Major findings. *Health Psychology, 5*(1), 45-69.

Sotile, W.M. (1992). *Heart illness and intimacy: How caring relationships aid recovery.* Baltimore: Johns Hopkins University Press

Suinn, R.M., & Bloom, L.J. (1978). Anxiety management training for pattern A behavior. *Journal of Behavior Medicine, 1,* 25-35.

Specific interventions that have been shown to be effective in changing components of TYABP include:

- **Retraining irrational beliefs that drive TYABP**

Jenni, M.A., & Wollersheim, J.P. (1979). Cognitive therapy, stress management training, and the Type A behavior pattern. *Cognitive Therapy and Research, 3,* 61-73.

Razin, A.M., Swencionis, C., & Zohman, L.R. (1986). Reduction of physiological, behavioral, and self-report responses in Type A behavior: A preliminary report. *International Journal of Psychiatric Medicine, 16*(1), 32-47.

- **Reframing Type B behaviors as opportunities to prove oneself as an effective environmental and emotional engineer**

Friedman, M., & Ulmer, D. (1984). *Treating Type A behavior and your heart.* New York: Knopf.

- **Aerobic exercise**

Blumenthal, J.A., Williams, R.S., Williams, R.B., & Wallace, A.G. (1980). Effects of exercise on the Type A (coronary prone) behavior pattern. *Psychosomatic Medicine, 42,* 289-296.

- **Coaching regarding the use of progressive muscle relaxation and self-monitoring in high-stress situations**

Roskies, E., Spevack, M., Surkis, A., Cohen, C., & Gilman, S. (1978). Changing the coronary-prone (Type A) behavior pattern in a nonclinical population. *Journal of Behavioral Medicine,* 201-216.

- **Anxiety management training (Suinn, 1975)**

Suinn, R.M. (1975). The cardiac stress management program for Type A patients. *Cardiac Rehabilitation, 5,* 13-15.

- **Stress management training**

Suinn, R.M. (1977). Type A behavior pattern. In R.B. Williams & W.D. Gentry (Eds.), Behavior approaches to medical treatment (pp. 55-65). Boston: Ballinger.

Suinn, R.M., & Bloom, L.J. (1978). Anxiety management training for pattern A behavior. *Journal of Behavior Medicine, 1,* 25-35.

- **Anger management training**

Thurman, C.W. (1985). Effectiveness of cognitive-behavioral treatments in reducing Type A behavior among university faculty. *Journal of Counseling Psychology, 32,* 74-83.

Sotile, W.M. (1992). *Heart illness and intimacy: How caring relationships aid recovery.* Baltimore: Johns Hopkins University Press.

More involved and specialized treatment of the psychosocial concerns of Type As almost always require coaching the Type A in effective ways to establish and maintain intimate connections with others, including effective sexual behaviors. A "secret" in the lives of many Type As is their discomfort with intimacy which is often due to a combination of unresolved psychodynamic issues (e.g., poor self-esteem based upon childhood experiences) and here-and-now interpersonal skill deficits (Sotile, 1992). Type As can be helped by discussion and normalization of their struggles to feel secure even if they slow down; to understand the opposite sex; to tolerate the meandering that is often necessary in order to maintain comfortable connections with loved ones; and to nurturingly tolerate differences from their loved ones in stress responsivity. In addition, coaching regarding specific sexual techniques is often helpful in promoting more comfort with physical affection and in promoting "relationship self-efficacy" which generalizes to other forms of interaction with one's sexual partner. Extensive guidelines for intervening in this area have been published elsewhere (i.e., Sotile, 1992).

Aggressive behavior and its effects on anger:
Ebbesen, E.B., Duncan, B., & Konecni, V.J. (1975). Effects of content of verbal aggression on future verbal aggression: A field experiment. *Journal of Experimental Social Psychology, 11,* 192-204.
Quanty, M.B. (1976). Aggression catharsis. In R.G. Green & E.C. O'Neal (Eds.), *Perspectives on aggression.* New York: Academic Press.

Definition of anger:
Biaggio, M.K. (1987). Therapeutic management of anger. *Clinical Psychology Review, 7,* 663-675.
Moon, J.R., & Eisler, R.M. (1983). Anger control: An experimental comparison of three behavioral treatments. *Behavior Therapy, 14,* 493-505.
Anger is an aversive state that motivates the individual to act with the goal of decreasing the anger or to terminate its source (Biaggio; Moon & Eisler).

Further research with the Recurrent Coronary Prevention Project model of treating TYABP:
Gill, J.J., Price, V.A., Friedman, M., Thoresen, C.E., Powerll, L.H., Ulmer, D., Brown, B., & Drews, F.R. (1985). Reduction in Type A behavior in healthy middle-aged American military officers. *American Heart Journal, 110,* 503-501.
The Gill et al. publication describes an 8-month, 21-session version of the RCPP treatment that was proven effective in reducing TYABP in healthy U.S. Army officers.

CHAPTER 8   Marital and Family Issues

Further information regarding marital/family factors in rehabilitation:
Bowers, J.E., & Kogan, H.N. (1984). Stress response contagion between spouses: Fact or fiction. *Family Systems Medicine, 2,* 420-427.
Doherty, W.J., & Whitehead, A. (1986). The social dynamics of cigarette smoking: a family systems perspective. *Family Process, 25,*453-459.
Sotile, W.M., Sotile, M.O., Ewen, G.S., & Sotile, L.J. (1993). Marriage and familyfactors relevant to effective cardiac rehabilitation: A review of risk factor literature. *Sports Medicine, Training and Rehabilitation, 4,* 115-128.
Sotile, W.M., Sotile, M.O., Sotile, L.J., & Ewen, G.S. (1993). Marital and family factors relevant to cardiac rehabilitation: An integrative review of the psychosocial literature. *Sports Medicine, Training and Rehabilitation, 4,* 217-236.

Family's effect on motivation for health behavior changes:
Barbarin, O.A., & Tirado, M. (1985). Enmeshment, family processes, and successful treatment of obesity. *Family Relations, 34,* 115-121.
Coyne, J.D., Ellard, J.H., & Smith, D.A. (1990). Unsupportive relationships, interdependence, and unhelpful exchanges. In I.G. Sarason, B.R. Sarason, & G. Pierce (Eds.), *Social support: An interactional view* (pp. 129-149). New York: Plenum Press.
Frenn, M.D., Borgeson, D.S., Lee, H.A., & Simandl, G. (1989). Life-style changes in a cardiac rehabilitation program: The client perspective. *Journal of Cardiovascular Nursing, 3*(2), 43-55.

Marital effect on self-efficacy for rehabilitation:
Antonucci, T.C., & Jackson, J.S. (1987). Social support, interpersonal efficacy, and health. In L. Carstensen & B.A. Edelstein (Eds.), *Handbook of clinical gerontology* (pp. 2391-311). New York: Pergamon Press.
Smith, D.A.F., & Coyne, J.C. (1988). Coping with a myocardial infarction: Determinants of patient self-efficacy. Symposium presentation at the 96th annual convention of the American Psychological Association, Atlanta.

Family and smoking cessation:
Coppotelli, H.C., & Orleans, C.T. (1985). Partner support and other determinants of smoking cessation maintenance among women. *Journal of Consulting and Clinical Psychology, 53,* 455-460.
McIntyre-Kingsolver, K., Lichtenstein, E., & Mermelstein, R.J. (1986). Spouse training in a multicomponent smoking cessation program. *Behavioral Therapy, 17,* 67-74.
Mermelstein, R., Lichtenstein, E., & McIntyre, K. (1983). Partner support and relapse in smoking cessation programs. *Journal of Consulting and Clinical Psychologists, 51,* 465-466.

Family perspectives on dietary changes:

Brownell, K.D., Heckerman, C.L., Westlake, R.J., Hayes, S.C., & Monti, P.M. (1978). The effect of couples training and partner cooperativeness in behavioral treatment of obesity. *Behavioral Research, 16,* 323-333.

Family systems and alcoholism:

Kaufman, E. (1984). Family system variables in alcoholism. *Alcoholism: Clinical and Experimental Research, 8,* 4-8.

Family systems and hypertension control:

Levin, D.M., Green, L.W., Deeds, S.G., Chwalow, J., Russell, R.P., & Finlay, J. (1979). Health education for hypertensive patients. *Journal of the American Medical Association, 241,* 1700-1703.

Morisky, D.E., Levine, D.M., Green, L.W., Shapiro, S., Russell, R.P., & Smith, C.R. (1983). Five-year blood pressure control and mortality following health education for hypertensive patients. *American Journal of Public Health, 73,* 153-162.

Adherence and family systems:

Andrew, G., & Parker, J. (1979). Factors related to dropout of post-myocardial infarction patients from exercise programs. *Medicine and Science in Sports and Exercise, 7,* 376-378.

Andrew, G.M., Oldridge, N.B., Parker, J.O., Cunningham, D.A., Rechnitzer, P.A., Jones, N.L., Buck, C., Kavanagh, T., Shepherd, R.J., Sutton, J.R., & McDonald, W. (1981). Reasons for dropout from exercise programs in postcoronary patients. *Medicine and Science in Sports and Exercise, 13,* 164-168.

Hilbert, G.A. (1985). Spouse support and myocardial infarction patient compliance. *Nursing Research, 34*(4), 217-220.

Miller, P., Wikoff, R., McMahon, M., Garrett, M.J., & Ringel, K. (1985). Indicators of medical regimen adherence for myocardial infarction patients. *Nursing Research, 34,* 268-272.

Stein, H.F., & Pontious, J.M. (1985). Family and beyond: The larger context of noncompliance. *Family Systems Medicine, 3,* 179-189.

The importance of spouse support in cardiac rehabilitation:

Ben-Sira, Z., & Eliezer, R. (1990). The structure of readjustment after heart attack. *Social Science & Medicine, 30*(5), 523-536.

Mayou, R. (1979). The course and determinants of reactions to myocardial infarction. *British Journal of Psychiatry, 143,* 588-594.

Mayou, R., Foster, A., & Williamson, B. (1978a). The psychological and social effects of myocardial infarction on wives. *British Medical Journal, 1,* 699-701.

Mayou, R., Foster, A., & Williamson, B. (1978b). Psychosocial adjustment in patients one year after myocardial infarction. *Journal of Psychosomatic Research, 22,* 447-453.

Mayou, R., Williamson, B., & Foster, A. (1978). Outcome two months after myocardial infarction. *Journal of Psychosomatic Research, 22,* 439-445.

Improved family functioning following cardiac illness:

Jenkins, C.D., Stanton, B.A., Savageau, J.A., Denlinger, P., & Klein, M.D. (1983). Coronary artery bypass surgery: Physical, psychological, social, and economic outcomes six months later. *Journal of the American Medical Association, 250,* 782-788.

Laerum, E., Johnsen, N., Smith, P., & Larsen, S. (1987). Can myocardial infarction induce positive changes in family relationships. *Family Practice, 4,* 302-305.

Effect of cardiac illness on patient's spouse:

Alonzo, A.A. (1986). The impact of the family and lay others on care-seeking during life-threatening episodes of suspected coronary artery disease. *Social Science & Medicine, 22*(12), 1297-1311.

Coyne, J.C., & Smith, D.A.F. (1991). Couples coping with a myocardial infarction: A contextual perspective on wives' distress. *Journal of Personality and Social Psychology, 61*(3), 404-412.

Fisher, L., & Ransom, D. (1990). Person-family transaction: Implications for stress and health. *Family Systems Medicine, 8,* 109-122.

Gillis, C.L. (1984). Reducing family stress during and after coronary artery bypass surgery. *Nursing Clinics of North America, 19,* 103-112.

Post, L., & Collins, C. (1981). The poorly coping chronic pulmonary disease patient: A psychotherapeutic perspective. *International Journal of Psychiatry in Medicine, 11*(2), 173-182.

Sotile, W.M., Sotile, M.O., Ewen, G.S., & Sotile, L.J. (1993). Marriage and family factors relevant to effective cardiac rehabilitation: A review of risk factor literature. *Sports Medicine, Training and Rehabilitation, 4,* 115-128.

Effect of marital quality on adjustment to unemployment:

Gore, S. (1978). The effect of social support in moderating the health consequences of unemployment. *Journal of Health and Social Behavior, 19,* 157-165.

Pearlin, L.I., Menaghan, E.G., Lieberman, M.A., & Mullan, J.T. (1981). The stress process. *Journal of Health and Social Behavior, 22,* 337-356.

Family stress management:

Patterson, J.M. (1988). Families experiencing stress: I. The Family Adjustment and Adaptation Response Model. II. Applying the FAAR Model to heal-related issues for intervention and research. *Family Systems Medicine, 6,* 202-237.

Long-range adjustment struggles of spouse and children of heart patients:

Honeyman, M.S., Rappaport, H., Reznikoff, M., Glueck, B.C., Jr., & Eisenberg, H. (1968). Psychological impact of heart disease in the family of the patient. *Psychosomatics, 9,* 34-37.

Family members' sense of responsibility for the patient's illness:

Reiss, D., & Oliveri, M.E. (1991). The family's conception of accountability and competence: A new approach to the conceptualization and assessment of family stress. *Family Processes, 30,* 193-214.

Complaints of family members of cardiopulmonary patients about their relationship with health care providers:

Coyne, J.C., & Smith, D.A.F. (1991). Couples coping with a myocardial infarction: A contextual perspective on wives' distress. *Journal of Personality and Social Psychology, 61*(3), 404-412.

The effect of medical diagnosis on coping choices:

Badger, T.A. (1992). Coping, life-style changes, health perceptions, and marital adjustment in middle-aged women and men with cardiovascular disease and their spouses. *Health Care for Women International, 13,* 43-55.

Referral patterns with aged female cardiac patients:

Ades, P.A., & Grunvald, M.H. (1990). Cardiopulmonary exercise testing before and after conditioning in older coronary patients. *American Heart Journal, 120*(3), 585-589.

Ades, P.A., Waldman, M.L., Polk, D., & Coflesky, J.T. (1992). Referral patterns and exercise response in the rehabilitation of female coronary patients aged 62 years. *American Journal of Cardiology, 69.*

Gender differences in reacting to stress:

Folkman, S., Lazarus, R.S., Dunkel-Schetter, C., DeLongis, A., & Gruen, R.J. (1986). Dynamics of a stressful encounter: Cognitive appraisal, coping and encounter outcomes. *Journal of Personality and Social Psychology, 50,* 992-1003.

Folkman, S., Lazarus, R.S., Pimley, S., & Novacek, J. (1987). Age differences in stress and coping processes. *Psychology and Aging, 2*(2), 171-184.

McCrae, R.R. (1984). Age differences in the use of coping mechanisms. *Journal of Gerontology, 37*(4), 454-460.

Effect of family stress levels at time of illness on reactions to illness:

Rejeski, W.J., Morley, D., & Sotile, W. (1985). Cardiac rehabilitation: A conceptual framework for psychologic assessment. *Journal of Cardiopulmonary Rehabilitation, 4,* 172-180.

Sotile, W.M. (1992). *Heart illness and intimacy: How caring relationships aid recovery.* Baltimore: Johns Hopkins University Press.

Family struggles in immediate posthospital stage:

Hoffman, L.A., Berg, J., & Rogers, R.M. (1989). Daily living with COPD: Self-help skills to improve functional ability. *Postgraduate Medicine, 86,* 153-166.

Crisis can be a mental health turning point for families:

Lipowski, Z.J. (1977). Psychosomatic medicine in the seventies: An overview. *American Journal of Psychiatry, 134,* 233-244.

CHAPTER 9   Controlling Cognitions

Seminal work on cognitive theory:

Beck, A.T. (1979). *Cognitive therapy and emotional disorders.* New York: New American Library.

Ellis, A., & Harper, R.A. (1975). *A new guide to rational living.* North Hollywood, CA: Wilshire Book.

CHAPTER 10   Positive Living

Extensive discussion of the significance of social support in the etiology of cardiopulmonary illnesses:

Blumenthal, J.A., Burg, M.M., Barefoot, J., Williams, R.B., Haney, T., & Zimet, G. (1987). Social support, Type A behavior and coronary artery disease. *Psychosomatic Medicine, 49,* 331-339.

Seeman, T.E., & Syme, S.L. (1987). Social networks and coronary artery disease: A comparison of the structure and function of social relations as predictors of disease. *Psychosomatic Medicine, 49,* 340-353.

Shumaker, S.A., & Czajkowski, S.M. (Eds.) (1994). *Social support and cardiovascular disease.* New York: Plenum Press.

Operationalization of the factors that have been proposed to define social support:

Berkman, L.F. (1984). Assessing the physical health effects of social networks and social support. *Annual Review of Public Health, 5,* 413-432.

Cobb, S. (1976). Social support as a moderator of life stress—presidential address. *Psychosomatic Medicine, 38,* 300-314.

Cohen, S., & Syme, S.L. (Eds.) (1985). *Social support and health.* New York: Academic Press.

Sarafino, E.P. (1990). *Health psychology: Biopsychosocial interactions.* New York: Wiley.

Effects of negative relationships:

Coyne, J.C., & DeLongis, A. (1986). Going beyond social support: The role of social relationships in adaptation. *Journal of Consulting and Clinical Psychology, 54,* 454-460.

Headey, B., Holmstrom, E., & Wearing, A. (1984). Well-being and ill-being: Different dimensions? *Social Indicators Research, 14,* 115-139.

Rook, K.S. (1984). The negative side of social interaction: Impact on psychological well-being. *Journal of Personality and Social Psychology, 46,* 1097-1108.

In her study of 120 widowed women (ages 60-89), Rook found that negative social interactions had more potent effects on well-being than positive social interactions. Coyne and DeLongis reviewed literature that suggested that unhappily married people are worse off than married people in terms of physical health and psychological well-being: "People who are unhappily married report more physical illness and depression, heavier drinking, and more isolation from persons outside their marriage than do happily married people" (Coyne & DeLongis, 1986, p. 455). In a long-term prospective study of well-being and ill-being in 942 Australians, Headey et al. found that the presence or absence of intimate attachments—and not just affiliation—is the key factor in determining whether being married enhances or detracts from well-being. It seems clear that if a marriage is not an intimate, sharing relationship, its effect on well-being may be negative.

Effects of positive social support on mortality:

Chandra, V., Szklo, M., Goldbert, R., & Tonascia, J. (1983). The impact of marital status on survival after acute myocardial infarction: A population-based study. *American Journal of Epidemiology, 117,* 320-325.

Chandra, Szklo, Goldberg, and Tonascia followed 1,401 patients for 10 years after their MI and found that those who were married at the time of their MI had a greatly decreased risk of dying both during their hospitalization and over the next 10 years. The distinction was greatest for women but also held for male patients.

Ruberman, W., Weinblatt, A.B., Goldberg, J.D., & Chaudhary, B.S. (1984). Psychosocial influences on mortality after myocardial infarction. *New England Journal of Medicine, 311,* 552-559.

Ruberman, Weinblatt, Goldberg, & Chaudhary demonstrated that increased stress and decreased support led to increased mortality from CHD or MI patients.

Case, R.B., Moss, A.J., Case, N., McDermott, M., & Eberly, S. (1992). Living alone after myocardial infarction: Impact on prognosis. *Journal of the American Medical Association, 267,* 515-519.

Williams, R.B., Barefoot, J.C., Califf, R.M., Haney, T.L., Saunders, W.B., Pryor, D.B., Hlatky, M.A., Siegler, I.C., & Mark, D.B. (1992). Prognostic importance of social and economic resources among medically treated patients with angiographically documented coronary artery disease. *Journal of the American Medical Association, 267,* 520-524.

Two recently published investigations (Case et al., 1992; Williams et al., 1992) lent further support to this finding when they demonstrated that being married, having fewer economic resources, being socially isolated, and lacking a confidant predicted poor survival for recovering CHD patients.

Effects of positive social support on morbidity:

Medalie, J.H., & Goldbourt, U. (1976). Angina pectoris among 10,000 men: II. Psychosocial and other risk factors as evidenced by a multivariate analysis of a five-year incidence study. *American Journal of Medicine, 60,* 910-921.

Seeman, T.E., & Syme, S.L. (1987). Social networks and coronary artery disease: A comparison of the structure and function of social relations as predictors of disease. *Psychosomatic Medicine, 49,* 340-353.

Jensen, P.S. (1983). Risk, protective factors, and supportive interventions in chronic airway obstruction. *Archives of General Psychiatry, 40,* 1203-1207.

In the Honolulu Heart Study, Medalie and Goldbourt showed that loving support from wives buffered the effect of anxiety on the incidence of angina.

Even the perception of support by a caring individual—the feeling of being loved and the belief that others would be available in times of need—have been found to predict the degree of coronary atherosclerosis in a study that investigated coronary angiographic findings (Seeman & Syme).

In a study of COPD patients (Jensen), high-risk patients with low social support were hospitalized significantly more frequently than low-risk patients or high-risk patients who were receiving increased social support.

Also see:

Friedman, E., Katcher, A.H., Lynch, J.J., & Thomas, S.A. (1980). Animal companions and one-year survival of patients after discharge from a coronary care unit. *Public Health Reports, 95,* 307-312.

Helsng, K.J., Szklo, M., & Komstock, G.W. (1981). Factors associated with mortality after widowhood. *American Journal of Public Health, 71,* 802-809.

Lowenthal, M.F., & Haven, C. (1968). Interaction and adaptation: Intimacy as a critical variable. *American Social Review, 33,* 20-30.

Lynch, J.J. (1977). *The broken heart: The medical consequences of loneliness.* New York: Basic Books.

Statistics regarding work return rates in cardiac populations:

Cay, E.L., Vetter, N., & Phillip, A. (1973). Return to work after a heart attack. *Journal of Psychosomatic Research, 17,* 231-243.

Miller, N.H., Taylor, C.B., Davidson, D.M., Hill, M.N., & Krantz, D.S. (1990). The efficacy of risk factor intervention and psychosocial aspects of cardiac rehabilitation. *Journal of Cardiac Rehabilitation, 10,* 198-209.

Work return with COPD patients:

Daughton, D.M., Fix, A.J., Kass, I., Patil, K.D., & Bell, C.W. (1979). Physiological-intellectual components of rehabilitation success in patients with chronic obstructive pulmonary disease (COPD). *Journal of Chronic Diseases, 32,* 405-409.

Kass, I., Dyksterhuis, J.E., Rubin, H., & Patil, K.D. (1975). Correlation of psychophysiological variables with vocational rehabilitation outcome in patients with chronic obstructive pulmonary disease. *Chest, 67,* 433-440.

Lertzman, M.M., & Cherniack, R.M. (1976). Rehabilitation of patients with chronic obstructive pulmonary disease. *American Review of Respiratory Diseases, 114,* 1145-1165.

Petty, T.L., MacIlroy, E.R., Swigert, M.A., & Brink, G.A. (1970). Chronic airway obstruction, respiratory insufficiency and gainful employment. *Archives of Environmental Health, 21,* 71-78.

Should work return be a standard of rehabilitation? See:

Cay, E.L., Vetter, N., & Phillip, A. (1973). Return to work after a heart attack. *Journal of Psychosomatic Research, 17,* 231-243.

Fletcher, A., Hunt, B., & Bulpitt, C. (1987). Evaluation of quality of life in trials of cardiovascular disease. *Journal of Chronic Disease, 40,* 557-566.

Johnson, J.L., & Morse, J.M. (1990). Regaining control: The process of adjustment after myocardial infarction. *Heart and Lung, 19,* 126-135.

Mayou, R. (1990). Quality of life in cardiovascular disease. *Psychotherapy and Psychosomatics, 54,* 99-109.

Ries, A.L. (1990). Position paper of the American Association of Cardiovascular and Pulmonary Rehabilitation: Scientific basis of pulmonary rehabilitation. *Journal of Cardiopulmonary Rehabilitation, 10,* 418-441.

Factors that affect work return in cardiac populations:

Bar-On, D., & Cristal, N. (1987). Causal attributions of patients, their spouses and physicians, and the rehabilitation of the patients after their first myocardial infarction. *Journal of Cardiopulmonary Rehabilitation, 7,* 285-298.

Barnes, G., Ray, M., Oberman, A., & Kouchoukos, N. (1977).Changes in working status of patients following coronary bypass surgery. *Journal of the American Medical Association, 238,* 1259-1262.

Dafoe, W.A., Franklin, B.A., & Cupper, L. (1993). Vocational issues and disability. In F.J. Pàshkow & W.A. Dafoe (Eds.), *Clinical cardiac rehabilitation: A cardiologist's guide* (pp. 227-241). Baltimore: Williams & Wilkins.

Daughton, D.M., Fix, A.J., Kass, I., Patil, K.D., & Bell, C.W. (1979). Physiological-intellectual components of rehabilitation success in patients with chronic obstructive pulmonary disease (COPD). *Journal of Chronic Diseases, 32,* 405-409.

Davidson, D.M. (1983). Return to work after cardiac events: A review. *Journal of Cardiac Rehabilitation, 3,* 60-69.

Dennis, C., Miller, H.N., Schwartz, R.G., Ahn, D.K., Kraemer, H.C., Gossard, D., Juneau, M., Taylor, C.B., & DeBusk, R.F. (1988). Early return to work after uncomplicated myocardial infarction: Results of a randomized trial. *Journal of the American Medical Association, 260,* 214-220.

Garrity, T.F. (1973b). Vocational adjustment after first myocardial infarction: Comparative assessment of several variables suggested in the literature. *Social Science & Medicine, 7,* 705-715.

Gundle, M.D., Reeves, B.R., & Tate, S. (1980). Psychosocial outcome after coronary artery surgery. *American Journal of Psychiatry, 137,* 1591-1594.

Kass, I., Dyksterhuis, J.E., Rubin, H., & Patil, K.D. (1975). Correlation of psychophysiological variables with vocational rehabilitation outcome in patients with chronic obstructive pulmonary disease. *Chest, 67,* 433-440.

Maeland, J.G., & Havik, O.E. (1987). Psychological predictors for return to work after a myocardial infarction. *Journal of Psychosomatic Research, 31,* 471-481.

Petty, T.L., MacIlroy, E.R., Swigert, M.A., & Brink, G.A. (1970). Chronic airway obstruction, respiratory insufficiency and gainful employment. *Archives of Environmental Health, 21,* 71-78.

Shanfield, S.B. (1990). Myocardial infarction and patients' wives. *Psychosomatics, 31,* 138-145.

Smith, G.R., & O'Rourke, D.F. (1988). Return to work after myocardial infarction: A test of multiple hypotheses. *Journal of the American Medical Association, 259,* 1673-1677.

Effects of early work return:

Mayou, R., Williamson, B., & Foster, A. (1978). Outcome two months after myocardial infarction. *Journal of Psychosomatic Research, 22,* 439-445.

Subjective perceptions of well-being:
Campbell, A., Converse, P., & Rogers, W. (1976). *The quality of American life*. New York: Russell Sage Foundation.
Religion, well-being, and health:
Blazer, D.G., & Palmore, E.B. (1976). Religion and aging. *Gerontologist, 16,* 82-85
Usui, W.M., Feil, T.J., & Durig, K.R. (1985). Socioeconomic comparisons and life satisfaction of elderly adults. *Journal of Gerontology, 40,* 110-114.
Zuckerman, D.M. (1984). Psychosocial predictors of mentality among the elderly poor. *American Journal of Epidemiology, 119,* 410-423.

PART III   SPECIAL TOPICS

CHAPTER 11   Sexual Aspects of Heart and Lung Illnesses

Sexual concerns of female cardiac patients:
Baggs, J., & Darch, A. (1987). Sexual counseling of women with coronary heart disease. *Heart and Lung, 16,* 154-158.
Papadopoulos, C., Beaumont, C., Shelley, S.I., & Larrimore, P. (1983). Myocardial infarction and sexual activity of the female patient. *Archives of Internal Medicine, 143,* 1528-1530.
Sexual concerns of wives of recovering cardiac patients:
Papadopoulos, C., Larrimore, P., Cardin, S., & Shelley, S. (1980). Sexual concerns and needs of the postcoronary patient's wife. *Archives of Internal Medicine, 140,* 38-41.
Shanfield, S.B. (1990). Myocardial infarction and patients' wives. *Psychosomatics, 31,* 138-145.
Sexual patterns during the first 3 years postillness:
Mann, S., Yates, J.G., & Raftery, E.B. (1981). The effects of myocardial infarction on sexual activity. *Journal of Cardiopulmonary Rehabilitation, 1,* 187-193.
Tuttle, W.B., Cook, W.L., & Fitch, E. (1964). Sexual behavior in post-myocardial infarction patients. *American Journal of Cardiology, 13,* 140-153.
Lack of information as an etiological factor in sexual problems for heart and lung patients:
Cole, C.M., Levin, E.M., Whitley, J.O., & Young, S.H. (1979). Brief sexual counselling during cardiac rehabilitation. *Heart and Lung, 8*(1), 124-129.
Hellerstein, H.F., & Friedman, E.H. (1969). Sexual activity and the post-coronary patient. *Medical Aspects of Human Sexuality, 3,* 70-96.
Johnston, B.L., Cantwell, J.D., Watt, E.W., & Fletcher, G.E. (1978). Sexual activity in exercising patients after myocardial infarction and revascularization. *Heart and Lung, 7,* 1026-1031.
Kravetz, H.M., & Pheatt, H. (1993). Sexuality in the pulmonary patient. In J.E. Hodgkin, G.L. Connors, & C.W. Bell (Eds.), *Pulmonary rehabilitation: Guidelines to success* (2nd ed., pp. 293-310). Philadelphia: Lippincott.
Papadopoulos, C. (1978). A survey of sexual activity after MI. *Cardiovascular Medicine, 3,* 821-826.
Sikorski, J.M. (1985). Knowledge, concerns and questions of wives of convalescent coronary artery bypass graft surgery patients. *Journal of Cardiac Rehabilitation, 5,* 74-85.
Diabetes and erectile dysfunction:
Kolodny, R.C., Kahn, C.B., Goldstein, H.H., & Barnett, D.B. (1974). Sexual dysfunction in diabetic men. *Diabetes, 23,* 306-309.
Sotile, W.M. (1979b). The penile prosthesis and diabetic impotence: Some caveats. *Diabetes Care, 2*(1), 26-30.
Orgasmic dysfunction in diabetic women:
Kolodny, R.C. (1971). Sexual dysfunction in diabetic females. *Diabetes, 20,* 557-559.
Diagnostic procedures regarding etiology of male sexual dysfunctions:
• **Nocturnal penile tumescence monitoring in laboratory (Karacan, 1982)**
Karacan, I. (1982). Nocturnal penile tumescence as a biological marker in assessing erectile dysfunction. *Psychosomatics, 23,* 349-360.

- **Nocturnal penile tumescence monitoring in home (Barry, Blank, & Boileau, 1980)**
  Barry, J.M., Blank, B.H., & Boileau, M. (1980). Nocturnal penile tumescence monitoring with stamps. *Urology, 15,* 171-172.
- **Doppler ultrasound of penile arteries (Jevtich, 1983)**
  Jevtich, M.J. (1983). Vascular noninvasive diagnostic techniques. In R.J. Krane, M.B. Siroky, & I. Goldstein (Eds.), *Male sexual dysfunction* (pp.139-164). Boston: Little, Brown.
- **Cavernography to detect penile venous leakage (Wespes, Delcour, Struyven, & Schulman, 1984)**
  Wespes, E., Delcour, C., Struyven, J., & Schulman, C.C. (1984). Cavernometry-cavernography: Its role in organic impotence. *European Urology, 10,* 229-232.

Problems from noninvasive diagnostic techniques for detecting vasculogenic impotency:
Mellinger, B.C., Vaughan, E.D., Thompson, S.L., & Goldstein, M. (1987). Correlation between intracavernous papaverine injection and Doppler analysis in impotent men. *Urology, 30,* 416-419.

Intracorporeal injections of papaverine:
Strachan, J.R., & Pryor, J.P. (1987). Diagnostic intracorporeal papaverine and erectile dysfunction. *British Journal of Urology, 59,* 264-266.

Intracorporeal injections of saline or radiographic contrast medium:
Newman, H.F., & Reiss, H. (1984). Artificial perfusion in impotence. *Urology, 24,* 469-471.

Use of stimulating electrodes to assess impotence:
Wagner, G., & Green, R. (1981). *Impotence: Physiological, psychological, and surgical diagnosis and treatment.* New York: Plenum Press.

Use of sacral electromyogram to assess sensory nervous system functions:
Ertekinm, C., & Reel, F. (1976). Bulbocavernosus reflex in normal men and in patients with neurogenic bladder and/or impotence. *Journal of the Neurological Sciences, 28,* 1-15.

Serum testosterone and serum prolactin assays:
Schover, L.R., & Jensen, S. (1988). *Sexuality and chronic illness a comprehensive approach.* New York: Guilford Press.

Physical assessments of female sexual functioning:
- **Vaginal photoplethysmograph (Semmlow & Lubowsky, 1983)**
  Semmlow, J.L., & Lubowsky, J. (1983). Sexual instrumentation. *IEEE Transactions on Biomedical Engineering, 6,* 309-319.
- **Heated oxygen electrodes (Amberson & Hoon, 1985)**
  Amberson, J.I., & Hoon, P. (1985). Hemodynamics of sequential orgasm. *Archives of Sexual Behavior, 14,* 351-360.

Risks of hormone replacement therapy for both sexes:
Schover, L.R. (1984). *Prime time: Sexual health for men over fifty.* New York: Holt Rinehart & Winston.

Penile prostheses:
Sotile, W.M. (1979a). The penile prosthesis: A review. *Journal of Sex and Marital Therapy, 5,* 90-102.

Prostaglandin E1 penile injections:
Stackl, W., Hasun, R., & Marberger, M. (1988). Intracavernous injection of prostaglandin E1 in impotent men. *Journal of Urology, 140,* 66-68.

Need to assess relationship dynamics before prescribing erection aids:
Beutler, L.E., Scott, F.B., Rogers, R.R., Karacan, I., Baer, P.E., & Gaines, J.A. (1986). Inflatable and noninflatable penile prostheses: Comparative follow-up evaluation. *Urology, 28,* 136-143.
Kramarsky-Binkhorst, S. (1978). Female partner perception of Small-Carrion implant. *Urology, 12,* 545-548.

Use of nasal prongs to inhale oxygen during intercourse:
Lyons, H.A. (1977). Sexual relations for male patients with chronic obstructive lung disease. *Medical Aspects of Human Sexuality, 11*(4), 119.

Effects of pulmonary rehabilitation on sexual functioning:

Pietropinto, A., & Arora, A. (1989). Chronic pulmonary disease and sexual functioning. *Medical Aspects of Human Sexuality, 23*, 78-82.

Effects of cardiac rehabilitation on sexual functioning:

Roviaro, A., Holmes, D.S., & Holsten, R.D. (1984). Influence of a cardiac rehabilitation program on the cardiovascular, psychological and social functioning of cardiac patients. *Journal of Behavioral Medicine, 7*, 61-81.

Sotile, W.M., Sotile, M.O., Sotile, L.J., & Ewen, G.S. (1993). Marital and family factors relevant to cardiac rehabilitation: An integrative review of the psychosocial literature. *Sports Medicine, Training and Rehabilitation, 4*, 217-236.

Sexual advice for recovering heart and lung patients:

Bonner, E.J., & Gendel, E.S. (1987). Sexual counseling for the elderly patient after myocardial infarction. *Aspects of Human Sexuality, 21*(3), 100-108.

Cole, C.M., Levin, E.M., Whitley, J.O., & Young, S.H. (1979). Brief sexual counselling during cardiac rehabilitation. *Heart and Lung, 8*(1), 124-129.

Conine, T., & Evans, J. (1981). Sexual adjustment in chronic obstructive pulmonary disease. *Respiratory Care, 26*(9), 871-874.

Kravetz, H.M., & Pheatt, H. (1993). Sexuality in the pulmonary patient. In J.E. Hodgkin, G.L. Connors, & C.W. Bell (Eds.), *Pulmonary rehabilitation: Guidelines to success* (2nd ed., pp. 293-310). Philadelphia: Lippincott.

Sotile, W.M. (1992). *Heart illness and intimacy: How caring relationships aid recovery.* Baltimore: Johns Hopkins University Press.

Sotile, W.M. (1993). The intimacy factor in cardiopulmonary rehabilitation: A practical model for structuring interventions. *Journal of Cardiopulmonary Rehabilitation, 13*(4), 237-242.

Walbroehl, G.S. (1992). Sexual concerns of the patient with pulmonary disease. *Postgraduate Medicine, 91*(5), 455-460.

Effects of relationship dynamics on sexual functioning in diabetics:

Jensen, S.B. (1985a). Emotional aspects in diabetes mellitus: A study of somatopsychological reactions in 51 couples in which one partner has insulin-treated diabetes. *Journal of Psychosomatic Research, 29*, 353-359.

Jensen, S.B. (1985b). Sexual relationships in couples with a diabetic partner. *Journal of Sex and Marital Therapy, 11*, 259-270.

CHAPTER 12   Helping Patients Stop Smoking

Smoking cessation rates following CHD:

Burling, T.A., Singleton, E.G., Bigelow, G.E., Baile, W.F., & Gottlieb, S.H. (1984). Smoking following myocardial infarction: A critical review of the literature. *Health Psychology, 3*, 83-96.

Ockene, J.K., Hosmer, D., Rippe, J., Williams, J., Goldberg, R.J., DeCosimo, D., Maher, P.M., & Dalen, J.E. (1985). Factors affecting cigarette smoking status in patients with ischemic heart disease. *Journal of Chronic Diseases, 38*(12), 985-994.

International literature regarding smoking cessation patterns in MI patients from New Zealand, London, Sweden, and Dundee:

Burt, A., Thornley, P., Illingworth, D., White, P., Shaw, T.R.D., & Turner, R. (1974). Stopping smoking after myocardial infarction. *Lancet, 1*, 304-306.

Long-term smoking cessation rates for CHD patients:

Hay, D.R., & Turnbott, S. (1970). Changes in smoking habits in men under sixty-five years after myocardial infarction and coronary insufficiency. *British Heart Journal, 32*, 738-740.

Werko, L. (1971). Can we prevent heart disease? *Annals of Internal Medicine, 74*, 278-288.

Posthospitalization relapse smoking rates for cardiopulmonary patients:

Baile, W.F., Gigelow, G.E., Gottlieb, S.H., Stitzer, M.L., & Sacktor, J.D. (1982). Rapid resumption of cigarette smoking following myocardial infarction: Inverse relation to MI severity. *Addictive Behavior, 7*, 373-380.

Poor long-term cessation rates with COPD populations:

Crowley, T.J., MacDonald, M.J., Zerbe, G.O., & Petty, T.L. (1991). Reinforcing breath carbon monoxide reductions in chronic obstructive pulmonary disease. *Drug and Alcohol Dependence, 29*(1), 47-62.

Pederson, L.L., Wanklin, J.M., & Lefcoe, N.M. (1991). The effects of counseling on smoking cessation among patients hospitalized with chronic obstructive pulmonary disease: A randomized clinical trial. *International Journal of the Addictions, 26*(1), 107-119.

Spontaneous quit rates following diagnosis of cardiopulmonary illness:

Burling, T.A., Singleton, E.G., Bigelow, G.E., Baile, W.F., & Gottlieb, S.H. (1984). Smoking following myocardial infarction: A critical review of the literature. *Health Psychology, 3,* 83-96.

Cohen, S., Lichtenstein, E., Prochaska, J.O., Rossi, J.S., Gritz, E.R., Carr, C.R., Orleans, C.T., Schoenbach, V.J., Biener, L., Abrams, D.B., DiClemente, C., Curry, S., Marlatt, G.A., Cummings, K.M., Emont, S.L., Giovino, G., & Ossip-Klein, D. (1989). Debunking myths about self-quitting: Evidence from ten prospective studies of persons who attempt to quit smoking by themselves. *American Psychologist, 44,* 1355-1365.

Concise summaries of the factors that should be emphasized in educating cardiopulmonary patients regarding the physiology of smoking and smoking cessation:

Glover, E.D. (Ed.) (1983). Nicotine withdrawal therapy [Special issue], *Health Values: The Journal of Health Behavior, Education & Promotion, 17*(2), 4-79.

McKool, K. (1987). Facilitating smoking cessation. *Journal of Cardiovascular Nursing, 1*(4), 28-41.

Support of the claim that brief intervention can promote smoking cessation:

Buist, A.S., Connett, J.E., Miller, R.D., Kanner, R.E., Owerns, G.R., & Voelker, H.I. (1993). Chronic obstructive pulmonary disease early intervention trial (Lung Health Study): Baseline characteristics of randomized participants. *Chest, 103*(6), 1863-1872.

Durkin, D.A., Kjelsberg, M.O., Buist, A.S., Connett, J.E., & Owens, G.R. (1993). Recruitment of participants in the Lung Health Study: I. Description of methods. *Controlled Clinical Trials, 14*(2) (Suppl.), 208-378.

Owens, G.R. (1991). Public screening for lung disease: Experience with the NIH Lung Health Study. *American Journal of Medicine, 91*(4A), 378-408.

See the ongoing study by the National Heart, Lung, and Blood Institute (NHLBI) that is investigating the long-term effects of an intervention that combines medical input, behavioral counseling, nicotine replacement therapy and group support in treating over 6,000 patients with abnormal pulmonary function. This investigation, called the NHLBI Health Study, is currently in its fifth year. Outcome data are still being gathered, but preliminary analysis has indicated support of the claim that personalized confrontation with information that smoking is leading to negative health consequences, followed by specific smoke-stopping counseling, can promote cessation for pulmonary patients. Four-month follow-up data has indicated an impressive 59% quit rate for the participants enrolled in this smoking-cessation program (Owens, 1991; Buist et al., 1993; Durkin, Kjelsberg, Buist, Connett, & Owens, 1993).

Information regarding various nicotine replacement agents can be obtained from the following:

Company name	Product	Toll-free number
Marion Merrell Dow	Nicoderm	1-800-NICODERM
Lederle	Prostep	1-800-334-3970
McNeil	Nicotrol	1-800-227-1616
Ciba Pharmaceuticals	Habitrol	1-800-631-1162
SmithKline Beecham	Nicorette	1-800-245-1040

CHAPTER 13   COPD and Aged Cardiopulmonary Patients

Discussion of the "emotional straight jacket" phenomenology:

Dudley, D.L., Glaser, E.M., Jorgenson, B.N., & Logan, D.L. (1980). Psychosocial concomitants to rehabilitation in chronic obstructive pulmonary disease: Part I. Psychosocial and psychological considerations. *Chest, 77*(3), 413-420.

Dudley, D.L., Holmes, T.H., & Martin, C.J. (1964). Changes in respiration associated with hypnotically induced emotion, pain and exercise. *Psychosomatic Medicine, 26,* 46-57.

Dudley, D.L., Martin, C.J., & Holmes, T.H. (1964). Psychophysiologic studies of pulmonary ventilation. *Psychosomatic Medicine, 26,* 645-660.

Dudley, D.L., Martin, C.J., & Holmes, T.H. (1968). Dyspnea: Psychological and physiologic observations. *Journal of Psychosomatic Research, 12,* 205-214.

Dudley, D.L., Martin, C.J., Masuda, M., & Holmes, T.H. (1969). *The psychophysiology of respiration in health and disease* (pp. 234-236). New York: Appleton-Century-Crofts.

Statistics regarding the aging population:

Bishop, D.S., Epstein, N.B., Baldwin, L.M., Miller, I.W., & Keitner, G.I. (1988). Older couples: The effect of health retirement and family functioning on morale. *Family Systems Medicine, 6*(2), 238-247.

Lancaster, J. (1981). Maximizing psychological adaptations in an aging population. *Advanced Nursing Science, 3,* 31-43.

Packa, D.R., Branyon, M.E., Kinney, M.R., Khan, S.H., Kelley, R., & Miers, L.J. (1989). Quality of life of elderly patients enrolled in cardiac rehabilitation. *Journal of Cardiovascular Nursing, 3*(2), 33-42.

The psychology of middle age:

Erikson, E. (1968). *Childhood and society* (2nd ed.). New York: Norton.

Levinson, D.J. (1978). *The seasons of a man's life.* New York: Ballantine.

Referral patterns of the aged to cardiopulmonary rehabilitation programs:

Ades, P.A., Hanson, J.S., Gunther, P.G., & Tonino, R.P. (1987). Exercise conditioning in the elderly coronary patient. *Journal of American Geriatric Society 35*(2), 121-124.

Lavie, C.J., Milani, R.V., & Littman, A.B. (1993). Benefits of cardiac rehabilitation and exercise training in secondary coronary prevention in the elderly. *Journal of American Coronary Care, 22*(3), 678-683.

Responses of the aged to formal cardiopulmonary rehabilitation:

Williams, M.A., Maresh, C.M., Esterbrook, D.J., Harbrecht, J.J., & Sketch, M.H. (1985). Early exercise training in patients older than age 65 years compared with that in younger patients after acute myocardial infarction or coronary artery bypass grafting. *American Journal of Cardiology, 55,* 263-266.

For further information about memory training in the elderly, see:

Yesavage, J.A. (1983). Imagery pretraining and memory training in the elderly. *Gerontology, 29,* 271-275.

Yesavage, J.A., Rose, T.L., and Spiegel, D. (1982). Relaxation training and memory improvement in elderly normals: Correlation of anxiety ratings and recall improvement. *Experimental Aging Research, 4,* 195-198.

A good source of information regarding the aged:

The National Association of Private Geriatric Care Managers, P.O. Box 6920, Yorkville Finance Station, New York, NY 10128

Excellent resources for aged patients:

Friedan B. (1993). *The Fountain of Age.* New York: Simon & Schuster.

Gutmann, D. (1987). *Reclaimed powers: Toward a new psychology of men and women in later life.* New York: Basic Books.

LeShan, E. (1986). *Oh, to be 50 again!* New York: Times Books.

CHAPTER 14 Improving Adherence and Structuring Interventions

Overview of adherence problems in several specific areas of rehabilitation:

- **Promoting exercise (Oldridge, 1988)**

Oldridge, N.B. (1988). Cardiac rehabilitation exercise programme: Compliance and compliance-enhancing strategies. *Sports Medicine, 6,* 42-55.

- **Modifying dietary behaviors and weight (Singh, Rastogi, Verma et al., 1992)**

Singh, R.B., Rastogi, S.S., Verma, R., Laxmi, B., Singh, R., Ghosh, S., & Niaz, M.A. (1992). Randomized controlled trial of cardioprotective diet in patients with recent acute myocardial infarction: Results of one-year follow-up. *British Medical Journal, 304,* 1689-1690.

- **Taking medications as prescribed, especially hypertensive medications (Hypertension Detection and Follow-up Program Cooperative Group, 1988)**
  Hypertension Detection and Follow-up Program Cooperative Group. (1988). Persistence of reduction in blood pressure and mortality of participants in the Hypertensive Detection and Follow-up Program. *Journal of the American Medical Association, 259,* 2113-2122.
- **Smoking cessation (Mulcahy, 1983)**
  Mulcahy, R. (1983). Influence of cigarette smoking on morbidity and mortality after myocardial infarction. *British Heart Journal, 49,* 410-415.

Obesity as a risk factor in CHD:
  Hubert, H.B., Feinleib, M., McNamara, P.M., & Castelli, W.P. (1983). Obesity as an independent risk factor for cardiovascular disease: A 26-year follow-up of participants in the Framingham Heart Study. *Circulation, 67,* 968-977.

Major investigations showing that dietary and medication interventions can decrease morbidity and mortality from CHD:
- **The Oslo Heart Study (Hjerman, Holme, Velve, Byer, & Leren, 1981)**
  Hjerman, L., Holme, I., Velve, M., Byer, K., & Leren, P. (1981). Effect of diet and smoking intervention on the incidence of coronary heart disease: Report from the Oslo Study Group of a randomized trial in healthy men. *Lancet, 2,* 1303-1310.
- **The Coronary Drug Project (Canner et al., 1986)**
  Canner, P.L., Berge, K.G., Wenger, N.K., Stamler, J., Friedman, L., Prineas, R.J., & Friedman, W. (1986). Fifteen-year mortality in coronary drug project patients: Long-term benefit with niacin. *Journal of the American College of Cardiology, 3,* 1245-1255.

Medical model of adherence:
  DiMatteo, M.R., & Friedman H.S. (1981). *Social psychology and medicine.* Cambridge, MA: Oelgeschlager, Gunn, & Hain.
  Stimson, G.V. (1974). Obeying doctor's orders: A view from the other side. *Social Sciences & Medicine, 8,* 97-104.

The Health Belief Model:
  Hochbaum, G.M. (1956). Why people seek diagnostic x-rays? *Public Health Reports, 71,* 377-380.
  Kegeles, S.S. (1963). Why people seek dental care: A test of a conceptual formulation. *Journal of Health and Human Behavior, 4,* 166-173.

Summary of adherence-enhancing strategies:
  Comoss, P.M. (1988). Nursing strategies to improve compliance with lifestyle changes in a cardiac rehabilitation population. *Journal of Cardiovascular Nursing, 2*(3), 23-36.
  Oldridge, N.B. (1986). Compliance with exercise programs. In M.L. Pollock & D.H. Schmidt (Eds.), *Heart disease and rehabilitation* (pp. 629-646). New York: Wiley.
  Oldridge, N.B., & Jones, N.L. (1983). Improving patient compliance in cardiac rehabilitation: Effects of written agreement and self-monitoring. *Journal of Cardiac Rehabilitation, 3,* 257-262.
  Oldridge, N.B., & Pashkow, F.J. (1993). Compliance and motivation in cardiac rehabilitation. In F.J. Pashkow & W.A. Dafoe (Eds.), *Clinical rehabilitation: A cardiologist's guide.* Baltimore: Williams & Wilkins.
  Rogers, K.R. (1987). Nature of spousal supportive behaviors that influence heart transplant patient compliance. *Journal of Heart Transplant, 60,* 90-95.
  Sackett, D.L, Haynes, R.B., Gibson, E.S., & Johnson, A. (1976). The problem of compliance with antihypertensive therapy. *Practical Cardiology, 2,* 35-39.
  Sotile, W.M. (1993). The intimacy factor in cardiopulmonary rehabilitation: A practical model for structuring interventions. *Journal of Cardiopulmonary Rehabilitation, 13*(4), 237-242.
  Southam, M.A., & Dunbar, J. (1986). Facilitating patient compliance with medical interventions. In K.A. Holroyd & T.L. Creer (Eds.), *Self-management of chronic disease* (pp. 163-187). New York: Academic Press.

Flagging patients at risk of low adherence:
  Blumenthal, J.A., Williams, R.S., Wallace, A.G., Williams, R.B., Jr., & Needels, T.L. (1982). Physiological and psychological variables predict compliance to prescribed exercise therapy in patients recovering from myocardial infarction. *Psychosomatic Medicine, 44,* 519-527.

Dhooper, S. (1984). Social networks and support during the crisis of heart attack. *Health Social Work, 9*, 294-303.

Oldridge, N.B. (1984). Compliance and dropout in cardiac exercise rehabilitation. *Journal of Cardiac Rehabilitation, 4*, 166-177.

Oldridge, N.B. (1986). Compliance with exercise programs. In M.L. Pollock & D.H. Schmidt (Eds.), *Heart disease and rehabilitation* (pp. 629-646). New York: Wiley.

Oldridge, N.B., & Pashkow, F.J. (1993). Compliance and motivation in cardiac rehabilitation. In F.J. Pashkow & W.A. Dafoe (Eds.), *Clinical rehabilitation: A cardiologist's guide*. Baltimore: Williams & Wilkins.

Sackett, D.L., & Haynes, R.B. (Eds.) (1976). *Compliance with therapeutic regimens*. Baltimore: Johns Hopkins University Press.

Siegrist, J., Siegrist, K., & Weber, I. (1986). Sociological concepts in the etiology of chronic disease: The case of ischemic heart disease. *Social Science & Medicine, 22*, 247-253.

Sirles, A.T., & Selleck, C.S. (1989). Cardiac disease and the family: Impact, assessment, and implications. *Journal of Cardiovascular Nursing, 3*(2), 23-32.

Multidisciplinary interventions for lowering lipids with use of lipid-lowering drugs:

DeBusk, R.F., Miller, N.H., Superko, H.R., Dennis, C.A., Thomas, R.J., Lew, H.T., Berger, W.E., III, Heller, R.S., Rompf, J., Gee, D., et al. (1994). A case management system for coronary risk factor modification following acute myocardial infarction. *Annals of Internal Medicine, 120*(9), 721-729.

Hamalainen, H., Luurila, O.J., Kallio, V., Knuts, L.R., Artila, M., & Hakkila, J. (1989). Long-term reduction in sudden deaths after a multifactorial intervention programme in patients with myocardial infarction: 10 year results of a controlled investigation. *European Heart Journal, 10*, 55-62.

Multidisciplinary interventions for lowering lipids without use of lipid-lowering drugs:

DeBusk, R.F., Miller, N.H., Superko, H.R., Dennis, C.A., Thomas, R.J., Lew, H.T., Berger, W.E., III, Heller, R.S., Rompf, J., Gee, D., et al. (1994). A case management system for coronary risk factor modification following acute myocardial infarction. *Annals of Internal Medicine, 120*(9), 721-729.

Hamalainen, H., Luurila, O.J., Kallio, V., Knuts, L.R., Artila, M., & Hakkila, J. (1989). Long-term reduction in sudden deaths after a multifactorial intervention programme in patients with myocardial infarction: 10 year results of a controlled investigation. *European Heart Journal, 10*, 55-62.

Karvetti, R.L., & Hamalainen, H. (1993). Long-term effect of nutrition education on myocardial infarction patients: A 10-year follow-up study. *Nutritional Metabolism and Cardiovascular Disease 16*(3), 185-192.

Ornish, D., Brown, S.E., Scherwitz, L.W., Billings, J.H., Armstrong, W.T., Ports, T.A., McLanahan, S.M., Kirkeeide, R.L., Brand, R.J., & Gould, K.L. (1990). Can lifestyle changes reverse coronary heart disease? *Lancet, 336*, 129-133.

Schuler, G., Hambrecht, J.R., Schlierf, G., Grunze, M., Methfessel, S., Hayer, K., & Kublen, W. (1992). Myocardial perfusion and regression of coronary artery disease in patients on a regimen of intensive physical exercise and low fat diet. *Journal of the American College of Cardiology, 19*, 34-42.

Problems with weight-reduction studies with cardiopulmonary populations:

Bengtsson, K. (1983). Rehabilitation after myocardial infarction—A controlled study. *Scandinavian Journal of Rehabilitation Medicine, 15*, 1-9.

Miller, N.H., Taylor, C.B., Davidson, D.M., Hill, M.N., & Krantz, D.S. (1990). The efficacy of risk factor intervention and psychosocial aspects of cardiac rehabilitation. *Journal of Cardiac Rehabilitation, 10*, 198-209.

Oldridge, N.B., & Pashkow, F.J. (1993). Compliance and motivation in cardiac rehabilitation. In F.J. Pashkow & W.A. Dafoe (Eds.), *Clinical rehabilitation: A cardiologist's guide*. Baltimore: Williams & Wilkins.

Vermeulen, A., Lie, K., & Burrer, D. (1983). Effects of cardiac rehabilitation after myocardial infarction: Changes in coronary risk factors and long-term prognosis. *American Heart Journal, 105*, 798-801.

Dietary intervention strategies:
- **General strategies (McAlister, Farquhar, Thoresen, & Maccoby, 1976)**
  McAlister, A.L., Farquhar, J.W., Thoresen, C.E., & Maccoby, N. (1976). Behavioral science applied to cardiovascular health: Progress and research needs in the modification of risk-taking habits in adult populations. *Health Education Monographs, 4,* 45-74.
- **Developing alternative behavioral responses to eating urges (Jeffery, 1987)**
  Jeffery, R.W. (1987). Behavioral treatment of obesity. *Annals of Behavioral Medicine, 9*(1), 20-24.
- **Teaching to cope differently in responding to urges to violate newly learned patterns of eating**
  Smith, T.W., & Leon, A.S. (1992). *Coronary heart disease: A behavioral perspective.* Champaign, IL: Research Press.
- **Involving the family of the patient in treatment (Bennett, 1986; Murphy et al., 1982; Perri, McAdoo, McAllister, Lauer, & Yancey, 1986; Sotile, Sotile, Ewen, & Sotile, 1993; Baranowski, Nader, Dunn, & Vanderpool, 1982)**
  Baranowski, T., Nader, P.R., Dunn, K., & Vanderpool, N.A. (1982). Family self-help: Promoting changes in health behavior. *Journal of Communication, 4,* 161-172.
  Bennett, G.A. (1986). Behavior therapy for obesity: A quantitative review of the effects of selected treatment characteristics on outcome. *Behavior Therapy, 17,* 554-562.
  Murphy, J.K., Williamson, A.E., Buxton, A.E., Moody, S.C., Absher, N., & Warner, M. (1982). The long-term effects of spouse involvement upon weight loss maintenance. *Behavioral Therapy, 13,* 681-693.
  Perri, M.G., McAdoo, W.G., McAllister, D.A., Lauer, J.B., & Yancey, D.Z. (1986). Enhancing the efficacy of behavior therapy for obesity: Effects of aerobic exercise and a multicomponent maintenance program. *Journal of Consulting and Clinical Psychology, 54,* 670-675.
  Sotile, W.M., Sotile, M.O., Ewen, G.S., & Sotile, L.J. (1993). Marriage and family factors relevant to effective cardiac rehabilitation: A review of risk factor literature. *Sports Medicine, Training and Rehabilitation, 4,* 115-128.
- **Incorporating physical exercise into a multicomponent program (Brownell & Wadden, 1986; Leon, 1989; Leon, Pollock, & Weltman, 1983)**
  Brownell, K.D., & Wadden, T.A. (1986). Behavior therapy for obesity: Modern approaches and better results. In K.D. Brownell & J.P. Foreyt (Eds.), Handbook of eating disorders (pp. 180-197). New York: Basic Books.
  Leon, A.S. (1989). The role of physical activity in the prevention and management of obesity. In A.J. Ryan & F.L. Allman (Eds.), *Sports medicine* (2nd ed., pp. 593-646). San Diego: Academic.
  Leon, A.S., Pollock, M.L., & Weltman, A. (1983). American College of Sports Medicine position statement on proper and improper weight loss programs. *Medicine and Science in Sports and Exercise, ix-xii,* 15.

Importance of using adherence-enhancing strategies in promoting weight loss:
  Brownell, K.D., & Jeffery, R.W. (1987). Improving long-term weight loss: Pushing the limits of treatment. *Behavioral Therapy, 18,* 353-374.
  In a review of the weight loss literature, Brownell and Jeffery (1987) mentioned eight studies that reported a 75% maintenance of posttreatment weight losses at 1-year follow-up. The authors also reported that the 21 studies reviewed claimed a mean weight loss of between 7 and 9 kg immediately after treatment. Furthermore, the amount of weight lost related more to length of participation in the program than to the technique used, and regardless of technique, regular exercise was universally associated with better maintenance of weight loss at follow-up. The emphasis in this research on the importance of length of participation in the program underscores the need to attend to adherence issues when intervening regarding diet or weight issues.

Interpersonal skill training for hypertensives:
  Ewart, C.K., Taylor, C.B., Kraemer, H.C., & Agras, W.S. (1984). Reducing blood pressure reactivity during interpersonal conflict: Effects of marital communication training. *Behavioral Therapy, 15,* 473-484.

Smith, T.W., & Sanders, J.D. (1986). Type A behavior, marriage, and the heart: Person-by-situation interactions and the risk of coronary disease. *Behavioral Medicine Abstracts, 7*, 59-62.

Multicomponent stress management interventions that have reported therapeutic effects of up to 5-15 mmHg reductions in blood pressures:

Crother, J.H. (1983). Stress management training and relaxation imagery in the treatment of essential hypertension. *Journal of Behavioral Medicine, 6*, 169-187.

Irvine, M.J., Johnston, D.W., Jenner, D.A., & Marie, G.V. (1986). Relaxation and stress management in the treatment of essential hypertension. *Journal of Psychosomatic Research, 30*, 437-450.

Patel, C., Marmot, M.G., Terry, D.J., Carruthers, M., Hunt, B., & Patel, M. (1985). Trial of relaxation in reducing coronary risk: Four-year follow-up. *British Medical Journal, 290*, 1103-1106.

Zurawski, R.M., Smith, T.W., & Houston, B.K. (1987). Stress management for essential hypertension: Comparison with a minimally effective treatment, predictors of response to treatment, and effects on reactivity. *Journal of Psychosomatic Research, 31*, 453-462.

Stress management interventions that reduced work site blood pressure levels among hypertensives:

Agras, W.S., Taylor, C.B., Kraemer, H.C., Southam, M.A., & Schneider, J.A. (1987). Relaxation training for essential hypertension at the worksite: Part 2. The poorly controlled hypertensive. *Psychosomatic Medicine, 49*, 264-273.

Charlesworth, E.A., Williams, B.J., & Baer, P.E. (1984). Stress management at the worksite for hypertension: Compliance, cost-benefit, health care, and hypertension-related variables. *Psychosomatic Medicine, 46*, 387-397.

Chesney, M.A., Black, G.W., Swan, G.E., & Ward, M.M. (1987). Relaxation training for essential hypertension and the worksite: Part I. The untreated mild hypertensive. *Psychosomatic Medicine, 49*, 250-263.

Lack of positive results from stress management interventions to reduce blood pressures:

Blackburn, H., & Leon, A.S. (1986). Preventive cardiology in practice: Minnesota studies on risk factor reduction. In M.L. Pollock & D.H. Schmidt (Eds.), *Heart disease and rehabilitation* (pp. 265-301). New York: Wiley.

General guidelines for structuring psychosocial interventions:

American Association of Cardiovascular and Pulmonary Rehabilitation. (1991). *Guidelines for cardiac rehabilitation programs*. Champaign, IL: Human Kinetics.

American Association of Cardiovascular and Pulmonary Rehabilitation. (1994). *Guidelines for cardiac rehabilitation programs* (2nd ed.). Champaign, IL: Human Kinetics.

Doherty, W.J., & Baird, M.A. (1983). *Family therapy and family medicine*. New York: Guilford Press.

My six levels of psychosocial intervention with cardiopulmonary patients is a modification of a similar model proposed by Doherty and Baird regarding ways to structure family-sensitive medical care.

Kolman, B.R. (1983). The value of group psychotherapy after myocardial infarction: A critical review. *Journal of Cardiac Rehabilitation, 3*, 360-366.

Rahe, R.M., Ward, H.W., & Hayes, V. (1979). Brief group therapy in myocardial infarction rehabilitation: Three to four year follow-up of a controlled trial. *Psychosomatic Medicine, 41*, 229-242.

Razin, A.M. (1982). Psychosocial intervention in coronary artery disease: A review. *Psychosomatic Medicine, 44*(4), 363-381.

Sotile, W.M. (1993). The intimacy factor in cardiopulmonary rehabilitation: A practical model for structuring interventions. *Journal of Cardiopulmonary Rehabilitation, 13*(4), 237-242.

Sotile, W.M., Sotile, M.O., Sotile, L.J., & Ewen, G.S. (1993). Marital and family factors relevant to cardiac rehabilitation: An integrative review of the psychosocial literature. *Sports Medicine, Training and Rehabilitation, 4*, 217-236.

Wallace, N., & Wallace, D.C. (1977). Group education after myocardial infarction. *Medical Journal of Australia, 2*, 245-247.

International literature on the effectiveness of formal rehabilitation programs:
- **United States**

  Agle, D.F., Baum, G.L., Chester, E.H., & Wendt, M. (1973). Multidiscipline treatment of chronic pulmonary insufficiency. 1. Psychological aspects of rehabilitation. *Psychosomatic Medicine, 35*(1), 41-49.

  DeBusk, R.F., Miller, N.H., Superko, H.R., Dennis, C.A., Thomas, R.J., Lew, H.T., Berger, W.E., III, Heller, R.S., Rompf, J., Gee, D., et al. (1994). A case management system for coronary risk factor modification following acute myocardial infarction. *Annals of Internal Medicine, 120*(9), 721-729.

  Emery, C.F., Leatherman, N.E., Burker, E.J., & MacIntrye, N.R. (1991). Psychological outcomes of a pulmonary rehabilitation program. *Chest, 100*, 613-619.

  Foster, S., & Thomas, H.M. (1990). Pulmonary rehabilitation in lung disease other than COPD. *American Review of Respiratory Diseases, 141*, 601-604.

  Oldridge, N.B., Guyatt, G., Jones, N., Corwe, J., Sincer, J., Feeny, D., McKelbie, R., Runions, J., Streiner, D., & Torrance, G. (1991). *American Journal of Cardiology, 67*, 1084-1089.

  Ornish, D., Scherwitz, L.W., Doody, R.S., Kerten, D., McLanahan, S.M., Brown, S.E., DePuey, G., Sonnemaker, R., Haynes, C., Lester, J., McAlister, G.K., Hall, R.J., Burdine, J.A., & Gotto, A.M. (1983). Effects of stress management training and dietary changes in treating ischemic heart disease. *Journal of the American Medical Association, 249*, 54-60.

  Squires, R.W., Allison, T.G., Miller, T.D., & Gan, G.T. (1991). Cardiopulmonary exercise testing after unilateral lung transplantation: A case report. *Journal of Cardiopulmonary Rehabilitation, 11*, 192-196.

- **Finland (Kaillio et al., 1979 Hamalainen et al., 1989; Engblom et al., 1992)**

  Engblom, E., Ronnemaa, T., Hamalainen, H., Kallio, V., Vanttinen, E., & Knuts, L.R. (1992). Coronary heart disease risk factors before and after bypass surgery: Results of a controlled trial on multifactorial rehabilitation. *European Heart Journal, 13*(8), 1053-1059.

  Hamalainen, H., Luurila, O.J., Kallio, V., Knuts, L.R., Artila, M., & Hakkila, J. (1989). Long-term reduction in sudden deaths after a multifactorial intervention programme in patients with myocardial infarction: 10 year results of a controlled investigation. *European Heart Journal, 10*, 55-62.

  Kallio, V., Hamalainen, H., Hakkila, J., & Laurila, O.J. (1979). Reduction in sudden deaths by a multifactorial intervention programme after acute myocardial infarction. *Lancet, 2*, 1091-1094.

- **The Netherlands**

  van Dixhoorn, J., Duivenvoorden, J.H., & Staal, H.A. (1989). Physical training and relaxation therapy in cardiac rehabilitation assessed through a composite criterion for training outcome. *American Heart Journal, 119*(3), 545-552.

- **Sweden (Bengstsson, 1983)**

  Bengtsson, K. (1983). Rehabilitation after myocardial infarction—A controlled study. *Scandinavian Journal of Rehabilitation Medicine, 15*, 1-9.

- **Australia**

  Goble, A.J., Hare, D.L., Macdonald, P.S., Oliver, R.G., Reid, M.A., & Worcester, M.C. (1991). Effect of early programmes of high and low intensity exercise on physical performance after transmural acute myocardial infarction. *British Heart Journal, 65*(3), 126-131.

For cutting-edge information on collaborative family health care, contact:

The Coalition for Collaborative Family Health Care, 40 West 12th Street, New York, NY 10011 (phone 202-966-5376).

REFERENCES AND
■ GENERAL BIBLIOGRAPHY ■

Achterberg, J. (1985). *Imagery in Healing*. Boston: Shambala Press.

Acosta, F. (1987). Weaning the anxious ventilator patient using hypnotic relaxation: Case reports. *American Journal of Clinical Hypnosis, 29*(4), 272-280.

Acosta-Austan, F. (1991). Tolerance of chronic dyspnea using a hypnoeducational approach: A case report. *American Journal of Clinical Hypnosis, 33*(4), 272-277.

Ades, P.A., & Grunvald, M.H. (1990). Cardiopulmonary exercise testing before and after conditioning in older coronary patients. *American Heart Journal, 120*(3), 585-589.

Ades, P.A., Hanson, J.S., Gunther, P.G., & Tonino, R.P. (1987). Exercise conditioning in the elderly coronary patient. *Journal of American Geriatric Society 35*(2), 121-124.

Ades, P.A., Waldman, M.L., Polk, D., & Coflesky, J.T. (1992, June 1). Referral patterns and exercise response in the rehabilitation of female coronary patients aged ≥ 62 years. *American Journal of Cardiology, 69*.

Agle, D.P., & Baum, G.L. (1977). Psychological aspects of chronic obstructive pulmonary disease. *Medical Clinics of North America, 61*, 749-758.

Agras, W.S., Taylor, C.B., Kraemer, H.C., Southam, M.A., & Schneider, J.A. (1987). Relaxation training for essential hypertension at the worksite: Part 2. The poorly controlled hypertensive. *Psychosomatic Medicine, 49*, 264-273.

Ahern, D.K., Gorkin, L., Anderson, J.L., Tierney, C., Hallstrom, A., & Ewart, C., for the Cardiac Arrhythmia Pilot Study (CAPS) Investigators. (1989, November). *Biobehavioral variables and mortality of cardiac arrest in the CAPS*. Paper presented at the annual meeting of the American Heart Association, New Orleans.

Aho, W.R. (1977). Relationship of wives' preventive health orientation to their beliefs about heart disease in husbands. *Public Health Reports, 92*, 65-71.

Aiken, L.H., & Henricks, T.F. (1971). Systematic relaxation as a nursing intervention technique with open heart surgery patients. *Nursing Research, 20*(3), 212-216.

Alberti, R., & Emmons, M. (1982). *A guide to assertive living: Your perfect right*. San Luis Obispo, California: Impact Publishers.

Alexander, A.B., Miklich, D., & Riff, H. (1972). The immediate effects of systematic relaxation training on peak expiratory flow rates in asthmatic children. *Psychosomatic Medicine, 34*(5), 388-393.

Allen, J.P., Eckardt, M.J., & Wallen, J. (1988). Screening for alcoholism: Techniques and issues. *Public Health Reports, 103*, 586-592.

Alonzo, A.A. (1986). The impact of the family and lay others on care-seeking during life-threatening episodes of suspected coronary artery disease. *Social Science & Medicine, 22*(12), 1297-1311.

Amberson, J.I., & Hoon, P. (1985). Hemodynamics of sequential orgasm. *Archives of Sexual Behavior, 14,* 351-360.

Ambrosino, N., Paggiaro, P.L., Macchi, M., Filieri, M., Toma, G., Lombardi, F.A., DelCesta, F., Parlanti, A., Loi, A.M., & Beschieri, L. (1981). A study of the short-term effect of rehabilitative therapy in chronic obstructive pulmonary disease. *Respiration, 41*(1), 40-44.

American Academy of Family Physicians (1987). *AAFP Stop Smoking Patient Guide.* Kansas City, Missouri: American Academy of Family Physicians.

American Association of Retired Persons and Administration on Aging. (1986). *A profile of older Americans, 1986.* Washington, D.C.: U.S. Department of Health and Human Resources.

American Council of Science and Health. (1983). *Postmenopausal estrogen therapy* (report). Summit, NJ: Author.

American Heart Association. (1989). *Heart facts.* Dallas: Author.

American Psychiatric Association. (1987). *Quick reference to the diagnostic criteria from DSM-III-R.* Washington, D.C.: Author.

American Psychiatric Association. (1994). *Diagnostic and statistical manual of mental disorders* (4th ed.). Washington, D.C.: Author.

American Thoracic Society. (1981). Official ATS Statement—pulmonary rehabilitation by the American Lung Association. *American Review of Respiratory Disease, 124,* 663-666.

American Thoracic Society. (1987). Standards for the diagnosis and care of patients with chronic obstructive pulmonary disease (COPD) and asthma. *American Review of Respiratory Diseases, 136,* 225-230.

Amick, T.L., & Ockene, J.K. (1994). The role of social support in the modification of risk factors for cardiovascular disease. In S.A. Shumaker & S.M. Cajkowski (Eds.), *Social support and cardiovascular disease* (pp. 259-280). New York: Plenum Press.

Anderson, D. (1988, July/August). The quest for meaningful old age. *The Family Therapy Networker,* 17-22, 72-74.

Anderson, E.A. (1987). Preoperative preparation for cardiac surgery facilitates recovery, reduces psychological distress, and reduces the incidence of acute post-operative hypertension. *Journal of Consulting and Clinical Psychology, 55,* 513-520.

Anderson, K.O., & Masur, F.T., III. (1983). Psychological preparation for invasive medical and dental procedures. *Journal of Behavioral Medicine, 6*(1), 1-40.

Anderson, K.O., & Masur, F.T. (1989). Psychologic preparation for cardiac catheterization. *Heart and Lung, 18,* 154-163.

Andrew, G., & Parker, J. (1979). Factors related to dropout of post-myocardial infarction patients from exercise programs. *Medicine and Science in Sports and Exercise, 11,* 376-378.

Andrew, G.M., Oldridge, N.B., Parker, J.O., Cunningham, D.A., Rechnitzer, P.A., Jones, N.L., Buck, C., Kavanagh, T., Shepherd, R.J., Sutton, J.R., & McDonald, W. (1981). Reasons for dropout from exercise programs in postcoronary patients. *Medicine and Science in Sports and Exercise, 13,* 164-168.

Andrew, J.M. (1970). Recovery from surgery, with and without preparatory instruction, for three coping styles. *Journal of Personality and Social Psychology, 15,* 223-226.

Annon, J.S., & Robinson, C.H. (1978). The use of vicarious learning models in treatment of sexual concerns. In J. LoPiccolo & L. LoPiccolo (Eds.), *Handbook of sex therapy* (pp. 35-60). New York: Plenum Press.

Antonucci, T.C., & Jackson, J.S. (1987). Social support, interpersonal efficacy, and health. In L. Carstensen & B.A. Edelstein (Eds.), *Handbook of clinical gerontology* (pp. 291-311). New York: Pergamon Press.

Antonucci, T.C., & Johnson, E.H. (1994). Conceptualization and methods in social support theory and research as related to cardiovascular disease. In S.A. Shumaker & S.M. Czajkowski (Eds.), *Social support and cardiovascular disease* (pp. 21-40). New York: Plenum Press.

Appleton, W.S. (1982). How depressed patients adversely affect their marriages. *Medical Aspects of Human Sexuality, 16,* 154-167.

Ashikaga, T., Vacek, P.M., & Lewis, S.O. (1980). Evaluation of a community-based education program for individuals with chronic obstructive pulmonary disease. *Journal of Rehabilitation Research and Development, 46,* 23-27.

Averill, J.R. (1992). *Anger and aggression: An essay on emotion.* New York: Springer-Verlag.

Badger, T.A. (1992). Coping, life-style changes, health perceptions, and marital adjustment in middle-aged women and men with cardiovascular disease and their spouses. *Health Care for Women International, 13,* 43-55.

Baggs, J., & Darch, A. (1987). Sexual counseling of women with coronary heart disease. *Heart and Lung, 16,* 154-158.

Baile, W.F., & Engel, B.T. (1978). A behavioral strategy for promoting treatment compliance following myocardial infarction. *Psychosomatic Medicine, 40,* 413-419.

Baile, W.F., Gigelow, G.E., Gottlieb, S.H., Stitzer, M.L., & Sacktor, J.D. (1982). Rapid resumption of cigarette smoking following myocardial infarction: Inverse relation to MI severity. *Addictive Behavior, 7,* 373-380.

Bandura, A. (1977a). Self-efficacy: Toward a unifying theory of behavioral change. *Psychological Review, 84,* 191-215.

Bandura, A. (1977b). *Social learning theory.* Englewood Cliffs, NJ: Prentice Hall.

Bandura, A. (1984). Recycling misconceptions of perceived self-efficacy. *Cognitive Therapy Research, 8,* 231-255.

Barach, A.L. (1955). Breathing exercises in pulmonary emphysema and allied chronic respiratory disease. *Archives of Physical Medicine and Rehabilitation, 36,* 379-390.

Baranowski, T., Nader, P.R., Dunn, K., & Vanderpool, N.A. (1982). Family self-help: Promoting changes in health behavior. *Journal of Communication, 4,* 161-172.

Barbach, L. (1984). *For each other.* New York: Signet.

Barbarin, O., & Gilbert, R. (1979). *Family process scales.* Ann Arbor, MI: Family Development Project.

Barbarin, O.A., & Tirado, M. (1985). Enmeshment, family processes, and successful treatment of obesity. *Family Relations, 34,* 115-121.

Barbarin, O.A., & Tirado, M.C. (1984). Family involvement and successful treatment of obesity: A review. *Family Systems Medicine, 2,* 37-45.

Barborowicz, P., Nelson, M., DeBusk, R.F., & Haskell, W.L. (1980). A comparison of in-hospital education approaches for coronary bypass patients. *Heart and Lung, 9,* 127.

Barefoot, J.C., Dahlstrom, W.C., & Williams, R.B. (1983). Hostility, CHD incidence, and total mortality: A 25-year follow-up study of 255 physicians. *Psychosomatic Medicine, 45,* 59-63.

Barnes, G., Ray, M., Oberman, A., & Kouchoukos, N. (1977).Changes in working status of patients following coronary bypass surgery. *Journal of the American Medical Association, 238,* 1259-1262.

Bar-On, D. (1987). Causal attributions and the rehabilitation of myocardial infarction victims. *Journal of Social and Clinical Psychology, 5,* 114-122.

Bar-On, D., & Cristal, N. (1987). Causal attributions of patients, their spouses and physicians, and the rehabilitation of the patients after their first myocardial infarction. *Journal of Cardiopulmonary Rehabilitation, 7,* 285-298.

Baron, R.A. (1979). Aggression, empathy and race: Effects of victim's pain cues, victim's race and level of instigation on physical aggression. *Journal of Applied Social Psychology, 9,* 103-114.

Barrera, M., Sandler, I.N., & Ramsay, T.B. (1981). Preliminary development of a scale of social support: Studies on college students. *American Journal of Community Psychology, 9,* 435-447.

Barry, J.M., Blank, B.H., & Boileau, M. (1980). Nocturnal penile tumescence monitoring with stamps. *Urology, 15,* 171-172.

Bartle, S.H., & Bishop, L.F. (1974). Psychological study of patients with coronary heart disease with unexpectedly long survival and high level functions. *Psychosomatics, 15,* 68-69.

Bass, C., & Wade, C. (1984). Chest pain with normal coronary arteries: A comparative study of psychiatric and social morbidity. *Psychological Medicine, 14,* 51-61.

Baum, G.L., Agle, D.F., Chester, E.N., & Wendt, M. (1973). Multidiscipline treatment of chronic pulmonary insufficiency: Functional status at one-year follow-up. In R.J. Johnston (Ed.), *Pulmonary Care* (pp. 355-362). New York: Crane & Stratton.

Beach, S.R., Sandeen, E.E., & O'Leary, K.D. (1990). *Depression in marriage.* New York: Guilford Press.

Beck, A.T. (1978). *Depression inventory.* Philadelphia: Center for Cognitive Therapy.

Beck, A.T. (1979). *Cognitive therapy and emotional disorders.* New York: New American Library.

Beck, A.T., Rush, A.J., Shaw, B.F., & Emery, G. (1979). *Cognitive therapy of depression.* New York: Guilford Press.

Becker, M.A., & Byrne, D. (1984). Type A behavior and daily activities of young married couples. *Journal of Applied Social Psychology, 14,* 82-88.

Becker, M.H. (1979). Patient perceptions and compliance: Recent studies of the health belief model. In R.B. Haynes, D.W. Taylor, & D.L. Sackett (Eds.), *Compliance in health care.* Baltimore: Johns Hopkins University Press.

Beckie, T. (1989). A supportive-educative telephone program: Impact on knowledge and anxiety after coronary artery bypass graft surgery. *Heart and Lung, 18,* 46-55.

Becklake, M.R., McGregor, M., Goldman, H.I., & Braudo, J.L. (1954). A study of the effects of physiotherapy in chronic hypertrophic emphysema using lung function tests. *Diseases of the Chest, 26,* 180-191.

Belman, M. (1986). Exercise in chronic obstructive pulmonary disease. *Clinical Chest Medicine, 7,* 585-597.

Beneke, W.M., & Paulsen, B.K. (1979). Long-term efficacy of a behavior modification weight loss program: A comparison of two follow-up maintenance strategies. *Behavioral Therapy, 10,* 8-13.

Bengtsson, K. (1983). Rehabilitation after myocardial infarction—A controlled study. *Scandinavian Journal of Rehabilitation Medicine, 15,* 1-9.

Bennett, G.A. (1986). Behavior therapy for obesity: A quantitative review of the effects of selected treatment characteristics on outcome. *Behavior Therapy, 17,* 554-562.

Benowitz, N.L. (1988). Pharmacologic aspects of cigarette smoking and nicotine addiction. *New England Journal of Medicine, 319,* 1318-1330.

Benowitz, N.L. (1991). Nicotine and coronary heart disease. *Trends in Cardiovascular Medicine, 1,* 315-321.

Ben-Sira, Z., & Eliezer, R. (1990). The structure of readjustment after heart attack. *Social Science & Medicine, 30*(5), 523-536.

Benson, H. (1975). *The relaxation response.* New York: William Morrow.

Berkman, L., & Seeman, T. (1986). The influence of social relationships on aging and the development of cardiovascular disease—A review. *Postgraduate Medical Journal, 62,* 805-807.

Berkman, L., & Syme, S.L. (1979). Social networks, host resistance, and mortality: A nine-year follow-up study of Alameda County residents. *American Journal of Epidemiology, 109,* 186-204.

Berkman, L.F. (1984). Assessing the physical health effects of social networks and social support. *Annual Review of Public Health, 5,* 413-432.

Berra, K. (1991, November). *Program design for the 21st century: Expanding the cardiopulmonary rehabilitation model to meet the needs of diverse patient populations.* Presented at the Sixth Annual Meeting of the American Association of Cardiovascular and Pulmonary Rehabilitation, Long Beach, CA.

Bertel, O., Buhler, F.R., Baitsch, G., Ritz, R., & Burkart, F. (1982). Plasma adrenaline and noradrenaline in patients with acute myocardial infarction: Relationship to ventricular arrhythmias of varying severity. *Chest, 82,* 64-68.

Beta-Blocker Heart Attack Trial Research Group. (1982). A randomized trial of propanolol in patients with acute myocardial infarction. I. Mortality results. *Journal of the American Medical Association, 247,* 1707-1714.

Beutler, L.E., Scott, F.B., Rogers, R.R., Karacan, I., Baer, P.E., & Gaines, J.A. (1986). Inflatable and noninflatable penile prostheses: Comparative follow-up evaluation. *Urology, 28,* 136-143.

Bharadwaj, L., & Wilkening, E. (1977). The prediction of perceived well-being. *Social Industrial Research, 4,* 421-439.

Biaggio, M.K. (1987). Therapeutic management of anger. *Clinical Psychology Review, 7,* 663-675.

Bilodeau, B.C., & Hackett, T.P. (1971). Issues raised in a group setting by patients recovering from myocardial infarction. *American Journal of Psychiatry, 128,* 73-78.

Bishop, D.S., Epstein, N.B., Baldwin, L.M., Miller, I.W., & Keitner, G.I. (1988). Older couples: The effect of health retirement and family functioning on morale. *Family Systems Medicine, 6*(2), 238-247.

Blackburn, H., & Leon, A.S. (1986). Preventive cardiology in practice: Minnesota studies on risk factor reduction. In M.L. Pollock & D.H. Schmidt (Eds.), *Heart disease and rehabilitation* (pp. 265-301). New York: Wiley.

Blake, R.L., Vandiver, T.A., Braun, S., Bertuso, D.D., & Straub, V. (1990). A randomized controlled evaluation of a psychosocial intervention in adults with chronic lung disease. *Family Medicine, 22*(5), 365-370.

Blaney, N.T., Brown, P., & Blaney, P.H. (1986). Type A, marital adjustment, and life stress. *Journal of Behavioral Medicine, 9*(5), 491-502.

Blazer, D.G. (1991). Spirituality and aging well. *Generations, 15(1),* 61-65.

Blazer, D.G., & Palmore, E.B. (1976). Religion and aging. *Gerontologist, 16,* 82-85.

Blumenthal, J., Williams, R.S., Needels, T., & Wallace, A. (1982). Psychological changes accompany aerobic exercise in healthy middle-aged adults. *Psychosomatic Medicine, 44,* 529-536.

Blumenthal, J.A. (1985). Psychological assessment in cardiac rehabilitation. *Journal of Cardiopulmonary Rehabilitation, 5,* 208-215.

Blumenthal, J.A., Burg, M.M., Barefoot, J., Williams, R.B., Haney, T., & Zimet, G. (1987). Social support, Type A behavior and coronary artery disease. *Psychosomatic Medicine, 49,* 331-339.

Blumenthal, J.A., Emery, C.F., Walsh, M.A., Cox, D.R., Kuhn, C.M., Williams, R.B., & Williams, R.S. (1988). Exercise training in healthy Type A middle-aged men: Effects on behavioral and cardiovascular responses. *Psychosomatic Medicine, 50,* 418-433.

Blumenthal, J.A., & Wei, J. (1993). Psychobehavioral treatment in cardiac rehabilitation. *Cardiology Clinics, 11*(2), 323-331.

Blumenthal, J.A., Williams, R.S., Wallace, A.G., Williams, R.B., Jr., & Needels, T.L. (1982). Physiological and psychological variables predict compliance to prescribed exercise therapy in patients recovering from myocardial infarction. *Psychosomatic Medicine, 44,* 519-527.

Blumenthal, J.A., Williams, R.S., Williams, R.B., & Wallace, A.G. (1980). Effects of exercise on the Type A (coronary prone) behavior pattern. *Psychosomatic Medicine, 42,* 289-296.

Bonner, E.J., & Gendel, E.S. (1987). Sexual counseling for the elderly patient after myocardial infarction. *Aspects of Human Sexuality, 21*(3), 100-108.

Boone, T., & Kelley, R. (1990). Sexual issues and research in counseling the post-myocardial infarction patient. *Journal of Cardiovascular Nursing, 4*(4), 65-75.

Borak, J., Silwinski, P., Piasecki, Z., & Zielinski, J. (1991). Psychological status of COPD patients on long-term oxygen therapy. *European Respiratory Journal, 4,* 59-62.

Borson, S., McDonald, G.J., Gayle, T., & Deffenbach, M. (1992). Improvement in mood, physical symptoms and function with nortriptyline for depression in patients with chronic obstructive pulmonary disease. *Psychosomatics, 33*(2), 190-201.

Bowers, J.E., & Kogan, H.N. (1984). Stress response contagion between spouses: Fact or fiction. *Family Systems Medicine, 2,* 420-427.

Boykoff, S.L. (1986). Visitation needs reported by patients with cardiac disease and their families. *Heart and Lung, 15*(6), 573-578.

Bramwell, L. (1986). Wives' experiences in the support role after husbands' first myocardial infarction. *Heart and Lung, 15,* 578-584.

Brownell, K.D., Heckerman, C.L., Westlake, R.J., Hayes, S.C., & Monti, P.M. (1978). The effect of couples training and partner cooperativeness in behavioral treatment of obesity. *Behavioral Research, 16,* 323-333.

Brownell, K.D., & Jeffery, R.W. (1987). Improving long-term weight loss: Pushing the limits of treatment. *Behavioral Therapy, 18,* 353-374.

Brownell, K.D., & Wadden, T.A. (1986). Behavior therapy for obesity: Modern approaches and better results. In K.D. Brownell & J.P. Foreyt (Eds.), *Handbook of eating disorders* (pp. 180-197). New York: Basic Books.

Bruhn, H., Wolf, S., & Philips B. (1971). Depression and death in myocardial infarction: A psychosocial study of screening male coronary patients over nine years. *Journal of Psychosomatic Research, 15,* 305-313.

Bryant, F.B., & Yarnold, P.R. (1990). The impact of Type A behavior on subjective life quality: Bad for the heart, good for the soul? In M.J. Strube (Ed.), Type A behavior [Special issue]. *Journal of Social Behavior and Personality, 5*(1), 369-404.

Buist, A.S., Connett, J.E., Miller, R.D., Kanner, R.E., Owens, G.R., & Voelker, H.I. (1993). Chronic obstructive pulmonary disease early intervention trial (Lung Health Study): Baseline characteristics of randomized participants. *Chest, 103*(6), 1863-1872.

Burgess, A.W., Lerner, D.J., D'Agostino, R.B., Vokonas, P.S., Hartman, C.R., & Gaccione, P. (1987). A randomized control trial of cardiac rehabilitation. *Social Science Medicine, 24,* 359-370.

Burke, R.J., & Weir, T. (1977a). Marital helping relationships: The moderators between stress and well-being. *Journal of Psychology, 95,* 121-130.

Burke, R.J., & Weir, T. (1977b). The husband-wife relationship: The "mental hygiene" function in marriage. *Psychology Report, 40,* 911-925.

Burke, R.J., Weir, T., & DuWors, R.E., Jr. (1979). Type A behavior of administrators and wives' reports of marital satisfaction and well-being. *Journal of Applied Psychology, 63*(1), 57-65.

Burling, T.A., Singleton, E.G., Bigelow, G.E., Baile, W.F., & Gottlieb, S.H. (1984). Smoking following myocardial infarction: A critical review of the literature. *Health Psychology, 3,* 83-96.

Burns, D. (1980). *Feeling good: The new mood therapy.* New York: New American Library.

Burt, A., Thornley, P., Illingworth, D., White, P., Shaw, T.R.D., & Turner, R. (1974). Stopping smoking after myocardial infarction. *Lancet, 1,* 304-306.

Buss, A.H., & Durkee, A. (1957). An inventory for assessing different kinds of hostility. *Journal of Consulting Psychology, 21,* 343-349.

Butts, W.C., Kucheman, M., & Widdowson, G.M. (1974). An automated method for determining serum thiocyanate to distinguish smokers from nonsmokers. *Clinical Chemistry, 20,* 1344-1348.

Buvat, J., Lemaire, A., Buvat-Herbaut, M., Guieu, J.D., Bailleul, J.P., & Fossati, P. (1985). Comparative investigations in 26 impotent and 26 nonimpotent diabetic patients. *Journal of Urology, 133,* 34-38.

Byrne, D., Barry, J., & Nelson, D. (1963). Relation of the revised repression-sensitization scale to measures of self-description. *Psychology Report, 13,* 323-334.

Byrne, D.G., Whyte, H.M., & Butler, K.L. (1981). Illness behaviour and outcome of survived myocardial infarction: A prospective study. *Journal of Psychosomatic Research, 25,* 97-107.

Campbell, A., Converse, P., & Rogers, W. (1976). *The quality of American life.* New York: Russell Sage Foundation.

Campbell, M.K., DeVeillis, B.M., Strecher, V.J., Ammerman, A.S., DeVellis, R.F., & Sandler, R.S. (in press). The impact of message tailoring on dietary behavior change for disease prevention in primary care settings. *American Journal of Public Health.*

Campbell, T.L. (1986). Family's impact on health: A critical review. *Family Systems Medicine, 4,* 135-323.

Canner, P.L., Berge, K.G., Wenger, N.K., Stamler, J., Friedman, L., Prineas, R.J., & Friedman, W. (1986). Fifteen-year mortality in coronary drug project patients: Long-term benefit with niacin. *Journal of the American College of Cardiology, 3,* 1245-1255.

Cannistra, L.B., Balady, G.J., O'Malley, C.J., Weiner, D.A., & Ryan, T.J. (1992). Comparison of the clinical profile and outcome of women and men in cardiac rehabilitation. *American Journal of Cardiology, 15,* 69.

Cannon, W.B. (1929). *Bodily changes in pain, hunger, fear and rage.* New York: Appleton.

Cantor, J.P., Zillman, D., & Day, K.D. (1978). Relationship between cardiovascular fitness and physiological responses to films. *Perceptive Motor Skills, 46,* 1123-1130.

Caplan, G. (1964). *Principles of Preventive Psychiatry.* New York: Basic Books.

Carmody, T.P., Fey, S.G., Pierce, D.K., Connor, W.E., & Matarazzo, J.D. (1982). Behavioral treatment of hyperlipidemia: Techniques, results, and future directions. *Journal of Behavioral Medicine, 5*(1), 91-116.

Carney, R.M., Rich, M.W., Freedland, K.E., Saini, J., Tevelde, A., Simeone, C., & Clark, K. (1988). Major depressive disorder predicts cardiac events in patients with coronary artery disease. *Psychosomatic Medicine, 50*, 627-633.

Carroll, M.E., & Melsch, R.A. (1984). Increased drug-reinforced behavior due to food deprivation. In T. Thompson, P.B. Dews, & J.E. Barrett (Eds.), *Advanced behavioral pharmacology* (pp. 4-47). New York: Academic Press.

Carroll, M.E., Sitzer, M.L., & Strain, E. (1990). The behavioral pharmacology of alcohol and other drugs. In M. Galanter (Ed.), *Recent developments in alcoholism* (pp. 5-46). New York: Plenum Press.

Carter, R.E. (1984). Family reactions and reorganization patterns in myocardial infarction. *Family Systems Medicine, 2*, 55-65.

Case, R.B., Heller, S.S., Case, N.B., Moss, A.J., & the Multicenter Post-Infarction Research Group. (1985). Type A behavior and survival after acute myocardial infarction. *New England Journal of Medicine, 312*, 737-741.

Case, R.B., Moss, A.J., Case, N., McDermott, M., & Eberly, S. (1992). Living alone after myocardial infarction: Impact on prognosis. *Journal of the American Medical Association, 267*, 515-519.

Cassata, D.M., & Kirkman-Liff, B. (1981). Mental health activities of family physicians. *Journal of Family Practice, 12*, 683-692.

Cassell, S. (1965). Effect of brief puppet therapy upon the emotional responses of children undergoing cardiac catheterization. *Consulting Psychology, 29*, 1-8.

Cassell, S., & Paul, M.H. (1967). The role of puppet therapy on the emotional responses of children hospitalized for cardiac catheterization. *Journal of Pediatrics, 71*, 233-239.

Cassem, N.H., & Hackett, T.P. (1971). Psychiatric consultation in a coronary unit. *Annals of Internal Medicine, 75*, 9-14.

Cassem, N.H., & Hackett, T.P. (1979). "Ego infarction." Psychological reactions to a heart attack. *Journal of Practicing Nurses, 29*, 17-39.

Cavenaugh, S.V., Clark, D.C., & Gibbons, R.D. (1984). Diagnosing depression in the hospitalized medically ill. *Psychosomatics, 24*, 809-815.

Cay, E.L., Vetter, N., & Phillip, A. (1973). Return to work after a heart attack. *Journal of Psychosomatic Research, 17*, 231-243.

Centers for Disease Control. (1989). *Reducing the health consequences of smoking: 25 years of progress.* A report of the Surgeon General (DHHS Publication No. CDC 89-8411). Rockville, MD: U.S. Department of Health and Human Services, Public Health Service.

Chambliss, C.A., & Murray, E.J. (1979). Efficacy attribution, locus of control, and weight loss. *Cognitive Therapy Research, 3*, 349-353.

Chandra, V., Szklo, M., Goldberg, R., & Tonascia, J. (1983). The impact of marital status on survival after acute myocardial infarction: A population-based study. *American Journal of Epidemiology, 117*, 320-325.

Charlesworth, E.A., Williams, B.J., & Baer, P.E. (1984). Stress management at the worksite for hypertension: Compliance, cost-benefit, health care, and hypertension-related variables. *Psychosomatic Medicine, 46*, 387-397.

Chatham, M.A. (1978). The effect of family involvement on patients' manifestations of postcardiotomy psychosis. *Heart and Lung, 7*, 995-999.

Chesney, M.A., Black, G.W., Swan, G.E., & Ward, M.M. (1987). Relaxation training for essential hypertension and the worksite: Part I. The untreated mild hypertensive. *Psychosomatic Medicine, 49*, 250-263.

Christie-Seely, J. (Ed.) (1984). *Working with the family in primary care.* New York: Praeger.

Christopherson, V. (1968). Role modification of the disabled male. *American Journal of Nursing, 68,* 290-293.

Clark, S. (1990). Nursing interventions for the depressed cardiovascular patient. *Journal of Cardiovascular Nursing, 5*(1), 54-64.

Cleary, P.D., Miller, M., Bush, B.T., Warburg, M.M., Delbanco, T.L., & Aronson, M.D. (1988). Prevalence and recognition of alcohol abuse in a primary care population. *American Journal of Medicine, 85,* 466-471.

Clough, P., Harnisch, L., Cebulski, P., & Ross, D. (1987). Method for individualizing patient care for obstructive pulmonary disease patients. *Health and Social Work, 12*(2), 127-133.

Cobb, S. (1976). Social support as a moderator of life stress—presidential address. *Psychosomatic Medicine, 38,* 300-314.

Cockcroft, A.E., Saunders, M.T., & Berry, G. (1981). Randomised controlled trial of rehabilitation in chronic respiratory disability. *Thorax, 36,* 200-203.

Coffman, C.B., Levine, S.B., Althof, S.E., & Stern, R.C. (1984). Sexual adaption among single young adults with cystic fibrosis. *Chest, 86,* 412-418.

Cohen, S., & Lichtenstein, E. (1990). Partner behaviors that support quitting smoking. *Journal of Consulting Clinical Psychologists, 58,* 304-309.

Cohen, S., Lichtenstein, E., Prochaska, J.O., Rossi, J.S., Gritz, E.R., Carr, C.R., Orleans, C.T., Schoenbach, V.J., Biener, L., Abrams, D.B., DiClemente, C., Curry, S., Marlatt, G.A., Cummings, K.M., Emont, S.L., Giovino, G., & Ossip-Klein, D. (1989). Debunking myths about self-quitting: Evidence from ten prospective studies of persons who attempt to quit smoking by themselves. *American Psychologist, 44,* 1355-1365.

Cohen, S., Mermelstein, R., Karmack, T., & Hoberman, H.N. (1985). Measuring the functional components of social support. In I.G. Sarason & B.R. Sarason (Eds.), *Social support: Theory, research and applications* (pp. 73-94). Dordrecht, Netherlands: Martinua Nijhoff.

Cohen, S., & Syme, S.L. (Eds.) (1985). *Social support and health.* New York: Academic Press.

Cole, C.M., Levin, E.M., Whitley, J.O., & Young, S.H. (1979). Brief sexual counseling during cardiac rehabilitation. *Heart and Lung, 8*(1), 124-129.

Colliton, M. (1981). The spiritual dimension of nursing. In J. Beland and L. Passois (Eds.), *Clinical nursing* (4th ed., pp. 492-501). New York: Macmillan.

Comoss, P.M. (1988). Nursing strategies to improve compliance with lifestyle changes in a cardiac rehabilitation population. *Journal of Cardiovascular Nursing, 2*(3), 23-36.

Condon, J.T. (1988). The assessment of Type A behaviour pattern: Results from a spouse-report approach. *Psychological Medicine, 18,* 747-755.

Condra, M., Morales, A., Owen, J.A., Surridge, D.H., & Fenemore, J. (1986). Prevalence and significance of tobacco smoking in impotence. *Urology, 27,* 495-498.

Conine, T., & Evans, J. (1981). Sexual adjustment in chronic obstructive pulmonary disease. *Respiratory Care, 26*(9), 871-874.

Connors, G., & Hilling, L. (1993). *Guidelines for pulmonary rehabilitation programs.* Champaign, IL: Human Kinetics.

Conroy, R.M., Mulcahy, R., Graham, I.M., Reid, V., & Cahill, S. (1986). Predictors of patient response to risk-factor modification advice after admission for unstable angina or myocardial infarction. *Journal of Cardiopulmonary Rehabilitation, 6,* 344-357.

Cook, W.W., & Medley, D.M. (1954). Proposed hostility and pharisaic virtue scales for the MMPI. *Journal of Applied Psychology, 38,* 414-418.

Cooney, J.L., & Zeichner, A. (1985). Selective attention to negative feedback in Type A and Type B individuals. *Journal of Personality and Social Psychology, 91,* 110-112.

Cooper, C.L., Faragher, E.B., Bray, C.L., & Ramsdale, D.R. (1985). The significance of psychosocial factors in predicting coronary disease in patients with valvular heart disease. *Social Science & Medicine, 20,* 315-318.

Coppotelli, H.C., & Orleans, C.T. (1985). Partner support and other determinants of smoking cessation maintenance among women. *Journal of Consulting and Clinical Psychology, 53,* 455-460.

Costa, P.T., Jr., Fleg, J.L., McCrae, R.R., & Lakatta, E.G. (1982). Neuroticism, coronary artery disease, and chest pain complaints: Cross-sectional and longitudinal studies. *Experimental Aging Research, 8,* 37-44.

Costa, P.T., Jr., & McCrae, R.R. (1985). *The NEO personality inventory manual.* Odessa, FL: Psychological Assessment Resources.

Covino, N.A., Dirks, J.F., Kinsman, R.A., & Seidel, J.A. (1982). Patterns of depression in chronic illness. *Psychotherapy and Psychosomatics, 37,* 144-153.

Cox, J.L. (1993). Algorithms for nicotine withdrawal therapy. *Health Values, 17*(2), 41-50.

Cox, J.P., Evans, J.F., & Jamieson, J.L. (1979). Aerobic power and tonic heart rate responses to psychosocial stressors. *Personal Social Psychology Bulletin, 5,* 160-163.

Coyne, J.C., & DeLongis, A. (1986). Going beyond social support: The role of social relationships in adaptation. *Journal of Consulting and Clinical Psychology, 54,* 454-460.

Coyne, J.C., Ellard, J.H., & Smith, D.A. (1990). Unsupportive relationships, interdependence, and unhelpful exchanges. In I.G. Sarason, B.R. Sarason, & G. Pierce (Eds.), *Social support: An interactional view* (pp. 129-149). New York: Plenum Press.

Coyne, J.C., & Smith, D.A.F. (1991). Couples coping with a myocardial infarction: A contextual perspective on wives' distress. *Journal of Personality and Social Psychology, 61*(3), 404-412.

Craig, J., & Craig, M. (1979). *Synergic power: Beyond domination, beyond permissiveness* (2nd ed.). Los Angeles, CA: Proactive Press.

Crisp, A.H., Desouza, M., & Queenan, M. (1981, September). *Myocardial infarction and the emotional climate.* Paper presented at the Sixth World Congress of the International College of Psychosomatic Medicine, Montreal, PQ.

Cromwell, R.L., Butterfield, E.C., Brayfield, T.M., & Curry, J.J. (1987). *Acute myocardial infarction: Reaction and recovery.* St. Louis, MO: Mosby.

Croog, S.H. (1983). Recovery and rehabilitation of heart patients: Psychosocial aspects. In D.S. Krantz, A. Baum, & J.S. Singer (Eds.), *Handbook of psychology and health. Vol. 3: Cardiovascular disorders and behavior.* London: Erlbaum.

Croog, S.H., & Fitzgerald, E. (1978). Subjective stress and serious illness of a spouse: Wives of heart patients. *Journal of Health and Social Behavior, 19,* 166-178.

Croog, S.H., & Levine, S. (1977). *The heart patient recovers.* New York: Human Sciences Press.

Croog, S.H., & Richards, N. (1977). Health beliefs and smoking patterns in heart patients and their wives: A longitudinal study. *American Journal of Public Health, 67,* 921-930.

Crowley, T.J., MacDonald, M.J., Zerbe, G.O., & Petty, T.L. (1991). Reinforcing breath carbon monoxide reductions in chronic obstructive pulmonary disease. *Drug and Alcohol Dependence, 29*(1), 47-62.

Curgian, L.M., & Gronkiewicz, C.A. (1988). Enhancing sexual performance in COPD. *Nurse Practitioner, 13,* 34-38.

Cutrona, C. (1986). Behavioral manifestations of social support: A microanalytic investigation. *Journal of Personality and Social Psychology, 51,* 201-208.

Dafoe, W.A., Franklin, B.A., & Cupper, L. (1993). Vocational issues and disability. In F.J. Pashkow & W.A. Dafoe (Eds.), *Clinical cardiac rehabilitation: A cardiologist's guide.* (pp. 227-241). Baltimore: Williams & Wilkins.

Dahlem, N.W., Kinsman, R.A., & Fukuhara, J.T. (1982). Medication usage patterns and medical decisions: Days hospitalized. *Psychological Reports, 51*(1), 169-170.

Dahlstrom, W., Walsh, G., & Dahlstrom, L. (1975). *An MMPI handbook.* Minneapolis, MN: University of Minnesota.

Dalack, G.W., & Roose, S.P. (1990). Perspectives on the relationship between cardiovascular disease and affective disorder. *Journal of Clinical Psychiatry, 51*(Suppl. 7), 4-9.

Dales, R.E., Spitzer, W.O., Schechter, M.T., & Suisa, S. (1989). *American Review of Respiratory Diseases, 139,* 1459-1463.

Daltroy, L.H. (1985). Improving cardiac patient adherence to exercise regimens: A clinical trial of health education. *Journal of Cardiac Rehabilitation, 5,* 40-49.

Daughton, D.M., Fix, A.J., Kass, I., Patil, K.D., & Bell, C.W. (1979). Physiological-intellectual components of rehabilitation success in patients with chronic obstructive pulmonary disease (COPD). *Journal of Chronic Diseases, 32,* 405-409.

Davidson, D.M. (1983). Return to work after cardiac events: A review. *Journal of Cardiac Rehabilitation, 3,* 60-69.

Davidson, D.M., & Shumaker, S.A. (1987). Social support and cardiovascular disease. *Arteriosclerosis, 7,* 101-104.

Davidson, M.J., Cooper, C.L., & Chamberlain, D. (1980). Type A coronary-prone behavior and stress in senior female managers and administrators. *Journal of Occupational Medicine, 22,* 801-805.

DeBruin, A., DeWitte, L., Stevens, F., & Diederiks, J. (1992). Sickness impact profile: The state of the art of a generic functional status measure. *Social Science & Medicine, 35,* 1003-1014.

DeBusk, R.F., Miller, N.H., Superko, H.R., Dennis, C.A., Thomas, R.J., Lew, H.T., Berger, W.E., III, Heller, R.S., Rompf, J., Gee, D. (1994). A case management system for coronary risk factor modification following acute myocardial infarction. *Annals of Internal Medicine, 120*(9), 721-729.

DeCenio, D.V., Leshner, M., & Leshner, B. (1968). Personality characteristics of patients with chronic obstructive pulmonary emphysema. *Archives of Physical Medicine and Rehabilitation, 10,* 471-475.

DeLaFuente, J.R., & Rosenbaum, A.H. (1981). Prolactin in psychiatry. *American Journal of Psychiatry, 138,* 1154-1160.

Delbanco, T.L. (1992). Enriching the doctor-patient relationship by inviting the patient's participation. *Annals of Internal Medicine, 116,* 414-418.

Dembroski, T.M., & Costa, P.T., Jr. (1987). Coronary-prone behavior: Components of the Type A pattern and hostility. *Journal of Personality and Social Psychology, 55,* 211-235.

Dennis, C., Miller, H.N., Schwartz, R.G., Ahn, D.K., Kraemer, H.C., Gossard, D., Juneau, M., Taylor, C.B., & DeBusk, R.F. (1988). Early return to work after uncomplicated myocardial infarction: Results of a randomized trial. *Journal of the American Medical Association, 260,* 214-220.

Denollet, J. (1993). Biobehavioral research on coronary heart disease: Where is the person? *Personality and Coronary Heart Disease, 16*(1), 115-141.

Derogatis, L., Abeloff, M., and Melisaratos, N. (1979). Psychological coping mechanisms and survival time in metastatic breast cancer. *Journal of the American Medical Association, 242*, 1504-1508.

Derogatis, L.R., Brand, R., & Jenkins, C. (1983). *Administration, scoring and procedures manual II*. Towson, MD: Clinical Psychometric Research.

Derogatis, L.R., & King, K.M. (1981). The coital coronary: A reassessment of the concept. *Archives of Sexual Behavior, 10*, 325-335.

Derogatis, L.R., & Lopez, M.C. (1983). *Psychosocial adjustment to illness scale*. Riderwood, MD: Clinical Psychometric Research.

Derogatis, L.R., & Spencer, P.M. (1982). *Brief symptom inventory*. Riderwood, MD: Clinical Psychometric Research.

Dhabuwala, C.B., Kumar, A., & Pierce, J.M. (1986). Myocardial infarction and its influence on male sexual function. *Archives of Sexual Behavior, 16*(6), 499-504

Dhooper, S. (1984). Social networks and support during the crisis of heart attack. *Health Social Work, 9*, 294-303.

Dhooper, S.S. (1983). Family coping with the crisis of heart attack. *Social Work and Health Care, 9*, 15-31.

Dhooper, S.S. (1990). Identifying and mobilizing social supports for the cardiac patient's family. *Journal of Cardiovascular Nursing, 5*(1), 65-73.

DiClemente, C.C., Prochaska, J.O., Fairhurst, S., Velicer, W.F., Velasquez, M.M., & Rossi, J.S. (1991). The process of smoking cessation: An analysis of precontemplation, contemplation and preparation stages of change. *Journal of Consulting and Clinical Psychology, 59*, 295-304.

Diener, E. (1984). Subjective well-being. *Psychology Bulletin, 95*, 542-575.

DiMatteo, M.R., & Friedman, H.S. (1981). *Social psychology and medicine*. Cambridge, MA: Oelgeschlager, Gunn, & Hain.

Dishman, R.K., Sallis, J.F., & Orenstein, D.R. (1985). The determinants of physical activity and exercise. *Public Health Reports, 199*(2), 158-171.

Doehrman, S.R. (1977). Psychosocial aspects of recovery from coronary heart disease: A review. *Social Science & Medicine, 11*, 199-218.

Doerr, B.C., & Jones, J.W. (1979). Effect of family preparation on the state anxiety level of the CCU patient. *Nursing Research, 28*, 315-316.

Doherty, W.J. (1986). Marital therapy and family medicine. In N. Jacobson & A. Gurman (Eds.), *A clinical handbook of marital therapy* (pp. 185-198). New York: Guilford Press.

Doherty, W.J., & Baird, M.A. (1983). *Family therapy and family medicine: Toward the primary care of families*. New York: Guilford Press.

Doherty, W.J., & Campbell, T.L. (1988). *Families and Health*. Newbury Park, CA: Sage.

Doherty, W.J., & Harkaway, J.E. (1990). Obesity and family systems: A family FIRO approach to assessment and treatment planning. *Journal of Marriage and Family Therapy, 16*, 287-298.

Doherty, W.J., Schrott, H.G., Metcalf, L., & Iasiello-Vailas, L. (1983). Effect of spouse support and health beliefs on medication adherence. *Journal of Family Practice, 17*(5), 837-841.

Dominick, K.L., Ribisil, P.M., Rejeski, W.J., Sotile, W.M., Brubaker, P.H., & Miller, H.S. (1994, October). Social support strategies improve physical activity outcomes in cardiac rehabilitation. Presented at the ninth annnual meeting of the Amereican Association of Cardiovascular and Pulmonary Rehabilitation, Portland, Oregon.

Dorbonne, A. (1966). Suicide among patients with cardiorespiratory illness. *Journal of the American Medical Association, 195*, 422-428.

Douglas, J.E., & Wilkes, T.D. (1975). Reconditioning cardiac patients. *American Family Physician, 11*(1), 123-129.

Dracup, K. (1994). Cardiac rehabilitation: The role of social support in recovery and compliance. In S.A. Shumaker & S.M. Czajkowski (Eds.), *Social support and cardiovascular disease* (pp. 333-354). New York: Plenum Press.

Dracup, K., & Breu, C.S. (1978). Using nursing findings to meet the needs of grieving spouses. *Nursing Research, 27*, 212-216.

Dracup, K., & Bryan-Brown, C.W. (1992). An open door policy in ICU. *American Journal of Critical Care, 1*(2), 16-18.

Dracup, K., Guzy, P.M., Taylor, S.E., & Barry, J. (1986). Cardiopulmonary resuscitation (CPR) training: Consequences for family members of high-risk cardiac patients. *Archives of Internal Medicine, 146*, 1757-1761.

Dracup, K., Meleis, A., Baker, K., & Edlefsen, P. (1984). Family-focused cardiac rehabilitation: A role supplementation program for cardiac patients and spouses. *Nursing Clinics of North America, 19*, 113-124.

Dracup, K., & Meleis, A.I. (1982). Compliance: An interactionist approach. *Nursing Research, 31*, 31-36.

Dracup, K., Moser, D.K., Marsden, C., Taylor, W.E., & Guzy, P.M. (1991). Effects of a multidimensional cardiopulmonary rehabilitation program on psychosocial function. *American Journal of Cardiology, 68*, 31-34.

Dracup, K., Taylor, S.E., Guzy, P.M., & Brecht, M.L. (1991). *Consequences of cardiopulmonary training for family members of cardiac patients* (final report to National Heart, Lung, and Blood Institute for Grant RO1 HL32171). Los Angeles: University of California at Los Angeles.

Dudley, D.L., Glaser, E.M., Jorgenson, B.N., & Logan, D.L. (1980). Psychosocial concomitants to rehabilitation in chronic obstructive pulmonary disease: Part I. Psychosocial and psychological considerations. *Chest, 77*(3), 413-420.

Dudley, D.L., Holmes, T.H., & Martin, C.J. (1964). Changes in respiration associated with hypnotically induced emotion, pain and exercise. *Psychosomatic Medicine, 26*, 46-57.

Dudley, D.L., Martin, C.J., & Holmes, T.H. (1964). Psychophysiologic studies of pulmonary ventilation. *Psychosomatic Medicine, 26*, 645-660.

Dudley, D.L., Martin, C.J., & Holmes, T.H. (1968). Dyspnea: Psychological and physiologic observations. *Journal of Psychosomatic Research, 12*, 205-214.

Dudley, D.L., Martin, C.J., Masuda, M., & Holmes, T.H. (1969). *The psychophysiology of respiration in health and disease* (pp. 234-236). New York: Appleton-Century-Crofts.

Dudley, D.L., & Pattison, E.M. (1969). Group psychotherapy in patients with severe diffuse obstructive pulmonary syndrome. *American Review of Respiratory Disease, 100*(4), 575-576.

Dudley, D.L., Wermuth, C., & Hague, W. (1973). Psychosocial aspects of care in the chronic obstructive pulmonary disease patient. *Heart and Lung, 2*, 289-303.

Durkin, D.A., Kjelsberg, M.O., Buist, A.S., Connett, J.E., & Owens, G.R. (1993). Recruitment of participants in the Lung Health Study: I. Description of methods. *Controlled Clinical Trials, 14* (Suppl.), 208-378.

Earnest, M.P., Yarnell, P.R., Merrill, S.L., & Knapp, G.L. (1980). Long-term survival and neurologic status after resuscitation from out-of-hospital cardiac arrest. *Neurology, 30,* 1298-1302.

Ebbesen, E.B., Duncan, B., & Konecni, V.J. (1975). Effects of content of verbal aggression on future verbal aggression: A field experiment. *Journal of Experimental Social Psychology, 11,* 192-204.

Egbert, L.D., Battit, G.E., Welch, C.E., & Bartlett, M.K. (1964). Reduction of postoperative pain by encouragement and instruction of patients. *New England Journal of Medicine, 270,* 825-827.

Eliot, R.S. (1993). Relationship of emotional stress to the heart. *Heart Disease & Stroke, 2*(3), 243-246.

Eliot, R.S., & Breo, D.L. (1984). *Is it worth dying for?* New York: Bantam.

Eliot, R.S., & Miles, R. (1973). What to tell the cardiac patient about sexual intercourse. *Resident-Intern Consultant, 2,* 14.

Ell, K., & Dunkel-Schetter, C. (1994). Social support and adjustment to myocardial infarction, angioplasty, and coronary artery bypass surgery. In S.A. Shumaker & S.M. Czajkowski (Eds.), *Social support and cardiovascular disease.* New York: Plenum Press.

Ellis, A. (1962). *Reason and emotion in psychotherapy.* New York: Lyle Stuart Press.

Ellis, A., & Harper, R.A. (1975). *A new guide to rational living.* North Hollywood, CA: Wilshire Book.

Emery, C.F. (1993). Psychosocial considerations among pulmonary patients. In J.E. Hodgkin, G.L. Connors, & C.W. Bell (Eds.), *Pulmonary rehabilitation: Guidelines to success* (2nd ed.) (pp. 279-292). Philadelphia: Lippincott.

Emery, C.F., Leatherman, N.E., Burker, E.J., & MacIntrye, N.R. (1991). Psychological outcomes of a pulmonary rehabilitation program. *Chest, 100,* 613-619.

Emery, C.F., Pinder, S.L., & Blumenthal, J.A. (1989). Psychological effects of exercise among elderly cardiac patients. *Journal of Cardiopulmonary Rehabilitation, 9,* 46-53.

Engblom, E., Ronnemaa, T., Hamalainen, H., Kallio, V., Vanttinen, E., & Knuts, L.R. (1992). Coronary heart disease risk factors before and after bypass surgery: Results of a controlled trial on multifactorial rehabilitation. *European Heart Journal, 13*(8), 1053-1059.

Engel, G.L. (1977). The need for a new medical model: A challenge to biomedicine. *Science, 196,* 129-136.

Epstein, N.B., Bishop, D.S., & Levin, S. (1983). The McMaster family assessment device. *Journal of Marriage and Family Therapy, 9,* 171-180.

Erickson, M. (1948). Hypnotic psychotherapy. *The Medical Clinics of North America* (pp. 571-584). New York: W.B. Saunders.

Erickson, M.H., Hershman, S., & Secter, I. (1961). *The practical application of medical and dental hypnosis.* New York: The Julian Press.

Erickson, M., Rossi, E., & Rossi, S. (1976). *Hypnotic realities.* New York: Wiley.

Erikson, E. (1968). *Childhood and society* (2nd ed.). New York: Norton.

Ertekin, C., & Reel, F. (1976). Bulbocavernosus reflex in normal men and in patients with neurogenic bladder and/or impotence. *Journal of the Neurological Sciences, 28,* 1-15.

Ewart, C.K. (1989). Psychological effects of resistive weight training: Implications for cardiac patients. *Medicine and Science in Sports and Exercise, 21*(6), 683-688.

Ewart, C.K., Taylor, C.B., Bandura, A., & DeBusk, R.F. (1980). Immediate psychological impact of exercise testing soon after myocardial infarction. *American Journal of Cardiology, 45,* 421.

Ewart, C.K., Taylor, C.B., Kraemer, H.C., & Agras, W.S. (1984). Reducing blood pressure reactivity during interpersonal conflict: Effects of marital communication training. *Behavioral Therapy, 15,* 473-484.

Ewart, C.K., Taylor, C.B., Reese, L.B., & DeBusk, R.F. (1983). Effects of early post-myocardial infarction exercise testing on self-perception and subsequent physical activity. *American Journal of Cardiology, 51,* 1076-1080.

Ewing, J.A. (1984). Detecting alcoholism: The CAGE questionnaire. *Journal of the American Medical Association, 252,* 1905-1907.

Fagerstrom, K.O. (1978). Measuring degree of physical dependency to tobacco smoking with reference to individualization of treatment. *Addictive Behaviors, 3,* 235-241.

Falger, P.R.J., Schouten, E.G.W., & Appels, A.W. (1988, April). Relationship between age, Type A behavior, life changes over the life-span, vital exhaustion, and first myocardial infarction: A case-referent study. *Proceedings of Society of Behavioral Medicine* (pp. 27-30). Boston: Society of Behavioral Medicine.

Farberow, N.L., McKelligott, J.W., Cohen S., & Dorbonne, A. (1966). Suicide among patients with cardiorespiratory illness. *Journal of the American Medical Association, 195,* 422-428.

Farquhar, J.W. (1987). *The American way of life need not be hazardous to your health.* Boston: Addison-Wesley.

Farquhar, J.W., Macoby, N., Wood, P.D., Alexander, J.K., Breitrose, H., Brown, B.W., Haskell, W.L., McAlister, A.L., Meyer, A.J., Nash, J.D., & Stern, M.P. (1977). Community education for cardiovascular health. *Lancet, 1,* 1192-1195.

Feuerstein, M., & Cohen, R. (1985). Arrhythmias: Evaluating and managing problems of heart rate and rhythm. In A.M. Razin (Ed.), *Helping cardiac patients: Behavioral and psychotherapeutic approaches* (pp. 55-111). San Francisco: Jossey-Bass.

Finlayson, A. (1976). Social networks as coping resource: Lay help and consultation patterns used by women in husbands' post-infarction career. *Social Science & Medicine, 10,* 97-103.

Finlayson, A., & McEwen, J. (1977). *Coronary heart disease and patterns of living.* New York: Prodist.

Finnegan, D.L., & Suler, J.R. (1985). Psychological factors associated with maintenance of improved health behaviors in post coronary patients. *Journal of Psychology, 119,* 87-94.

Fiore, J., Becker, J., & Coppel, D.B. (1983). Social network interactions: A buffer or a stress. *American Journal of Community Psychology, 11,* 423-439.

Fiore, M.C. (1991). The new vital sign: Assessing and documenting smoking status. *Journal of the American Medical Association, 266,* 3183-3184.

Fisher, L., & Ransom, D. (1990). Person-family transaction: Implications for stress and health. *Family Systems Medicine, 8,* 109-122.

Fletcher, A., Hunt, B., & Bulpitt, C. (1987). Evaluation of quality of life in trials of cardiovascular disease. *Journal of Chronic Disease, 40,* 557-566.

Fletcher, E.C. (1984). Sexual dysfunction in men with chronic obstructive pulmonary disease. *Medical Aspects of Human Sexuality, 5,*151-157.

Fletcher, E.C., & Martin, R.J. (1982). Sexual dysfunction and erectile impotence in chronic obstructive pulmonary disease. *Chest, 81,* 413-421.

Foley, J.L., Sivarajan, E.S., & Woods, F.N. (1983). Differences between men and women in recovery from myocardial infarction. *Circulation, 68*(Suppl. III), 124.

Folkman, S., Lazarus, R.S., Dunkel-Scheltter, C., DeLongis, A., & Gruen, R.J. (1986). Dynamics of a stressful encounter: Cognitive appraisal, coping and encounter outcomes. *Journal of Personality and Social Psychology, 50,* 992-1003.

Folkman, S., Lazarus, R.S., Pimley, S., & Novacek, J. (1987). Age differences in stress and coping processes. *Psychology and Aging, 2*(2), 171-184.

Follick, M.J., Gorkin, L., Capone, R.J., Smith, T.W., Ahern, D.K., Stablein, D., Niaura, R., & Visco, J. (1988). Psychological distress as a predictor of ventricular arrythmias in a post-myocardial infarction population. *American Heart Journal, 116,* 32-36.

Folstein, M.F., Folstein, S.E., & McHugh, P.E. (1975). Mini mental state: A practical method for the clinician. *Journal of Psychiatry Research, 12,* 189-198.

Fontana, A.F., Kerns, R.D., Rosenberg, R.L., & Colonese, K.L. (1989). Support, stress, and recovery from coronary heart disease: A longitudinal causal model. *Health Psychology, 8*(2), 175-193.

Forbes, B. (1977). *Dame Edith Evans.* Boston: Little, Brown. Quoted in E.C. Taylor (Ed.) (1984), *Growing on: Ideas about aging* (p. 14). New York: Van Nostrand.

Forshee, T. (1988). *The influence of family visits on physiologic responses in coronary care patients.* Unpublished dissertation, University of Washington School of Nursing, Seattle.

Foster, S., & Thomas, H.M. (1990). Pulmonary rehabilitation in lung disease other than COPD. *American Review of Respiratory Diseases, 141,* 601-604.

Foxall, M.J., Ekbert, J.Y., & Griffith, N. (1987). Comparative study of adjustment patterns of chronic obstructive pulmonary disease patients and peripheral vascular disease patients. *Heart and Lung, 16,* 354-363.

Frank, E. (1978). Frequency of sexual dysfunction in "normal" couples. *New England Journal of Medicine, 299,* 111-115.

Frasure-Smith, N. (1991). In-hospital symptoms of psychological stress as predictors of long-term outcome after acute myocardial infarction in men. *American Journal of Cardiology, 67,* 121-127.

Frasure-Smith, N., Lesperance, F., & Talajic, M. (1993). Depression following myocardial infarction. *Journal of the American Medical Association, 270*(15), 1819-1825.

Frasure-Smith, N., & Prince, R. (1985). The ischemic heart disease life stress monitoring program: Impact on mortality. *Psychosomatic Medicine, 47,* 431-445.

Frasure-Smith, N., & Prince, R. (1989). Long-term follow-up of the ischemic heart disease life stress monitoring program. *Psychosomatic Medicine, 51,* 485-513.

Frenn, M.D., Borgeson, D.S., Lee, H.A., & Simandl, G. (1989). Life-style changes in a cardiac rehabilitation program: The client perspective. *Journal of Cardiovascular Nursing, 3*(2), 43-55.

Friedman, H.S. (1990). Patient-physician interaction. In S. Shoemaker (Ed.), *The handbook of health behavior changes* (pp. 85-101). New York: Springer.

Friedman, J. (1978). Sexual adjustment of the postcoronary male. In J. LoPiccolo & L. LoPiccolo (Eds.), *Handbook of sex therapy* (pp. 373-386). New York: Plenum Press.

Friedman, M., & Rosenman, R.H. (1974). *Type A behavior and your heart.* New York: Knopf.

Friedman, M., Thoresen, C.E., Gill, J.J., Ulmer, D., Powell, L.H., Price, V.A., Brown, B., Thompson, L., Robin, D., Breall, W.S., Bourg, E., Levy, R., & Dixon, T. (1986). Alteration of Type A behavior and its effect on cardiac recurrences in post-myocardial infarction patients: Summary results of the recurrent coronary prevention project. *American Heart Journal, 112,* 653-665.

Friedman, M., & Ulmer, D. (1984). *Treating Type A behavior and your heart.* New York: Knopf.

Friis, R., & Taff, G.A. (1986). Social support and social networks and coronary heart disease and rehabilitation. *Journal of Cardiopulmonary Rehabilitation, 6,* 132-147.

Frodi, E.B., Macaulay, J., & Thome, P.R. (1977). Are women always less aggressive than men? A review of the experimental literature. *Psychological Bulletin, 84,* 634-660.

Fuentes, R.J., Rosenberg, J.M., & Marks, R.G. (1983, February). Sexual side effects: What to tell your patients, what not to say. *RN,* 35-41.

Fuller, B.F., & Foster, G.M. (1982). The effects of family/friend visits vs. staff interaction on stress/arousal of surgical intensive care patients. *Heart and Lung, 11,* 457-463.

Gallagher, W. (1993). Midlife myths. *The Atlantic, 271*(5), 51-58.

Garrity, T.F. (1973a). Social involvement and activeness as predictors of morale six months after first myocardial infarction. *Social Science & Medicine, 7,* 199-207.

Garrity, T.F. (1973b). Vocational adjustment after first myocardial infarction: Comparative assessment of several variables suggested in the literature. *Social Science & Medicine, 7,* 705-715.

Garrity, T.F., & Klein, R.F. (1975). Emotional response and clinical severity as early determinants of six-month mortality after myocardial infarction. *Heart and Lung, 4,* 730-737.

Gatchel, R.J., Gaffney, F.A., & Smith, J.E. (1986). Comparative efficacy of behavioral stress management versus propranolol in reducing psychophysiological reactivity in post-myocardial infarction patients. *Journal of Behavioral Medicine, 9,* 503-513.

Gayle, R.C., Spitler, D.L., Karper, W.B., Jaeger, R.M., & Rice, S.N. (1988). Psychological changes in exercising COPD patients. *International Journal of Rehabilitation Research, 11,* 335.

Gianetti, V.J., Reynolds, J., & Rihn, T. (1985). Factors which differentiate smokers from ex-smokers among cardiovascular patients: A discriminant analysis. *Social Science & Medicine, 20,* 241-245.

Gift, A.G., & Cahill, C. (1990). Psychophysiologic aspects of dyspnea in chronic obstructive pulmonary disease: A pilot study. *Heart and Lung, 19,* 252-257.

Gift, A.G., & McCrone, S.H. (1993). Depression in patients with COPD. *Heart and Lung, 22*(4), 289-297.

Gift, A.G., Moore, T., & Soeken, K. (1992). Relaxation to reduce dyspnea and anxiety in COPD patients. *Nursing Research, 41*(4), 242-246.

Gift, A.G., Palut, S.M., & Jacox, A. (1986). Psychologic and physiologic factors related to dyspnea in subjects with chronic obstructive pulmonary disease. *Heart and Lung, 15*(4), 595-601.

Gilchrist, P.N., Phillips, P.J., Odgers, C.L., & Hoogendorp, J. (1985). The psychological aspects of artificial nutritional support. *Australian & New Zealand Journal of Psychiatry, 19,* 54-59.

Gill, J.J., Price, V.A., Friedman, M., Thoresen, C.E., Powell, L.H., Ulmer, D., Brown, B., & Drews, F.R. (1985). Reduction in Type A behavior in healthy middle-aged American military officers. *American Heart Journal, 110,* 503-514.

Gillis, C.L. (1984). Reducing family stress during and after coronary artery bypass surgery. *Nursing Clinics of North America, 19,* 103-112.

Gillum, R.F. (1989). Sudden coronary death in the United States: 1980-1985. *Circulation, 79,* 756-765.

Ginsberg, D., Hall, S.M., & Rosinski, M. (1991). Partner interaction and smoking cessation: A pilot study. *Addictive Behavior, 16,* 195-202.

Glasgow, R.E., & Rosen, G.M. (1987). Behavioral bibliotherapy: A review of self-help behavior therapy manuals. *Psychology Bulletin, 85,* 1-23.

Glass, D.C. (1977). *Behavior patterns, stress, and coronary disease.* Hillsdale, NJ: Erlbaum.

Glover, E.D. (Ed.). (1983). Nicotine withdrawal therapy [Special issue]. *Health Values: The Journal of Health Behavior, Education & Promotion, 17*(2), 4-79.

Glover, E.D. (1993). What can we expect from the nicotine transdermal patch? A theoretical/practical approach. *Health Values, 17*(2), 69-79.

Glover, P.N. (1993). Smoking intervention: A combination therapy approach to cessation. *Health Values, 17*(2), 51-58.

Glynn, T.J., & Manley, M.W. (1992). *How to help your patients stop smoking: A National Cancer Institute manual for physicians* (DHHS Publication No. NIH 92-3064). Bethesda, MD: National Institutes of Health.

Goble, A.J., Hare, D.L., Macdonald, P.S., Oliver, R.G., Reid, M.A., & Worcester, M.C. (1991). Effect of early programmes of high and low intensity exercise on physical performance after transmural acute myocardial infarction. *British Heart Journal, 65*(3), 126-131.

Gochros, H., & Fisher, J. (1986). *Treat yourself to a better sex life.* Englewood Cliffs, NJ: Spectrum.

Godin, G. (1989). The effectiveness of interventions in modifying behavioral risk factors of individuals with coronary heart disease. *Journal of Cardiopulmonary Rehabilitation, 9,* 223-236.

Goff, D., & Dimsdale, J.K. (1985). The psychologic effects of exercise. *Journal of Cardiopulmonary Rehabilitation, 5,* 274-290.

Goldberg, D.P., & Blackwell, B. (1970). Psychiatric illness in general practice. A detailed study using a new method of case identification. *British Medical Journal, 11,* 439-443.

Goldberg, J.R. (1992). The new frontier: Marriage and family therapy with aging families. *Family Therapy News, 23*(4), 14.

Goldman, L.S., & Kimball, C.P. (1985). Cardiac surgery: Enhancing postoperative outcomes. In A.M. Razin (Ed.), *Helping cardiac patients: Behavioral and psychotherapeutic approaches* (pp. 113-155). San Francisco: Jossey-Bass.

Goldstein, I. (1987). Penile revascularization. *Urologic Clinics of North America, 14,* 805-813.

Gordon, G.H., Michiels, T.M., Mahutte, C.K., & Light, R.W. (1985). Effect of desipramine on control of ventilation and depression scores in patients with severe chronic obstructive pulmonary disease. *Psychiatric Research, 15*(1), 25-37.

Gore, S. (1978). The effect of social support in moderating the health consequences of unemployment. *Journal of Health and Social Behavior, 19,* 157-165.

Gore, S. (1981). Stress-buffering function of social supports: An appraisal and clarification of research models. In B.S. Dohrenwend & B.P. Dohrenwend (Eds.), *Stressful events and their contexts* (pp. 202-222). New Brunswick, NJ: Rutgers University Press.

Gorkin, L., Follick, M.J., Wilkin, D.L., & Niaura, R. (1994). Social support and the progression and treatment of cardiovascular disease. In S.A. Shumaker & S.M. Czajkowski (Eds.), *Social support and cardiovascular disease* (pp. 281-300). New York: Plenum Press.

Gorlin, R. (1992). Must cardiology lose his heart? *Journal of the American College of Cardiology, 19,* 1635-1640.

Gottlieb, B.H. (1985). Assessing and strengthening the impact of social support on mental health. *Social Work, 30,* 293-300.

Granger, J.W. (1974). Full recovery from myocardial infarction: Psychosocial factors. *Heart and Lung, 3,* 600-610.

Green, R.G., & Quanty, M.B. (1977). The catharsis of aggression: An evaluation of a hypothesis. In L. Berkowitz (Ed.), *Advances in experimental social psychology* (Vol. 10, pp. 45-62). New York: Academic Press.

Greenberg, G.D., Ryan, J.J., & Bourlier, P.E. (1985). Psychological and neuropsychological aspects of COPD. *Psychosomatic Medicine, 26,* 29.

Greer, H.S., Morris, T., & Pettingale, K.W. (1979). Psychological response to breast cancer: Effect on outcome. *Lancet, 2,* 785-787.

Greist, J.H., Jefferson, J.W., & Marks, I.M. (1986). Anxiety and its treatment. New York: Warner Books.

Grinder, J., & Bandler, R. (1981). *Trance-formations: Neuro-linguistic programming and the structure of hypnosis.* Moab, UT: Real People Press.

Gruen, W. (1975). Effects of brief psychotherapy during the hospitalization period on the recovery process in heart attacks. *Journal of Consulting Clinical Psychology, 43,* 252-270.

Guba, C.J., & McDonald, J.L., Jr. (1993). Epidemiology of smoking. *Health Values, 17*(2), 4-11.

Gundle, M.D., Reeves, B.R., & Tate, S. (1980). Psychosocial outcome after coronary artery surgery. *American Journal of Psychiatry, 137,* 1591-1594.

Guyatt, G.H., Berman, L.B., & Townsend, M. (1987). Long-term outcome after respiratory rehabilitation. *Canadian Medical Association Journal, 137,* 1089-1095.

Haaga, D.A. (1987). Treatment for the Type A behavior pattern. *Clinical Psychology Review, 7,* 557-574.

Haas, Z., & Cardon, H. (1969). Rehabilitation in chronic obstructive pulmonary disease: A 5 year study of 252 male patients. *Medical Clinics of North America, 53,* 593-606.

Hackett, T.P. (1985). Depression following myocardial infarction. *Psychosomatics, 26*(Suppl.), 23-28.

Hackett, T.P., & Cassem, N.H. (1969). Factors contributing to delay in responding to the signs and symptoms of acute myocardial infarction. *American Journal of Cardiology, 24,* 651-656.

Hackett, T.P., & Cassem, N.H. (1974). Development of a quantitative rating scale to assess denial. *Journal of Psychosomatic Research, 18,* 93-100.

Hackett, T.P., Cassem, N.H., & Wishnie, H.A. (1968). The coronary care unit: An appraisal of its psychological hazards. *New England Journal of Medicine, 279,* 1365-1370.

Hall, L. (1994a). The future of health care: Implications for cardiac and pulmonary rehabilitation. *Journal of Cardiopulmonary Rehabilitation, 14*(4), 228-231.

Hall, R.G., Sachs, D.P.L., Hall, S.M., & Benowitz, N.L. (1984). Two-year efficacy and safety of rapid smoking therapy in patients with cardiac and pulmonary disease. *Journal of Consulting and Clinical Psychology, 52,* 574-580.

Halpern, J. (1987). *Helping your aging parents: A practical guide for adult children.* New York: McGraw-Hill.

Halstead, W.C., & Wepman, J.M. (1959). The Halstead-Wepman aphasia screening test. *Journal of Speech and Hearing Disorders, 14,* 9-14.

Hamalainen, H., Luurila, O.J., Kallio, V., Knuts, L.R., Artila, M., & Hakkila, J. (1989). Long-term reduction in sudden deaths after a multifactorial intervention programme in patients with myocardial infarction: 10 year results of a controlled investigation. *European Heart Journal, 10,* 55-62.

Hanson, B.S., Isacsson, S.O., & Janzon, L. (1990). Social support and quitting smoking for good. Is there an association? Results from the population study, "Men born in 1914," Malmo, Sweden. *Addictive Behavior, 15,* 221-223.

Hanson, C.D., Klesges, R.C., Eck, L.H., Cigrang, J.A., & Carle, D.L. (1990). Family relations, coping styles, stress, and cardiovascular disease risk factors among children and their parents. *Family Systems Medicine, 8,* 387-400.

Hanson, E.I. (1982). Effects of chronic lung disease on life in general and on sexuality: Perceptions of adult patients. *Heart and Lung, 11,* 435-441.

Harding, A.L., & Morefield, M.A. (1976). Group intervention for wives of myocardial infarction patients. *Nursing Clinics of North America, 11,* 339-347.

Harkaway, J., & Madsen, W.C. (1989). A systemic approach to medical non-compliance: The case of chronic obesity. *Family Systems Medicine, 7,* 42-65.

Hart, K.E. (1988). Association of Type A behavior and its components to ways of coping with stress. *Journal of Psychosomatic Research, 32,* 213-219.

Hatch, J.P., Klatt, K.D., & Supik, J.D. (1985). Combined behavioral pharmacological treatment of essential hypertension. *Biofeedback & Self-Regulation, 10,* 119-138.

Hathaway, S.R., & McKinley, J.C. (1989). *The Minnesota Multiphasic Personality Inventory-2.* Minneapolis, MN: University of Minnesota Press.

Hatsukami, D.K., & Lando, H. (1993). Behavioral treatment for smoking cessation. *Health Values, 17*(2), 32-40.

Havik, O.E., & Maeland, J.G. (1988). Verbal denial and outcome in myocardial infarction patients. *Journal of Psychosomatic Research, 32,* 145-157.

Hay, D.R., & Turnbott, S. (1970). Changes in smoking habits in men under sixty-five years after myocardial infarction and coronary insufficiency. *British Heart Journal, 32,* 738-740.

Haynes, R.B. (1976). A critical review of the determinants of patient compliance with therapeutic regimens. In D.L. Sackett & R.B. Haynes (Eds.), *Compliance with therapeutic regimens* (pp. 38-54). Baltimore: Johns Hopkins University Press.

Haynes, R.B. (1979). Determinants of compliance: The disease and the mechanics of treatment. In R.B. Haynes, D.W. Taylor, & D.L. Sackett (Eds.), *Compliance in health care* (pp. 112-130). Baltimore: Johns Hopkins University Press.

Haynes, S.G., Eaker, E.D., & Feinleib, M. (1983). Spouse behavior and coronary heart disease in men: Prospective results from the Framingham Heart Study: I. Concordance of risk factors and the relationship of psychosocial status to coronary incidence. *American Journal of Epidemiology, 118,* 1-22.

Haynes, S.G., Feinleib, M., & Kannel, W.B. (1980). The relationship of psychosocial factors to coronary heart disease in the Framingham Study: Part 3. 8-year incidence of CHD. *American Journal of Epidemiology, 111,* 37-58.

Haynes, S.G., & Matthews, K.A. (1988). Review and methodologic critique of recent studies on Type A behavior and cardiovascular disease. *Annals of Behavior Medicine, 10,* 47-59.

Haywood, J., & Obier, K. (1971). Psychosocial problems of coronary care unit patients. *Journal of the National Medical Association, 63,* 425-428.

Hazaleus, S.L., & Deffenbacher, J.L. (1986). Relaxation and cognitive treatments of anger. *Journal of Consulting and Clinical Psychology, 54*(2), 222-226.

Headey, B., Holmstrom, E., & Wearing, A. (1984). Well-being and ill-being: Different dimensions? *Social Indicators Research, 14,* 115-139.

Heatherton, T.F., Kozlowski, L.Y., Frecker, R.C., & Fagerstrom, K.O. (1991). The Fagerstrom test for nicotine dependence: A revision of the Fagerstrom Tolerance Questionnaire. *British Journal of Addiction, 86,* 1119-1127.

Hecker, M.H.L., Chesney, M.A., Black, G.W., & Frautschi, N. (1988). Coronary-prone behaviors in the Western Collaborative Group Study. *Psychosomatic Medicine, 2,* 153-164.

Heiman, J., LoPiccolo, L., & LoPiccolo, J. (1976). *Becoming orgasmic: A sexual growth program for women.* New York: Prentice Hall.

Heimberger, R.F., & Reitan, R.M. (1961). Easily administered written test for lateralizing brain lesions. *Journal of Neurosurgery, 181,* 301-312.

Heitzmann, C.A., & Kaplan, R.M. (1988). Assessment of the methods for measuring social support. *Health Psychology, 7,* 75-109.

Helgeson, V.X. (1989). The origin, development, and current state of the literature on Type A behavior. *Journal of Cardiovascular Nursing, 3*(2), 59-73.

Heller, S., Frank, K., Kornfeld, D., Malm, J.R., & Bowman, F.O., Jr. (1974). Psychological outcome following open-heart surgery. *Archives of Internal Medicine, 135,* 908-914.

Hellerstein, H.F., & Friedman, E.H. (1969). Sexual activity and the post-coronary patient. *Medical Aspects of Human Sexuality, 3,* 70-96.

Henderson, S., Byrne, D.G., Duncan-Jones, P., & Scott, R. (1980). Measuring social relationships: The interview schedule for social interactions. *Psychological Medicine, 10,* 723-734.

Higgins, C., & Schweiger, M. (1983). Smoking termination patterns in a cardiac rehabilitation program. *Journal of Cardiac Rehabilitation, 3,* 55-59.

Higgins, M.W. (1989). Chronic airways disease in the United States: Trends and determinants. *Chest, 96*(Suppl.), 328-334.

Hilbert, G.A. (1985). Spouse support and myocardial infarction patient compliance. *Nursing Research, 34*(4), 217-220.

Hjerman, L., Holme, I., Velve, M., Byer, K., & Leren, P. (1981). Effect of diet and smoking intervention on the incidence of coronary heart disease: Report from the Oslo Study Group of a randomized trial in healthy men. *Lancet, 2,* 1303-1310.

Hlatky, M.A., Haney, T., & Barefoot, J.C. (1986). Medical, psychological, and social correlates of work disability among men with coronary artery disease. *American Journal of Cardiology, 58,* 911-915.

Hobson, K.G. (1984). The effects of aging on sexuality. *Health and Social Work, 9*(1), 25-35.

Hochbaum, G.M. (1956). Why people seek diagnostic x-rays? *Public Health Reports, 71,* 377-380.

Hodgkin, J.E. (1988). Pulmonary rehabilitation: Structure, components, and benefits. *Journal of Cardiopulmonary Rehabilitation, 11,* 423-434.

Hodgkin, J.E., Connors, G.L., & Bell, C.W. (Eds.) (1993). *Pulmonary rehabilitation: Guidelines to success* (2nd ed.). Philadelphia: Lippincott.

Hodson, M.E. (1989). Managing adults with cystic fibrosis. *British Medical Journal, 298,* 471-472.

Hoffman, L.A., Berg, J., & Rogers, R.M. (1989). Daily living with COPD: Self-help skills to improve functional ability. *Postgraduate Medicine, 86,* 153-166.

Holland, W.W. (1989). Chronic airways disease in the United Kingdom. *Chest, 96*(Suppl.), 318-321.

Hollis, J.F., Lichtenstein, E., Mount, K., Bogt, T.M., Stevens, V.J., & Biglan, A. (1993). Nurse-assisted counseling for smokers in primary care. *Annals of Internal Medicine, 118,* 521-525.

Holmes, D., & Roth, D. (1985). Association of aerobic fitness with pulse rate and subjective responses to psychological stress. *Psychophysiology, 22*, 525-529.

Holmes, T.H., & Rahe, R.H. (1967). The Social Readjustment Scale. *Journal of Psychosomatic Research, 11*, 213-218.

Holohan, C.J., & Moos, R.H. (1986). Personality coping, and family resources in stress resistance: A longitudinal analysis. *Journal of Personality and Social Psychology, 51*, 389-395.

Holub, D., Eklund, P., & Keenan, P. (1975). Family conferences as an adjunct to total coronary care. *Heart and Lung, 4*, 767-769.

Honeyman, M.S., Rappaport, H., Reznikoff, M., Glueck, B.C., Jr., & Eisenberg, H. (1968). Psychological impact of heart disease in the family of the patient. *Psychosomatics, 9*, 34-37.

Hoop, J.W., & Maddox, S.E. (1984). Education of patients and their families. In J.E. Hodgkin, E.G. Zorn, & G.L. Connors (Eds.), *Pulmonary rehabilitation: Guidelines to success* (pp. 50-62). Philadelphia: Lippincott.

Hooyman, N.R., & Lustbader, W. (1986). *Taking care: Supporting older people and their families.* New York: The Free Press.

Horwitz, R.I., Viscoli, C.M., Berkman, L., Donaldson, R.M., Horwitz, S.M., Murray, C.J., Ransohoff, D.F., & Sindelar, J. (1990). Treatment adherence and risk of death after a myocardial infarction. *Lancet, 336*, 1002-1003.

Hosay, P.M. (1977). The unfulfilled promise of health education. *New York University Education Quarterly, 2*, 16-22.

House, J.S. (1981). *Work, stress and social support.* Boston: Addison-Welsey.

Houston, B.K., & Kelly, K.E. (1989). Hostility in employed women: Relation to work and marital experiences, social support, stress, and anger expression. *Personality and Social Psychology Bulletin, 15*, 175-182.

Houston-Miller, N. (1990, March). *Behavior modification and its effect on cardiac rehabilitation.* Paper presented to the Eleventh Annual North Carolina Cardiopulmonary Rehabilitation Symposium, Pinehurst, NC.

Houston-Miller, N., Taylor, C.B., Davidson, D.M., Hill, M.N., & Krantz, D.S. (1990). The efficacy of risk factor intervention and psychosocial aspects of cardiac rehabilitation. *Journal of Cardiac Rehabilitation, 10*, 198-209.

Howe, R.L. (1983, Fall). Spiritual dimensions of aging. *Generations*, 38-41.

Howell, R.H., & Krantz, D.S. (1994). The role of mental stress in the pathogenesis of coronary atherosclerosis and acute coronary events. *Medicine, Exercise, Nutrition and Health, 3*, 131-140.

Howland, J., Nelson, E.C., Barlow, P.B., McHargue, G., Maier, P.A., Brent, P., Laser-Wolston, N., & Parker, H.W. (1986). Chronic obstructive airway disease: Impact of health education. *Chest, 90*, 233-238.

Hubert, H.B., Feinleib, M., McNamara, P.M., & Castelli, W.P. (1983). Obesity as an independent risk factor for cardiovascular disease: A 26-year follow-up of participants in the Framingham Heart Study. *Circulation, 67*, 968-977.

Hughes, J.R. (1984). Psychological effects of habitual aerobic exercise. A critical review. *Preventive Medicine, 13*, 66-78.

Hughes, J.R. (1989). Dependence potential and abuse liability of nicotine replacement therapies. *Biomedical Pharmacotherapy, 43*, 11-17.

Hughes, J.R., & Glaser, M. (1993). Transdermal nicotine for smoking cessation. *Health Values, 17*(2), 25-31.

Hull, E.M., Young, S.H., & Ziegler, M.G. (1984). Aerobic fitness affects cardiovascular and catecholamine responses to stressors. *Psychophysiology, 21,* 353-360.

Hunt, S., McEwen, J., & McKenna, S. (1980). A quantitative approach to perceived health. *Journal of Epidemiology and Community Health, 34,* 281-295.

Hunt, W.A., Barrett, W., & Branch, L.G., (1971). Relapse rates in addiction programs. *Journal of Clinical Psychology, 4,* 455-456.

Hurley, M. (1986). *Classification of Nursing Diagnosis: Proceedings of the Sixth Conference,* 543. St. Louis, MO: CV Mosby.

Hypertension Detection and Follow-up Program Cooperative Group. (1979). Five-year findings of the Hypertension Detection and Follow-up Program: I. Reduction in mortality of persons with high blood pressure, including mild hypertension. *Journal of the American Medical Association, 242,* 2562-2571.

Hypertension Detection and Follow-up Program Cooperative Group. (1988). Persistence of reduction in blood pressure and mortality of participants in the Hypertension Detection and Follow-up Program. *Journal of the American Medical Association, 259,* 2113-2122.

Ibrahim, M., Feldman, J., Sultz, H., Staiman, M., Young, L., & Dean, D. (1974). Management after myocardial infarction: A controlled trial of the effect of group psychotherapy. *International Journal of Psychiatry Medicine, 5*(3), 253.

Inaba-Roland, K.E., & Maricle, R.A. (1992). Assessing delirium in the acute care setting. *Heart and Lung, 21*(1), 48-55.

Irvine, M.J., Johnston, D.W., Jenner, D.A., & Marie, G.V. (1986). Relaxation and stress management in the treatment of essential hypertension. *Journal of Psychosomatic Research, 30,* 437-450.

Janis, I.L. (1958). *Psychological stress: Psychoanalytic and behavioral studies of surgical patients.* New York: Wiley.

Jasnoski, M., & Holmes, D. (1981). Influence of initial aerobic fitness, aerobic training and changes in aerobic fitness on personality functioning. *Journal of Psychosomatic Research, 25,* 553-556.

Jasnoski, M., Holmes, D., Soloman, S., & Aguiar, C. (1981). Exercise, changes in aerobic capacity and changes in self-perceptions: An experimental investigation. *Journal of Research in Personality, 15,* 460-466.

Jeffery, R.W. (1987). Behavioral treatment of obesity. *Annals of Behavioral Medicine, 9*(1), 20-24.

Jenkins, C.D. (1971). Psychologic and social precursors of coronary disease. *New England Journal of Medicine, 284,* 244-255.

Jenkins, C.D. (1983). Psychosocial and behavioral risk factors. In N. Kaplan & J. Stamler, (Eds.), *Prevention of coronary heart disease* (pp. 98-112). Philadelphia: W.B. Saunders.

Jenkins, C.D., Rosenman, R.H., & Zyzanski, S.J. (1974). Prediction of clinical coronary heart disease by a test for the coronary-prone behavior pattern. *New England Journal of Medicine, 23,* 1271-1279.

Jenkins, C.D., Stanton, B.A., Savageau, J.A., Denlinger, P., & Klein, M.D. (1983). Coronary artery bypass surgery: Physical, psychological, social, and economic outcomes six months later. *Journal of the American Medical Association, 250,* 782-788.

Jenkins, C.D., Stanton, B.A., Savageau, J.A., Ockene, J., Kenlinger, P., & Klein, M.D. (1983). Physical, psychologic, social and economic outcomes after cardiac valve surgery. *Archives of Internal Medicine, 132,* 2107-2113.

Jenkins, L.S. (1987). Self-efficacy: New perspectives in caring for patients recovering from myocardial infarction. *Progressive Cardiovascular Nursing, 2*, 32-35.

Jenni, M.A., & Wollersheim, J.P. (1979). Cognitive therapy, stress management training, and the Type A behavior pattern. *Cognitive Therapy and Research, 3*, 61-73.

Jensen, P.S. (1983). Risk, protective factors, and supportive interventions in chronic airway obstruction. *Archives of General Psychiatry, 40*, 1203-1207.

Jensen, S.B. (1985a). Emotional aspects in diabetes mellitus: A study of somatopsychological reactions in 51 couples in which one partner has insulin-treated diabetes. *Journal of Psychosomatic Research, 29*, 353-359.

Jensen, S.B. (1985b). Sexual relationships in couples with a diabetic partner. *Journal of Sex and Marital Therapy, 11*, 259-270.

Jensen, S.B. (1986). Sexual dysfunction and diabetes mellitus: A six-year follow-up study. *Archives of Sexual Behavior, 15*, 271-284.

Jevtich, M.J. (1983). Vascular noninvasive diagnostic techniques. In R.J. Krane, M.B. Siroky, & I. Goldstein (Eds.), *Male sexual dysfunction* (pp.139-164). Boston: Little, Brown.

Johnson, J.L., & Morse, J.M. (1990). Regaining control: The process of adjustment after myocardial infarction. *Heart and Lung, 19*, 126-135.

Johnson, W.L. (1974). *Adjustment to the crisis of coronary heart disease.* New York: National League for Nursing.

Johnston, B.L., Cantwell, J.D., Watt, E.W., & Fletcher, G.E. (1978). Sexual activity in exercising patients after myocardial infarction and revascularization. *Heart and Lung, 7*, 1026-1031.

Johnston, D.W. (1985). Psychological interventions in cardiovascular disease. *Journal of Psychosomatic Research, 29*, 447-456.

Jones, N.F., Kinsman, R.A., Dirks, J.F., & Dahlem, N.W. (1979). Psychological contributions to chronicity in asthma: Patient response styles influencing medical treatment and its outcome. *Medical Care, 17*(11), 1103-1118.

Kahn, D. (1990). The dichotomy of drugs and psychotherapy. *Psychiatric Clinical Nurses of America, 13*, 197-208.

Kahn, J.P., Kornfeld, D.S., Frank, K.A., Heller, S.C., & Hoar, P.F. (1980). Type A behavior and blood pressure during coronary artery bypass surgery. *Psychosomatic Medicine, 42*, 407-414.

Kamerow, D.B., Pincus, H.A., & MacDonald, D.I. (1986). Alcohol abuse, other drug abuse, and mental disorders in medical practice. *Journal of the American Medical Association, 255*, 2054-2057.

Kaplan, H.S. (1974). *The new sex therapy.* New York: Brunner/Mazel.

Kaplan, H.S. (1983). *The evaluation of sexual disorders.* New York: Brunner/Mazel.

Kaplan, R., Atkins, C., & Timms, R. (1984). Validity of a quality of well-being scale as an outcome measure in chronic obstructive pulmonary disease. *Journal of Chronic Disease, 37*, 85-95.

Kaplan, R.M., Atkins, C.J., & Reinsch, S. (1984). Specific efficacy expectations mediate exercise compliance in patients with COPD. *Health Psychology, 3*, 223-242.

Kaplan, R.M., Ries, A.L., Prewitt, L.M., & Eakin, E. (1994). Self-efficacy expectations predict survival for patients with chronic obstructive pulmonary disease. *Health Psychology, 13*(4), 366-368.

Kaplan, R.M., & Simon, H.J. (1990). Compliance in medical care: Reconsideration of self-predictions. *Annals of Behavioral Medicine, 12*, 66-71.

Karacan, I. (1982). Nocturnal penile tumescence as a biological marker in assessing erectile dysfunction. *Psychosomatics, 23,* 349-360.

Karajgee, B., Rifkin, A., Doddi, S., & Kolli, R. (1990). The prevalence of anxiety disorders in patients with chronic obstructive pulmonary disease. *American Journal of Psychiatry, 147,* 200-201.

Karvetti, R.L., & Hamalainen, H. (1993). Long-term effect of nutrition education on myocardial infarction patients: A 10-year follow-up study. *Nutritional Metabolism and Cardiovascular Disease 16*(3), 185-192.

Kass, I., Dyksterhuis, J.E., Rubin, H., & Patil, K.D. (1975). Correlation of psycho-physiological variables with vocational rehabilitation outcome in patients with chronic obstructive pulmonary disease. *Chest, 67,* 433-440.

Kass, I., Updegraff, K., & Muffly, R.B. (1972). Sex in chronic obstructive pulmonary disease. *Medical Aspects of Human Sexuality, 6*(2), 33-42.

Katon, W., & Sullivan, M.D. (1990). Depression and chronic medical illness. *Journal of Clinical Psychiatry, 51*(Suppl. 6), 3-11.

Kaufman, E. (1984). Family system variables in alcoholism. *Alcoholism: Clinical and Experimental Research, 8,* 4-8.

Kavanagh, D.J., & Bower, G.H. (1985). Mood and self-efficacy: Impact of joy and sadness on perceived capabilities. *Cognitive Therapy Research, 9,* 507-525.

Kazdin, A.E. (1974). Covert modeling, model similarity, and reduction of avoidance behavior. *Behavior Therapy, 5,* 325-340.

Keefe, F.J., & Blumenthal, J.A. (Eds.) (1982). *Assessment strategies in behavioral medicine.* New York: Grune & Stratton.

Kegeles, S.S. (1963). Why people seek dental care: A test of a conceptual formulation. *Journal of Health and Human Behavior, 4,* 166-173.

Kellner, R. (1987). *Manual of the symptom questionnaire.* Albuquerque, NM: University of New Mexico.

Kellner, R., Samet, J., & Pathak, D. (1992). Dyspnea, anxiety, and depression in chronic respiratory impairment. *General Hospital Psychiatry, 14*(1), 20-28.

Kelly, K., & Houston, B.K. (1985). Type A behavior in employed women: Relation to work, marital and leisure variables, social support, stress, tension and health. *Journal of Personality and Social Psychology, 48,* 1067-1079.

Kemp, B.J. (1993). Psychologic care of the older rehabilitation patient. *Geriatric Rehabilitation, 9*(4), 841-857.

Kendall, P.C., & Watson, D. (1981). Psychological preparation for stressful medical procedures. In C.K. Prokop & L.A. Bradley (Eds.), *Medical psychology: Contributions to behavioral medicine* (pp. 197-221). New York: Academic.

Kendall, P.C., Williams, L., Pechacek, T.F., Graham, L.E., Shisslak, C., & Herzoll, N. (1979). Cognitive-behavioral and patient education interventions in cardiac catheterization procedures: The Palo Alto Medical Psychology Project. *Journal of Consulting and Clinical Psychology, 47,* 49-58.

Kersten, L. (1990a). Changes in self-concept during pulmonary rehabilitation, part 1. *Heart and Lung, 19*(5), 456-462.

Kersten, L. (1990b). Changes in self-concept during pulmonary rehabilitation, part 2. *Heart and Lung, 19*(5), 463-470.

Kersten, L.D. (1989). Patient motivation. *Comprehensive respiratory nursing—a decision making approach* (pp. 453-471). Pittsburgh: Saunders.

Kiecolt-Glaser, J.K., & Glaser, R. (1988). Psychological influences on immunity: Implications for AIDS. *American Psychologist, 43,* 892-898.

Killen, J.D., Fortmann, S.P., Newman, B., & Varady, A. (1990). Evaluation of a treatment approach combining nicotine gum with self-guided behavioral treatments for smoking relapse prevention. *Journal of Consulting and Clinical Psychology, 58,* 85-92.

Kilmann, P.R., Wagner, M.K., & Sotile, W.M. (1977). The differential impact of self-monitoring on smoking behavior: An exploratory study. *Journal of Clinical Psychology, 33*(3), 912-914.

Kimball, C.P. (1978). Interviewing and therapy in the acute situation. In T.B. Karasu & R.I. Steinmuller (Eds.), *Psychotherapeutics in medicine* (pp. 203-231). New York: Grune & Stratton.

King, K.B. (1985). Measurement of coping strategies, concerns, and emotional response in patients undergoing coronary artery bypass grafting. *Heart and Lung, 14,* 579-586.

Kinsman, R., Fernandez, E., Schocket, M., Dirks, J., & Covino, N. (1982). Multidimensional analysis of the symptoms of chronic bronchitis and emphysema. *Journal of Behavioral Medicine, 6*(4), 339-357.

Kleges, R.C., & Shumaker, S.A. (1992). Understanding the relations between smoking and body weight and their importance to smoking cessation and relapse. *Health Psychology, 11*(Suppl.), 1-3.

Kleman, M., Bickert, A., Karpinski, A., Wantz, D., Jacobsen, B., Lowery, B., & Menapace, F. (1993). Physiologic responses of coronary care patients to visiting. *Journal of Cardiovascular Nursing, 7*(3), 52-62.

Kline, N.W., & Warren, B.A. (1983). The relationship between husband and wife perceptions of the prescribed health regimen and level of function in the marital couple post-myocardial infarction. *Family Practice Research Journal, 2*(4), 271-280.

Knapp, D., & Blackwell, B. (1985). Emotional and behavioral problems in cardiac rehabilitation patients. *Journal of Cardiac Rehabilitation, 5,* 112-123.

Kobasa, S.C.O., Maddi, S.R., Puccetti, M.C., & Zola, M.A. (1985). Effectiveness of hardiness, exercise and social support as resources against illness. *Journal of Psychosomatic Research, 29,* 525-533.

Koch, A.Y. (1983). Family adaptation to medical stressors. *Family Systems Medicine, 1*(4), 74-87.

Koenig, H.G., Smiley, M., & Gonzales, J.P. (1988). *Religion, health and aging: A review and theoretical integration.* New York: Greenwood Press.

Kolman, P. (1983). The value of group psychotherapy after myocardial infarction: a critical review. *Journal of Cardiac Rehabilitation, 3,* 360-366.

Kolman, P. (1984). Sexual dysfunction in the post-MI patient. *Journal of Cardiac Rehabilitation, 4,* 334-340.

Kolodny, R., Masters, W., & Johnson, V. (1979). *Textbook of sexual medicine.* Boston: Little, Brown.

Kolodny, R.C. (1971). Sexual dysfunction in diabetic females. *Diabetes, 20,* 557-559.

Kolodny, R.C., Kahn, C.B., Goldstein, H.H., & Barnett, D.B. (1974). Sexual dysfunction in diabetic men. *Diabetes, 23,* 306-309.

Kottke, T.E., & Solbert, L.I. (1993). Smoking intervention during cardiac rehabilitation. In F.J. Pashkow & W.A. Dafoe (Eds.), *Clinical cardiac rehabilitation: A cardiologist's guide* (pp. 243-247). Baltimore: Williams & Wilkins.

Kramarsky-Binkhorst, S. (1978). Female partner perception of Small-Carrion implant. *Urology, 12,* 545-548.

Krantz, D., & Manuck, S. (1984). Acute psychophysiologic reactivity and risk of cardiovascular disease: A review and methodologic critique. *Psychology Bulletin, 96,* 435-464.

Krantz, D.S. (1980). Cognitive processes and recovery from heart attack: A review and theoretical analysis. *Journal of Human Stress, 6,* 27-38.

Krantz, D.S. (1993, October). *Stress and myocardial ischemia: New insights.* Presented to the Eighth Annual Meeting of the American Association of Cardiovascular and Pulmonary Rehabilitation, Orlando, FL.

Krantz, D.S., Arabian, J.M., Davia, J.E., & Parker, J.S. (1982). Type A behavior and coronary artery bypass surgery: Intraoperative blood pressure and perioperative complications. *Psychosomatic Medicine, 44,* 273-284.

Krantz, D.S., & Durel L.A. (1983). Psychobiological substrates of Type A behavior pattern. *Health Psychology, 2,* 393-411.

Krantz, D.S., Durel, L.A., Davia, J.E., Shaffer, R.T., Arabian, J.M., Dembroski, T.M., & MacDougal, J.M. (1982). Propranolol medication among coronary patients: Relationship to Type A behavior and cardiovascular response. *Journal of Human Stress, 8*(3), 4-12.

Krantz, D.S., & Hedges, S.M. (1987). Some cautions for research on personality and health. *Journal of Personal Health, 55,* 351-357.

Kravetz, H.M. (1982a). Sexual counseling for the COPD patient: Clinical challenge in cardiopulmonary medicine. *Monograph of the American College of Chest Physicians, 4*(1).

Kravetz, H.M. (Author and Narrator). (1982b). *A visit with Harry* [slide-tape program]. Phoenix: The Pulmonary Foundation.

Kravetz, H.M. (Author and Narrator). (1982c). *A visit with Helen* [slide-tape program]. Phoenix: The Pulmonary Foundation.

Kravetz, H.M., & Pheatt, H. (1993). Sexuality in the pulmonary patient. In J.E. Hodgkin, G.L. Connors, & C.W. Bell (Eds.), *Pulmonary rehabilitation: Guidelines to success* (2nd ed., pp. 293-310). Philadelphia: Lippincott.

Kravetz, H.M., Weiss, M., & Meadows, S.R. (1980). *Sexual counseling for the male pulmonary patient* [slide-tape program]. Phoenix: The Pulmonary Foundation.

Krupnick, S. (1993, October). *Clinical anxiety management.* Presented at Trends in Critical Care Nursing '93: Southeastern Chapter of the American Association of Critical Care Nursing Conference.

Kubler-Ross, E. (1969). *On death and dying.* New York: Macmillan.

Kulik, J.A., & Mahler, H.I.M. (1987). Effects of preoperative roommate assignment on preoperative anxiety and recovery from coronary-bypass surgery. *Health Psychology, 6*(6), 525-543.

Kulik, J.A., & Mahler, I.M. (1989). Social support and recovery from surgery. *Health Psychology, 8,* 221-238.

Kurosawa, H., Shimizu, Y., Nishimatsu, Y., Hiruse, S., & Takano, T. (1980). The relationship between mental distress and physical severities in patients with acute myocardial infarction. *Japanese Circulation Journal, 47,* 723-278.

Laerum, E., Johnsen, N., Smith, P., & Arnesen, H. (1991). Positive psychological and life-style changes after myocardial infarction: A follow-up study after 2-4 years. *Family Practice, 8,* 229-233.

Laerum, E., Johnsen, N., Smith, P., & Larsen, S. (1987). Can myocardial infarction induce positive changes in family relationships. *Family Practice, 4,* 302-305.

Laffrey, S.C., & Crabtree, M.K. (1988). Health and health behavior of persons with chronic cardiovascular disease. *International Journal of Nursing Studies, 25*(1), 41-52.

Lake, B.W., Suarez, E.C., Schneiderman, N., & Tocci, N. (1985). The Type A behavior pattern, physical fitness, and psychophysiological reactivity. *Health Psychology, 4,* 169.

Lancaster, J. (1981). Maximizing psychological adaptations in an aging population. *Advanced Nursing Science, 3,* 31-43.

Lando, H.A., Hellerstedt, W.L., Pirie, P.I., & McGovern, P.G. (1992). Brief supportive telephone outreach as a recruitment and intervention strategy for smoking cessation. *American Journal of Public Health, 82,* 41-46.

Lane, C., & Hobfoll, S.E. (1992). How loss affects anger and alienates potential supporters. *Journal of Consulting and Clinical Psychology, 60*(6), 935-942.

Langosch, W., Seer, P., Brodner, G., Kallinke, D., Kulick, B., & Heim, F. (1982). Behavior therapy with coronary heart disease patients: Results of a comparative study. *Journal of Psychosomatic Research, 26*(5), 475-484.

Larson, J.L., McNaughton, M.W., Kennedy, J.W., & Mansfield, L.W. (1980). Heart rate and blood pressure responses to sexual activity and a stair-climbing test. *Heart and Lung, 9*(6), 1025-1030.

Lavie, C.J., Milani, R.V., & Littman, A.B. (1993). Benefits of cardiac rehabilitation and exercise training in secondary coronary prevention in the elderly. *Journal of American Coronary Care, 22*(3), 678-683.

Layne, O.L., & Yudofsky, S.C. (1971). Postoperative psychosis in cardiotomy patients. *New England Journal of Medicine, 284,* 518-520.

Lazarus, A. (1976). *Multimodal behavior therapy.* New York: Springer.

Lazarus, R.S. (1966). *Psychological stress and the coping process.* New York: McGraw-Hill.

Lazarus, R.S., & Folkman, S. (1984). *Stress, appraisal, and coping.* New York: Springer.

Lebovitis, B.Z., Shekelle, R.B., Ostfeld, A.M., & Paul, O. (1967). Prospective and retrospective psychological studies of coronary heart disease. *Psychosomatic Medicine, 29*(3), 265-272.

Lebowitz, B.D. (1978). Old age and family functioning. *Journal of Gerontological Social Work, 1*(2), 111-118.

Lehman, D.R., Ellard, J.H., & Wortman, J.H. (1986). Social support for the bereaved: Recipients' and providers' perspectives on what is helpful. *Journal of Consulting and Clinical Psychology, 54,* 438-446.

Leigh, H., Hofer, M.A., Cooper, J., & Reiser, M.F. (1972). A psychological comparison of patients in "open" and "closed": Coronary care units. *Journal of Psychosomatic Research, 16,* 449-458.

Leiker, M., & Hailey, B.J. (1988). A link between hostility and disease: Poor health habits? *Behavioral Medicine, 3,* 129-133.

Lenfant, C. (1982). Lung research: Government and community. *American Review of Respiratory Diseases, 126,* 753-757.

Leon, A.S. (1989). The role of physical activity in the prevention and management of obesity. In A.J. Ryan & F.L. Allman (Eds.), *Sports medicine* (2nd ed., pp. 593-646). San Diego: Academic.

Leon, A.S., Pollock, M.L., & Weltman, A. (1983). American College of Sports Medicine position statement on proper and improper weight loss programs. *Medicine and Science in Sports and Exercise, ix-xii,* 15.

Leriche, A., & Morel, A. (1948). The syndrome of thrombotic obliteration of the aortic bifurcation. *Annals of Surgery, 127,* 193-208.

Leserman, J., Stuart, E.M., Mamish, M.E., & Benson, H. (1989). The efficacy of the relaxation response in preparing for cardiac surgery. *Behavioral Medicine, 2*, 111-117.

Levenkron, J.C., Goldstein, J.G., Adamides, O., & Greenland, P. (1985). Chronic chest pain with normal coronary arteries: A behavioral approach to rehabilitation. *Journal of Cardiopulmonary Rehabilitation, 5*, 475-479.

Levenson, J.L., Kay, R., Monteperrante, J., & Herman, M.W. (1984). Denial predicts favorable outcome in unstable angina pectoris. *Psychosomatic Medicine, 46*, 25-32.

Levenson, R.W., & Gottman, J.M. (1983). Marital interaction: Physiological linkage and affective exchange. *Journal of Personality and Social Psychology, 45*, 587-597.

Levenson, R.W., & Gottman, J.M. (1985). Physiological and affective predictors of change in relationship satisfaction. *Journal of Personality and Social Psychology, 49*, 85-94.

Leventhal, H., Zimmerman, R., & Gutman, M. (1984). Compliance: A self-regulation perspective. In W.D. Gentry (Ed.), *Handbook of behavioral medicine* (pp. 369-346). New York: Guilford Press.

Levin, R. (1987). *Heartmates: A survival guide for the cardiac spouse.* New York: Pocket Books.

Levine, J., Warrenburg, S., Kerns, R.D., Schwartz, G., Delaney, R., Fontana, A., Gradman, A., Smith, S., Allen, S., & Cascione, R. (1987). The role of denial in recovery from coronary heart disease. *Psychosomatic Medicine, 49*, 109-117.

Levinson, D.J. (1978). *The seasons of a man's life.* New York: Ballantine.

Levitan, H. (1983). Suicidal trends in patients with asthma and hypertension: A case study. *Psychotherapy and Psychosomatics, 39*(3), 165-170.

Levy, S.M., Lee, J., Gagley, C., & Lippman, M. (1988). Survival hazards analysis in first recurrent breast cancer patients: Seven-year follow-up. *Psychosomatic Medicine, 50*, 520-528.

Lewin, B., Robertson, I.H., Cay, E.L., Irving, J.B., & Campbell, M. (1992). Effects of self-help post-myocardial-infarction rehabilitation on psychological adjustment and use of health services. *Lancet, 339*, 1036-1040.

Lewis, J.M., Beavers, W.R., Gossett, J.T., & Phillips, V.A. (1976). *No single thread.* New York: Brunner/Mazel.

Lichtenstein, E., & Mermelstein, R.J. (1986). Some methodological cautions in the use of the tolerance questionnaire. *Addictive Behaviors, 11*, 439-442.

Light, R.W., Merrill, E.J., Despers, J.A., Gordon, G.H., & Mutalipassi, L.R. (1985). Prevalence of depression and anxiety in patients with COPD: Relationship to functional capacity. *Chest 87*, 35-43.

Lipowski, Z.J. (1977). Psychosomatic medicine in the seventies: An overview. *American Journal of Psychiatry, 134*, 233-244.

Lloyd, G.G., & Cawley, R.M. (1983). Distress or illness? A study of psychological symptoms after myocardial infarction. *British Journal of Psychiatry, 142*, 120-125.

Locke, H.J., & Wallace, K.M. (1959). Short-term marital adjustment and prediction tests: Their reliability and validity. *Journal of Marriage and Family Living, 21*, 251-255.

Longworth, J.C.D. (1982). Psychophysiological effects of slo stroke back massage in normotensive females. *Advances of Nursing Science, 4*, 44-61.

LoPiccolo, J., & LoPiccolo, L. (Eds.) (1978). *Handbook of sex therapy.* New York: Plenum Press.

Lovibond, S.H., Birrell, P.C., & Langeluddecke, P. (1985). Changing coronary heart disease risk-factor status: The effects of three behavioral programs. *Journal of Behavioral Medicine, 9*(5), 415-437.

Lowenthal, M.F., & Haven, C. (1968). Interaction and adaptation: Intimacy as a critical variable. *American Social Review, 33,* 20-30.

Lowery, B.J. (1991). Psychological stress, denial and myocardial infarction outcomes. *Image: Journal of Nursing Scholarship, 23,* 51-55.

Lown, B., & Verrier, R.L. (1976). Neural activity and ventricular fibrillation. *New England Journal of Medicine, 294,* 1165-1170.

Lown, B., Verrier, R.L., & Rabinowitz, S.H. (1977). Neural and psychological mechanisms and the problem of sudden death. *American Journal of Cardiology, 39,* 890-902.

Lynch, J.J. (1977). *The broken heart: The medical consequences of loneliness.* New York: Basic Books.

Lynch, J.J., Thomas, S.A., Paskewitz, D.A., Datcher, A.H., & Weir, L.O. (1977). Human contact and cardiac arrhythmias in a coronary care unit. *Psychosomatic Medicine, 39,* 188-192.

Lyons, H.A. (1977). Sexual relations for male patients with chronic obstructive lung disease. *Medical Aspects of Human Sexuality, 11*(4), 119.

MacDonald, A.J.D. (1986). Do general practitioners 'miss' depression in elderly patients? *British Medical Journal, 292,* 1365-1367.

MacDougall, J.M., Dembroski, T.M., Dimsdale, J.E., & Hackett, T.P. (1985). Components of Type A, hostility, and anger. *Health Psychology, 4,* 137-152.

Mackenzie, T.B., & Popkin, M.K. (1980). Stress response syndrome occurring after delirium. *American Journal of Psychiatry, 137*(11), 1433-1435.

Maeland, J.G., & Havik, O.E. (1987). Psychological predictors for return to work after a myocardial infarction. *Journal of Psychosomatic Research, 31,* 471-481.

Maes, S. (1992). Psychosocial aspects of cardiac rehabilitation in Europe. *British Journal of Clinical Psychology, 31,* 473-483.

Maguire, L. (1983). *Understanding social networks.* Beverly Hills, CA: Sage.

Mahler, D., Faryniarz, K., Tomlinson, E., Colice, G.L., Robins, A.G., Olmstead, E.M., & Conner, G.T. (1992). Impact of dyspnea and physiologic function on general health status in patients with chronic obstructive pulmonary disease. *Chest, 102,* 395-401.

Malan, S.S. (1992), Psychosocial adjustment following MI: Current views and nursing implications. *Journal of Cardiovascular Nursing, 6*(4), 57-70.

Mall, R., & Medeiros, M. (1988). Objective evaluation of results of a pulmonary rehabilitation program in a community hospital. *Chest, 94,* 1156-1160.

Mann, S., Craig, M.W.M., Gould, B.A., Melville, D.I., & Raftery, E.B. (1982). Coital blood pressure in hypertensives: Cephalgia, syncope, and effects of beta-blockade. *British Heart Journal, 47,* 84-89.

Mann, S., Yates, J.G., & Raftery, E.B. (1981). The effects of myocardial infarction on sexual activity. *Journal of Cardiopulmonary Rehabilitation, 1,* 187-193.

Marks, I.M. (1986). *Fears, phobias, and rituals: An interdisciplinary perspective.* Cambridge, MA: Oxford University Press.

Marlatt, G.A. (1985). Relapse prevention: Theoretical. In R. Gordon (Ed.), *Relapse prevention* (pp. 3-70). New York: Guilford Press.

Marlatt, G.A., Curry, S., & Gordon, J.R. (1988). A longitudinal analysis of unaided smoking cessation. *Journal of Consulting and Clinical Psychology, 56,* 715-720.

Marlatt, G.A., & Gordon, J.R. (1980). Determinant of relapse: Implications for the maintenance of behavior change. In P.O. Davidson & S.M. Davidson (Eds.), *Behavioral medicine: Changing health lifestyles* (pp. 410-452). New York: Brunner/Mazel.

Marsden, C., & Dracup, K. (1991). Different perspectives: The effect of heart disease on patients and spouses. *AACN Clinical Issues, 2,* 285-292.

Marsland, C.P., & Logan, R.L. (1984). Coronary care and rehabilitation: Patient and spouse responses. *New Zealand Medical Journal, 97,* 406-408.

Martin, J.E., & Dubbert, P.M. (1984). Behavioral management strategies for improving health and fitness. *Journal of Cardiac Rehabilitation, 4,* 200-208.

Massey, M.A. (1994). Assessment, intervention, and referral of patients suffering from alcoholism. *Journal of Cardiopulmonary Rehabilitation, 14,* 27-29.

Masters, W.H., & Johnson, V.E. (1966). *Human sexual response.* Boston: Little, Brown.

Masters, W.H., & Johnson, V.E. (1970). *Human sexual inadequacy.* Boston: Little, Brown.

Matano, R.A., & Bronstone, A.B. (1994). Assessment, intervention, and referral of patients suffering from alcoholism. *Journal of Cardiopulmonary Rehabilitation, 14,* 27-29.

Matthews, K.A. (1982). Psychological perspectives on the Type A behavior pattern. *Psychological Bulletin, 91,* 293-323.

Matthews, K.A. (1988). Coronary heart disease and Type A behaviors: Update on and alternative to the Booth-Kewley and Friedman (1987) quantitative review. *Psychology Bulletin, 104,* 373-380.

Matthews, K.A., Glass, D.C., Rosenman, R.H., & Bortner, R.W. (1977). Competitive drive, pattern A and coronary heart disease: A further analysis of some data from the Western Collaborative Group study. *Journal of Chronic Diseases, 31,* 489-498.

Matthews, K.A., Rosenman, R.H., Dembroski, T.M., Harris, E.L., & MacDougall, J.M. (1984). Familial resemblance in components of the Type A behavior pattern: A reanalysis of the California Type A twin study. *Psychosomatic Medicine, 46,* 512-522.

Matthews, K.A., & Siegel, J.M. (1983). Type A behaviors by children, social comparison, and standards for self-evaluation. *Developmental Psychology, 19,* 135-140.

Matthews, K.A., & Woodall, L.K. (1988). Childhood origins of overt Type A behaviors and cardiovascular reactivity to behavioral stressors. *Annals of Behavioral Medicine, 10,* 71-77.

Mayou, R. (1979). The course and determinants of reactions to myocardial infarction. *British Journal of Psychiatry, 143,* 588-594.

Mayou, R. (1990). Quality of life in cardiovascular disease. *Psychotherapy and Psychosomatics, 54,* 99-109.

Mayou, R., & Bryant, B. (1987). Quality of life after coronary artery surgery. *Quarterly Journal of Medicine, 62,* 239-248.

Mayou, R., Foster, A., & Williamson, B. (1978b). Psychosocial adjustment in patients one year after myocardial infarction. *Journal of Psychosomatic Research, 22,* 447-453.

Mayou, R., Williamson, B., & Foster, A. (1976). Attitude and advice after myocardial infarction. *British Medical Journal, 1,* 1577-1579.

Mayou, R., Williamson, B., & Foster, A. (1978). Outcome two months after myocardial infarction. *Journal of Psychosomatic Research, 22,* 439-445.

McAlister, A.L., Farquhar, J.W., Thoresen, C.E., & Maccoby, N. (1976). Behavioral science applied to cardiovascular health: Progress and research needs in the modification of risk-taking habits in adult populations. *Health Education Monographs, 4,* 45-74.

McCaffrey, R.J., & Blanchard, E.B. (1985). Stress management approaches to the treatment of essential hypertension. *Annals of Behavioral Medicine, 7*(11), 5-12.

McConnaughy, E.A., DiClemente, C.C., Prochaska, J.O., & Velicer, W.F. (1989). Stages of change in psychotherapy: A follow-up report. *Psychotherapy: Theory, Research and Practice, 4,* 494-503.

McConnaughy, E.A., Prochaska, J.O., & Velicer, W.F. (1983). Stages of change in psychotherapy: Measurement and sample profiles. *Psychotherapy: Theory, Research and Practice, 20,* 368-375.

McCrae, R.R. (1984). Age differences in the use of coping mechanisms. *Journal of Gerontology, 37*(4), 454-460.

McCulloch, D.K., Young, R.J., Prescott, R.J., Campbell, I.W., & Clark, B.V. (1984). The natural history of impotence in diabetic men. *Diabetologia, 26,* 437-440.

McDaniel, S.H., Hepworth, J., & Doherty, W.J. (1992). *Medical family therapy: A biopsychosocial approach to families with health problems.* New York: Basic Books.

McGann, M. (1976). Group sessions for the families of post-coronary patients. *Supervisor Nurse, 1,* 17-19.

McGrath, F.J., & Robinson, J.C. (1973). The medical social worker in the coronary care unit. *Medical Journal of Australia, 2,* 1113-1118.

McIntyre-Kingsolver, K., Lichtenstein, E., & Mermelstein, R.J. (1986). Spouse training in a multicomponent smoking cessation program. *Behavioral Therapy, 17,* 67-74.

McKay, M., Rogers, P.D., & McKay, J. (1989). *When anger hurts: Quieting the storm within.* Oakland, California: New Harbinger Publications, Inc.

McKenna, J.P. (Ed.) (1992). *The Beaver guide to common outpatient problems* (2nd ed.). New Castle, PA: Brindle Printing.

McKool, K. (1987). Facilitating smoking cessation. *Journal of Cardiovascular Nursing, 1*(4), 28-41.

McNair, D.M., Lorr, M., & Droppleman, L.F. (1971). *Profile of mood states.* San Diego: Educational and Industrial Testing Service.

McPherson, B., Paivio, A., Yhasz, M., Rechnitzer, P.A., Pickard, H.A., & Lefcoe, N.M. (1967). Psychological effects of an exercise program for postinfarction and normal adult men. *Journal of Sports Medicine and Physical Fitness, 7,* 95-102.

McSweeney, A., Grant, I., Heaton, R., Adams, K., & Timms, R. (1982). Life quality of patients with chronic obstructive pulmonary disease. *Archives of Internal Medicine, 142,* 473-478.

Medalie, J., Snyder, M., & Groen, J. (1973). Angina pectoris among 10,000 men: 5-year incidence and univariate analysis. *American Journal of Medicine, 55,* 583-594.

Medalie, J.H., & Goldbourt, U. (1976). Angina pectoris among 10,000 men: II. Psychosocial and other risk factors as evidenced by a multrivariate analysis of a five-year incidence study. *American Journal of Medicine, 60,* 910-921.

Meissner, W.W. (1973). Family process and psychosomatic disease. In J.G. Howells (Ed.), *Advances in family psychiatry* (Vol. 1, pp. 112-127). New York: International Universities Press.

Mellinger, B.C., Vaughan, E.D., Thompson, S.L., & Goldstein, M. (1987). Correlation between intracavernous papaverine injection and Doppler analysis in impotent men. *Urology, 30,* 416-419.

Melzak, R. (1975). The McGill pain questionnaire: Major properties and scoring methods. *Pain, 1,* 277-299.

Mermelstein, R., Lichtenstein, E., & McIntyre, K. (1983). Partner support and relapse in smoking cessation programs. *Journal of Consulting and Clinical Psychologists, 51,* 465-466.

Michal, V. (1982). Arterial disease as a cause of impotence. *Clinics in Endocrinology and Metabolism, 11,* 725-748.

Michela, J.L. (1987). Interpersonal and individual impacts of a husband's heart attack. In A. Baum & J.E. Singer (Eds.), *Handbook of psychology and health: Vol. 5. Stress* (pp. 255-301). Hillsdale, NJ: Erlbaum.

Milani, R.V., Littman, A.B., & Lavie, C.J. (1993). Depressive symptoms predict functional improvement following cardiac rehabilitation and exercise program. *Journal of Cardiopulmonary Rehabilitation 13*, 406-411.

Miller, P., Johnson, N., Garrett, M.J., Wikoff, R., & McMahon, M. (1982). Health beliefs and adherence to the medical regimen of ischemic heart disease patients. *Heart and Lung, 11*(4), 332-339.

Miller, P., Wikoff, R., McMahon, M., Garrett, M., & Ringel, K. (1988). Influence of a nursing intervention on regimen adherence and societal adjustments post-myocardial infarction. *Nursing Research, 37*, 297-302.

Miller, P., Wikoff, R., McMahon, M., Garrett, M.J., & Ringel, K. (1985). Indicators of medical regimen adherence for myocardial infarction patients. *Nursing Research, 34*, 268-272.

Miller, P.J., & Wikoff, R. (1989). Spouses' psychosocial problems, resources, and marital functioning postmyocardial infarction. *Progress in Cardiovascular Nursing, 4*, 71-76.

Miller, R.S., & Lefcourt, H.M. (1982). The assessment of social intimacy. *Journal of Personality Assessment, 46*, 514-518.

Millon, T., Green, C.J., & Meagher, R.B. (1982). *Millon behavioral health inventory manual*. Minneapolis, MN: National Computer Systems.

Minuchin, S., Baker, L., Rosman, B., Liebman, R., Milman, L., & Todd, T. (1979). A conceptual model of psychosomatic illness in children: Family organization and family therapy. In J.G. Howells (Ed.), *Advances in family psychiatry* (Vol. 1). New York: International Universities Press.

Moberg, D.O. (1971). *Spiritual well-being: Background and issues*. Washington, D.C.: White House Conference on Aging.

Mohr, D.C., & Beutler, L.E. (1990). Erectile dysfunction: A review of diagnostic and treatment procedures. *Clinical Psychology Review, 10*, 123-150.

Moon, J.R., & Eisler, R.M. (1983). Anger control: An experimental comparison of three behavioral treatments. *Behavior Therapy, 14*, 493-505.

Moos, R.H. (1982). Coping with acute health crisis. In T. Millon, C. Green, & R. Maegher (Eds.), *Handbook of clinical health psychology* (pp. 76-90). New York: Plenum Press.

Moos, R.H., Finney, J.W., & Gamble, W. (1982). The process of recovery from alcoholism: II. Comparing spouses of alcoholic patients and matched community controls. *Journal Studies of Alcohol, 43*, 888-909.

Moos, R.H., & Moos, B.S. (1981). *Family environment scale manual*. Palo Alto, CA: Consulting Psychologists Press.

Moran, M.G. (1991). Psychological factors affecting pulmonary and rheumatologic diseases: A review. *Psychosomatics, 32*(1), 14-23.

Morisky, D.E., Levine, D.M., Green, L.W., Shapiro, S., Russell, R.P., & Smith, C.R. (1983). Five-year blood pressure control and mortality following health education for hypertensive patients. *American Journal of Public Health, 73*, 153-162.

Moss, G.E., Dielman, T.E., Campanelli, P.C., Leech, S.L., Harian, W.R., VanHarrison, R., & Horvath, W.J. (1986). Demographic correlates of 51 assessments of Type A behavior. *Psychosomatic Medicine, 4*, 564-674.

Mossey, J.M., & Shapiro, M. (1982). Self-rated health: a predictor of mortality among the elderly. *American Journal of Public Health, 72*, 800-808.

Mueller, C., & Donnerstein, E. (1977). The effects of humor-induced arousal upon aggressive behavior. *Journal of Research in Personality, 11*, 73-82.

Mulcahy, R. (1983). Influence of cigarette smoking on morbidity and mortality after myocardial infarction. *British Heart Journal, 49,* 410-415.

Mullen, P.D., Green, L.W., & Persinger, G. (1985). Clinical trials of patient education for chronic conditions: A comparative meta-analysis of intervention types. *Preventive Medicine, 14,* 753-781.

Mumford, E., Schlesinger, H.J., & Glass, G.V. (1982). The effects of psychological intervention on recovery from surgery and heart attacks: An analysis of the literature. *American Journal of Public Health, 72,* 141-152.

Munro, B.H., Creamer, A.M., Haggerty, M.R., & Cooper, F.S. (1988). Effect of relaxation therapy of post-myocardial infarction patients' rehabilitation. *Nursing Research, 37*(4), 231-235.

Murphy, J.K., Williamson, A.E., Buxton, A.E., Moody, S.C., Absher, N., & Warner, M. (1982). The long-term effects of spouse involvement upon weight loss maintenance. *Behavioral Therapy, 13,* 681-693.

Myrtek, M. (1987). Life satisfaction, illness behavior, and rehabilitation outcome: Results of a one year follow-up study with cardiac patients. *International Journal of Rehabilitation Research, 10,* 373-382.

Nadig, P.W., Ware, J.C., & Blumoff, R. (1986). Noninvasive device to produce and maintain an erection-like state. *Urology, 27,* 126-131.

Nagle, R., Gangola, R., & Picton-Robinson, L. (1971). I: Factors influencing return to work after myocardial infarction. *Lancet, 2,* 454-456.

Naismith, L.D., Robinson, J.R., Shaw, G.B., & MacIntyre, M.M.J. (1979). Psychosocial rehabilitation after myocardial infarction. *British Medical Journal, 1,* 439-442.

Naparstek, B. (1995). *Staying well with guided imagery.* New York: Warner.

National Heart, Lung, and Blood Institute. (1982). Management of patient compliance in the treatment of hypertension. *Hypertension, 4,* 415-423.

National Interfaith Coalition on Aging. (1975, August). Spiritual well-being definition: A model of ecumenical work product. *NICA Inform, 1,* p. 4.

Neish, C.M., & Hopp, J.W. (1988). The role of education in pulmonary rehabilitation. *Journal of Cardiopulmonary Rehabilitation, 11,* 439-441.

Nemec, E., Mansfield, L., & Kennedy, J.W. (1976). Heart rate and blood pressure response during sexual activity in normal males. *American Heart Journal, 92*(3), 274-277.

Nett, L.M. (1992, October). *Bedside nicotine counseling.* Paper presented to Seventh Annual Meeting, American Association of Cardiovascular and Pulmonary Rehabilitation, Chicago.

Nett, L.M., & Petty, T.L. (1985). Reconciliary ethical principles and new technology: A commentary on critical care medicine and mechanical ventilation. *Respiratory Care, 30,* 610-620.

Newman, H.F., & Reiss, H. (1984). Artificial perfusion in impotence. *Urology, 24,* 469-471.

Newmark, C.S., Cook, L., Clarke, M., & Faschingbauer, T.R. (1973). Application of Faschingbauer's abbreviated MMPI to psychiatric inpatients. *Journal of Consulting and Clinical Psychologists, 41,* 416-421.

Nickel, J.T., Brown, K.J., & Smith, B.A. (1990). Depression and anxiety among chronically ill heart patients: Age differences in risk and predictors. *Research Nursing Health, 13,* 87-97.

Novaco, R. (1975). *Anger control: The development and evaluation of an experimental treatment.* Lexington, MA: Heath.

Novaco, R.W. (1976a). The functions and regulation of arousal of anger. *American Journal of Psychiatry, 133,* 1124-1128.

Novaco, R.W. (1976b). Treatment of chronic anger through cognitive and relaxation controls. *Journal of Consulting and Clinical Psychology, 44,* 681.

Nunes, E., Frank, K.A., & Kornfeld, D.S. (1987). Psychologic treatment for the Type A behavior pattern and for coronary heart disease: A metanalysis of the literature. *Psychosomatic Medicine, 48,* 159-173.

Nyamathi, A., Dracup, K., & Jacoby, A. (1988). Development of a spousal coping instrument. *Progress in Cardiovascular Nursing, 3,* 1-6.

Nyamathi, A.M. (1988). Perceptions of factors influencing the coping of wives of myocardial infarction patients. *Journal of Cardiovascular Nursing, 2,* 65-76.

Ockene, J.K., Benfari, R.C., Nuttall, R.L., Hurwitz, I.S., & Ockene, I.S. (1982). Relationship of psychosocial factors to smoking behavior change in an intervention program. *Preventive Medicine, 11,* 13-28.

Ockene, J.K., Hosmer, D., Rippe, J., Williams, J., Goldberg, R.J., DeCosimo, D., Maher, P.M., & Dalen, J.E. (1985). Factors affecting cigarette smoking status in patients with ischemic heart disease. *Journal of Chronic Diseases, 38*(12), 985-994.

O'Farrell, T.J. (1989). Marital and family therapy in alcoholism treatment. *Journal of Substance Abuse Treatment, 6,* 23-29.

O'Keefe, J.L., & Smith, T.W. (1988). Self-regulation and Type A behavior. *Journal of Research in Personality, 22,* 232-251.

Oldenburg, B., Perkins, R.J., & Andrews, G. (1985). Controlled trial of psychological intervention in myocardial infarction. *Journal of Consulting and Clinical Psychology, 53,* 852-859.

Oldridge, N.B. (1982). Compliance and exercise in primary and secondary prevention of coronary heart disease: A review. *Preventive Medicine, 11,* 56-70.

Oldridge, N.B. (1984). Compliance and dropout in cardiac exercise rehabilitation. *Journal of Cardiac Rehabilitation, 4,* 166-177.

Oldridge, N.B. (1986). Compliance with exercise programs. In M.L. Pollock & D.H. Schmidt (Eds.), *Heart disease and rehabilitation* (pp. 629-646). New York: Wiley.

Oldridge, N.B. (1988). Cardiac rehabilitation exercise programme: Compliance and compliance-enhancing strategies. *Sports Medicine, 6,* 42-55.

Oldridge, N.B., Guyatt, G., Jones, N., Corwe, J., Sincer, J., Feeny, D., McKelbie, R., Runions, J., Streiner, D., & Torrance, G. (1991). Effects on quality of life with comprehensive rehabilitation after acute myocardial infarction. *American Journal of Cardiology, 67,* 1084-1089.

Oldridge, N.B., & Jones, N.L. (1983). Improving patient compliance in cardiac rehabilitation: Effects of written agreement and self-monitoring. *Journal of Cardiac Rehabilitation, 3,* 257-262.

Oldridge, N.B., & Pashkow, F.J. (1993). Compliance and motivation in cardiac rehabilitation. In F.J. Pashkow & W.A. Dafoe (Eds.), *Clinical rehabilitation: A cardiologist's guide,* Baltimore: Williams & Wilkins.

Oldridge, N.B., & Rogowski, B.L. (1990). Self-efficacy and inpatient cardiac rehabilitation. *American Journal of Cardiology, 66,* 362-365.

Oldridge, N.B., & Spencer, J. (1985). Exercise habits and perceptions before and after graduating or dropout from supervised cardiac exercise rehabilitation. *Journal of Cardiopulmonary Rehabilitation, 5,* 313-319.

O'Leary, A. (1985). Self-efficacy and health. *Behavioral Research Therapy, 23*(4), 437-451.

Oliveri, M.E., & Reiss, D. (1981). A theory-based empirical classification of family problem-solving behaviors. *Family Process, 20,* 409-418.

Olson, D.H., & Ryder, R.G. (1975). *Marital and family interaction.* St. Paul, MN: Family Social Science.

O'Malley, P.A., & Menke, R. (1988). Relationship of hope and stress after myocardial infarction. *Heart and Lung, 17,* 184-190.

Ornish, D., Brown, S.E., Scherwitz, L.W., Billings, J.H., Armstrong, W.T., Ports, T.A., McLanahan, S.M., Kirkeeide, R.L., Brand, R.J., & Gould, K.L. (1990). Can lifestyle changes reverse coronary heart disease? *Lancet, 336,* 129-133.

Ornish, D., Scherwitz, L.W., Doody, R.S., Kerten, D., McLanahan, S.M., Brown, S.E., DePuey, G., Sonnemaker, R., Haynes, C., Lester, J., McAlister, G.K., Hall, R.J., Burdine, J.A., & Gotto, A.M. (1983). Effects of stress management training and dietary changes in treating ischemic heart disease. *Journal of the American Medical Association, 249,* 54-60.

Ornstein, R., & Sobel, D. (1987). *The healing brain.* New York: Simon & Schuster.

Orzeck, S.A., & Staniloff, H.M. (1987). Comparison of patients' and spouses' needs during the posthospital convalescence phase of a myocardial infarction. *Journal of Cardiopulmonary Rehabilitation, 7,* 59-67.

Ostfeld, A.M., Lebovitis, B.Z., Shekelle, R.B., & Paul, O. (1964). A prospective study of the relationship between personality and coronary heart disease. *Journal of Chronic Diseases, 17,* 265-276.

Ott, C.R., Sivarajan, E.S., Newton, K.M., Almes, M.J., Bruce, R.A., Bergren, M., & Gibson, B. (1983). A controlled randomized study of early cardiac rehabilitation: The Sickness Impact Profile as an assessment tool. *Heart and Lung, 12,* 162-170.

Owens, G.R. (1991). Public screening for lung disease: Experience with the NIH Lung Health Study. *American Journal of Medicine, 91*(4A), 378-408.

Owens, J.F., & Hutelmyer, C.M. (1982). The effect of preoperative intervention on delirium in cardiac surgical patients. *Nursing Research, 31*(1), 60-62.

Packa, D. (1989). Quality of life of cardiac patients: A review. *Journal of Cardiovascular Nursing, 3*(2), 1-11.

Packa, D.R., Branyon, M.E., Kinney, M.R., Khan, S.H., Kelley, R., & Miers, L.J. (1989). Quality of life of elderly patients enrolled in cardiac rehabilitation. *Journal of Cardiovascular Nursing, 3*(2), 33-42.

Paine, R., & Make, B.J. (1986). Pulmonary rehabilitation for the elderly. *Clinical Geriatric Medicine, 2,* 213-235.

Pancheri, P., Bellaterra, M., Matteoli, S., Christofari, M., Polizzi, C., & Puletti, M. (1978). Infarct as a stress agent: Life history and personality characteristics in improved versus not-improved patients after severe heart attack. *Journal of Human Stress, 4,* 16-22.

Papadopoulos, C. (1978). A survey of sexual activity after MI. *Cardiovascular Medicine, 3,* 821-826.

Papadopoulos, C., Beaumont, C., Shelley, S.I., & Larrimore, P. (1983). Myocardial infarction and sexual activity of the female patient. *Archives of Internal Medicine, 143,* 1528-1530.

Papadopoulos, C., Larrimore, P., Cardin, S., & Shelley, S. (1980). Sexual concerns and needs of the postcoronary patient's wife. *Archives of Internal Medicine, 140,* 38-41.

Parker, S.R. (1988). Behavioral science aspects of COPD: Current status and future directions. In A.J. McSweeny & I. Grant (Eds.), *Chronic obstructive pulmonary disease: A behavioral perspective* (pp. 118-132). New York: Marcel Dekker.

Pashkow, P. (1994, May). Outcome measurement in cardiac and pulmonary rehabilitation. Committee Report to Board of Directors, American Association of Cardiovascular and Pulmonary Rehabilitation, Chicago, IL.

Patel, C., Marmot, M.G., & Terry, D.J. (1981). Controlled trial of biofeedback-aided behavioural methods in reducing mild hypertension. *British Medical Journal, 282,* 2005-2008.

Patel, C., Marmot, M.G., Terry, D.J., Carruthers, M., Hunt, B., & Patel, M. (1985). Trial of relaxation in reducing coronary risk: Four-year follow-up. *British Medical Journal, 290,* 1103-1106.

Patterson, J.M. (1988). Families experiencing stress: I. The Family Adjustment and Adaptation Response Model. II. Applying the FAAR Model to heal-related issues for intervention and research. *Family Systems Medicine, 6,* 202-237.

Patterson, J.M. (1989). Illness beliefs as a factor in patient-spouse adaptation to treatment for coronary artery disease. *Family Systems Medicine, 7,* 428-442.

Paul, G.L. (1969). Physiological effects of relaxation training and hypnotic suggestion. *Journal of Abnormal Psychology, 74,* 425-437.

Pearce, J.W., LeBow, M.D., & Orchard, J. (1981). Role of spouse involvement in the behavioral treatment of overweight women. *Journal of Consulting and Clinical Psychology, 49,* 236-244.

Pearlin, L.I., & Johnson, J.S. (1977). Marital status, life strains, and depression. *American Social Review, 42,* 704-715.

Pearlin, L.I., Menaghan, E.G., Lieberman, M.A., & Mullan, J.T. (1981). The stress process. *Journal of Health and Social Behavior, 22,* 337-356.

Pennebaker, J.W., Kiecolt-Glaser, J.K., & Glaser, R. (1988). Disclosure of traumas and immune function: Health implications for psychotherapy. *Journal of Consulting and Clinical Psychology, 56,* 239-245.

Perkins, K.A. (1988). Maintaining smoking abstinence after myocardial infarction. *Journal of Substance Abuse, 1,* 91-107.

Perkins, K.A., Dubbert, P.M., Martin, J.E., Faulstich, M.E., & Harris, J.K. (1988). Cardiovascular reactivity to psychological stress in aerobically trained versus untrained mild hypertensives and normotensives. *Health Psychology, 7,* L329-340.

Perls, F.S. (1969). *Gestalt therapy verbatim.* New York: Bantam.

Perri, M.G., McAdoo, W.G., McAllister, D.A., Lauer, J.B., & Yancey, D.Z. (1986). Enhancing the efficacy of behavior therapy for obesity: Effects of aerobic exercise and a multicomponent maintenance program. *Journal of Consulting and Clinical Psychology, 54,* 670-675.

Peterson, C., Seligman, M.E.P., & Vaillant, G.E. (1988). Pessimistic explanatory style is a risk factor for physical illness: A thirty-five year longitudinal study. *Journal of Personality and Social Psychology, 55,* 23-27.

Petty, T. (1981). Home oxygen in advanced obstructive pulmonary disease. *The Medical Clinics of North America, 65(3),* 615-627.

Petty, T.L., MacIlroy, E.R., Swigert, M.A., & Brink, G.A. (1970). Chronic airway obstruction, respiratory insufficiency and gainful employment. *Archives of Environmental Health, 21,* 71-78.

Pietropinto, A., & Arora, A. (1989). Chronic pulmonary disease and sexual functioning. *Medical Aspects of Human Sexuality, 23,* 78-82.

Pimm, J.B., & Feist, J.R. (1984). *Psychological risks of coronary artery bypass surgery.* New York: Plenum Press.

Popkin, M.K., Callies, A.L., & Mackenzie, T.B. (1985). The outcome of antidepressant use in the medically ill. *Archives of General Psychiatry, 42,* 1160-1163.

Porzelius, J., Vest, M., & Nochomovitz, M. (1992). *Behaviour Research and Therapy, 30*(1), 75-77.

Post, L., & Collins, C. (1981). The poorly coping chronic pulmonary disease patient: A psychotherapeutic perspective. *International Journal of Psychiatry in Medicine, 11*(2), 173-182.

Pozen, M.W., Stechmiller, J.A., Harris, W., Smith, S., Fried, D.D., & Voigt, G.C. (1977). A nurse rehabilitator's impact on patients with myocardial infarction. *Medical Care, 15,* 830-837.

Price, V.A. (1982). *Type A behavior patterns: A model for research and practice.* New York: Academic.

Price, V.A. (1988). Research and clinical issues in treating Type A behavior. In B.K. Houston & C.R. Snyder (Eds.), *Type A behavior pattern: Research, theory, and intervention* (pp. 275-311). New York: Wiley.

Prigatano, G., Wright, E., & Levin, D. (1984). Quality of life and its predictors in patients with mild lypoxemia and chronic obstructive pulmonary disease. *Archives of Internal Medicine, 144,* 1613-1619.

Pritikin, E., & Reece, T. (1993). *Parentcare survival guide: Helping your folks through the not-so-golden years.* Hauppauge, NY: Barron's Educational Series, Inc.

Prochaska, J.O., & DiClemente, C.C. (1983). Stages and processes of self-change of smoking: Toward an integrative model of change. *Journal of Clinical and Consulting Psychology, 51,* 390-395.

Prochaska, J.O., & DiClemente, C.C. (1984). *The transtheoretical approach: Crossing the traditional boundaries of therapy.* Homewood, IL: Dow Jones-Irwin.

Prochaska, J.O., & DiClemente, C.C. (1992). Stages of change in the modification of problem behaviors. In. M. Hersen, R.M. Eisler, & P.M. Miller (Eds.), *Progress in behavior modification* (pp. 184-218). Newbury Park, CA: Sage.

Prochaska, J.O., DiClemente, C.C., & Norcross, J.C. (1992). In search of how people change: Applications to addictive behaviors. *American Psychologist, 47*(9), 1102-1114.

Prochaska, J.O., DiClemente, C.C., Velicer, W.F., Ginpil, S., & Norcross, J.C. (1985). Predicting change in smoking status for self-changers. *Addictive Behavior, 10,* 395-406.

Prochaska, J.O., Velicer, W.F., Rossi, J.S., Goldstein, M.G., Marcus, B.H., Rakowski, W., Fiore, C., Harlow, L., Redding, C.A., Rosenbloom, D., & Rossi, S.R. (1994). Stages of change and decisional balance for 12 problem behaviors. *Health Psychology, 13*(1), 39-46.

Procidano, M.E., & Heller, K. (1983). Measures of perceived social support from friends and from family: Three validation studies. *American Journal of Community Psychology, 11,* 1-24.

Pruyser, P.W. (1975). Aging: Downward, upward or forward? In S. Hiltner (Ed.), *Toward a theology of aging* (pp. 102-118). New York: Human Sciences Press.

Psaty, B.M., Koepsell, T.D., Wagner, E.H., LoGerfo, J.P., & Inui, T.S. (1990). The relative risk of incident coronary heart disease associated with recently stopping the use of beta-blockers. *Journal of the American Medical Association, 263,* 1653-1657.

Quanty, M.B. (1976). Aggression catharsis. In R.G. Green & E.C. O'Neal (Eds.), *Perspectives on aggression* (pp. 211-221). New York: Academic Press.

Rabinowitz, B., & Florian, V. (1992). Chronic obstructive pulmonary disease—psychosocial issues and treatment goals. *Social Work in Health Care, 16*(4), 69-86.

Radloff, L.S. (1977). The CES-D Scale: A self-report depression scale for research in the general population. *Applied Psychological Measure, 1,* 385-401.

Ragland, D.R., & Brand, R.J. (1988). Type A behavior and mortality from coronary heart disease. *New England Journal of Medicine, 318,* 65-69.

Rahe, R.M., Ward, H.W., & Hayes, V. (1979). Brief group therapy in myocardial infarction rehabilitation: Three to four year follow-up of a controlled trial. *Psychosomatic Medicine, 41,* 229-242.

Rankin, S.H. (1990). Differences in recovery from cardiac surgery: A profile of male and female patients. *Heart and Lung, 19*(5), 481-485.

Raphael, B. (1977). Preventive intervention with the recently bereaved. *Archives of General Psychiatry 34*(Dec), 1450-1454

Rapp, S.R., Parisi, S.A., Walsh, D.A., & Wallace, C.E. (1988). Detecting depression in the elderly inpatient. *Journal of Consulting and Clinical Psychology, 56,* 509-513.

Razin, A.M. (1982). Psychosocial intervention in coronary artery disease: A review. *Psychosomatic Medicine, 44*(4), 363-381.

Razin, A.M., Swencionis, C., & Zohman, L.R. (1986). Reduction of physiological, behavioral, and self-report responses in Type A behavior: A preliminary report. *International Journal of Psychiatric Medicine, 16*(1), 32-47.

Rechnitzer, P.A., Pickard, H.A., Paivio, A.U., Yuhasz, M.S., & Cunningham, D. (1972). Long-term follow-up study of survival and recurrence rates following myocardial infarction in exercising and control subjects. *Circulation, XLV,* 203-207.

Reed, D., McGee, D., Katshuhiko, Y., & Feinleib, M. (1983). Social networks and coronary heart disease among Japanese men in Hawaii. *American Journal of Epidemiology, 117,* 384-396.

Reich, P., Regestein, Q.R., Murawski, B.J., DeSilva, R.A., & Lown, B. (1983). Unrecognized organic mental disorders in survivors of cardiac arrest. *American Journal of Psychiatry, 140*(9), 1194-1197.

Reiger, D., Goldberg, I., & Taube, C. (1978). The de facto U.S. mental health services system. *Archives of General Psychiatry, 35,* 685-693.

Reiss, D., & Oliveri, M.E. (1991). The family's conception of accountability and competence: A new approach to the conceptualization and assessment of family stress. *Family Processes, 30,* 193-214.

Reitan, R.M. (1958). Validity of the trail making test as an indicator of organic brain damage. *Perceptive Motor Skills, 8,* 271-276.

Rejeski, W.J. (1983). Rehabilitation and prevention of coronary heart disease: An overview of the Type A behavior pattern. *Quest, 33*(2), 154-165.

Rejeski, W.J., & Kenney, E.A. (1988). *Fitness motivation: Preventing participant dropout.* Champaign, IL: Human Kinetics.

Rejeski, W.J., Morley, D., & Miller, H.S. (1983). Coronary prone behavior as a moderator of GTX performance. *Journal of Cardiac Rehabilitation, 3,* 339-346.

Rejeski, W.J., Morley, D., & Miller, H.S. (1984). The Jenkins Activity Survey: Exploring its relationship with compliance to exercise prescription and MET gain within a cardiac rehabilitation setting. *Journal of Cardiac Rehabilitation, 4,* 90-94.

Renfroe, K.L. (1988). Effect of progressive relaxation on dyspnea and state anxiety in patients with chronic obstructive pulmonary disease. *Heart & Lung, 17,* 408-413.

Rennard, S., Daughton, D., Fortmann, S., Killan, J., Petty, T., Silvers, W., Repsher, L., Stillman, D., Cansey, D., Knowles, M., & Rolf, C. (1991). Transdermal nicotine enhances smoking cessation in coronary artery disease patients. *Chest, 100,* 5S.

Reynolds, W.M., & Gould, J.W. (1981). A psychometric investigation of the standard and short form Beck Depression Inventory. *Journal of Consulting and Clinical Psychology, 49,* 306-307.

Rhodewalt, F., & Fairfield, M. (1990). An alternative approach to Type A behavior and health: Psychological reactance and medical noncompliance. In M.J. Strube (Ed.), Type A behavior [Special issue]. *Journal of Social Behavior and Personality, 5*(1), 323-342.

Ribisl, P.M., Smalley, M.B., Brubaker, P.H., Rejeski, W.J., Sotile, W.M., & Miller, H.S., Jr. (1994). Contrast in social support between men and women with coronary artery disease. Presented to the National Meeting of the American College of Sports Medicine, Indianapolis, IN.

Ries, A.L. (1990). Position paper of the American Association of Cardiovascular and Pulmonary Rehabilitation: Scientific basis of pulmonary rehabilitation. *Journal of Cardiopulmonary Rehabilitation, 10,* 418-441.

Rifkin, B.G. (1968). The treatment of cardiac neurosis using systematic desensitization. *Behavioral Research Therapy, 6,* 239-241.

Rimer, B.K., & Orleans, C.T. (1993). *Nicotine addiction.* New York: Oxford University Press.

Rogers, K.R. (1987). Nature of spousal supportive behaviors that influence heart transplant patient compliance. *Journal of Heart Transplant, 60,* 90-95.

Rook, K.S. (1984). The negative side of social interaction: Impact on psychological well-being. *Journal of Personality and Social Psychology, 46,* 1097-1108.

Roose, S.P., Dalack, G.W., & Woodring, S. (1991). Death, depression and heart disease. *Journal of Clinical Psychiatry, 52*(Suppl. 6), 34-39.

Rose, G., Heller, R.F., Pedoc, H.T., & Christie, D.G. (1980). Heart disease prevention project: A randomised controlled trial in industry. *British Medical Journal, 279,* 747-751.

Rose, M.I., & Robbins, B. (1993). Psychosocial recovery issues and strategies in cardiac rehabilitation. In F.J. Pashkow & W.A. Dafoe (Eds.), *Clinical cardiac rehabilitation: A cardiologist's guide* (pp. 248-261). Baltimore: Williams & Wilkins.

Rosen, J.L., & Bibring, G.L. (1966). Psychological reaction of male patients to heart attack. *Psychosomatic Medicine, 28,* 808-820.

Rosenberg, L., Kaufman, D.W., Helmrich, S.P., & Shapiro, S. (1985). The risk of myocardial infarction after quitting smoking in men under 55 years of age. *New England Journal of Medicine, 313,* 1511-1514.

Rosenman, R.H. (1978). The interview method of assessment of the coronary-prone behavior pattern. In T.M. Dembroski, J. Weiss, J.L. Shields, S.G. Haynes, & M. Feinleib (Eds.), *Coronary-prone behavior* (pp. 55-69). New York: Springer-Verlag.

Rosenman, R.H. (1990). Type A behavior pattern: A personal overview. In M.J. Strube (Ed.). *Journal of Social and Behavioral and Personality, 5*(1), 1-4.

Rosenthal, S. (1987). *Sex over forty.* Los Angeles: Tarcher.

Roskies, E. (1987). *Stress management for the healthy Type A: Theory and practice.* New York: Guilford Press.

Roskies, E., Seraganian, P., Oseasohn, R., Hanley, J.A., Collu, R., Martin, N., & Smilga, C. (1986). The Montreal Type A intervention project: Major findings. *Health Psychology, 5*(1), 45-69.

Roskies, E., Spevack, M., Surkis, A., Cohen, C., & Gilman, S. (1978). Changing the coronary-prone (Type A) behavior pattern in a nonclinical population. *Journal of Behavioral Medicine, 1,* 201-216.

Ross, C.E., & Hayes, D. (1988). Exercise and psychologic well-being in the community. *American Journal of Epidemiology, 127*, 762-771.

Ross, H.L., & Phipps, E. (1986). Physician-patient power struggles: Their role in noncompliance. *Family Medicine, 18*(2), 99-101.

Ross, J., Monro, L., Diwell, A., Mackean, J.M., Marsh, J., & Barker, O.J. (1978). Wessex cardiac surgery follow-up survey: The quality of life after operation. *Thorax, 33*, 3-9.

Rotter, J.B. (1972). *Application of a social learning theory of personality.* New York: Holt Rinehart & Winston.

Roviaro, A., Holmes, D.S., & Holsten, R.D. (1984). Influence of a cardiac rehabilitation program on the cardiovascular, psychological and social functioning of cardiac patients. *Journal of Behavioral Medicine, 7*, 61-81.

Rowe, J.W., & Kahn, R.L. (1987). Human aging: Usual and successful. *Science, 237*(July 10), 143-149.

Rozanski, A., Bairey, C.N., Krantz, D.S., Friedman, J., Resser, K.J., Morell, M., Hilton-Chalfer, S., Hestrin, L., Bietendorf, J., & Berman, D.S. (1988). Mental stress and the induction of silent myocardial ischemia in patients with coronary artery disease. *New England Journal of Medicine, 318*, 118-145.

Ruberman, W., Weinblatt, A.B., Goldberg, J.D., & Chaudhary, B.S. (1984). Psychosocial influences on mortality after myocardial infarction. *New England Journal of Medicine, 311*, 552-559.

Ruzbarsky, V., & Michal, V. (1977). Morphologic changes in the arterial bed of the penis with aging: Relationship to the pathogenesis of impotence. *Investigative Urology, 15*, 194-199.

Rydon, P., Redman, S., Sanson-Fisher, R.W., & Reid, A.L.A. (1992). Detection of alcohol-related problems in general practice. *Journal of Studies of Alcohol, 53*, 197-202.

Sackett, D.L., & Haynes, R.B. (Eds.) (1976). *Compliance with therapeutic regimens.* Baltimore: Johns Hopkins University Press.

Sallis, J.F., Flora, J.A., & Formann, S.P. (1981). Mediated smoking cessation programs in the Stanford Five-City Project. *Addictive Behaviors, 10*, 441-443.

Sandhu, H.S. (1986). Psychosocial issues in chronic obstructive pulmonary disease. *Clinics in Chest Medicine, 7*(4), 629-642.

Sarafino, E.P. (1990). *Health psychology: Biopsychosocial interactions.* New York: Wiley.

Sarason, B.R., & Sarason, I.G. (1994). Assessment of social support. In S.A. Shumaker & S.M. Czajkowski (Eds.), *Social support and cardiovascular disease* (pp. 41-64). New York: Plenum Press.

Sarason, I.G., Levine, H.M., Basham, R.B., & Sarason, B.R. (1983). Assessing social support: The social support questionnaire. *Journal of Personality and Social Psychology, 44*, 127-139.

Satir, V. (1964). *Conjoint Family Therapy.* Palo Alto, CA: Science and Behavior Books.

Sawyer, J.D. (1983). Suicide in cases of chronic obstructive pulmonary disease. *Journal of Psychiatric Treatment and Evaluation, 5*(2-3), 281-283.

Scalzi, C., Burke, L., & Greenland, S. (1980). Evaluation of an inpatient education program for coronary patients and families. *Heart and Lung, 9*, 846-853.

Schaie, K.W., & Willis, S.L. (1986). Can decline in adult intellectual functioning be reversed? *Developmental Psychology 22*(2), 223-232.

Schindler, B.A., Shook, J., & Schwartz, G.M. (1989). Beneficial effects of psychiatric intervention on recovery after coronary artery bypass graft surgery. *General Hospital Psychiatry, 11*, 358-364.

Schleifer, S.J., Macari-Hinson, M.M., Coyle, D.A., Slater, W.R., Kahn, M., Gorlin, R., & Zucker, H.A. (1989). The nature and course of depression following myocardial infarction. *Archives of Internal Medicine, 149,* 1785-1789.

Schockern, D.D., Green, A.F., Worden, T.J., Harrison, E.E., & Spielberger, D.C. (1987). Effects of age on the relationship between anxiety and coronary artery disease. *Psychosomatic Medicine, 49,* 118-126.

Schover, L.R. (1984). *Prime time: Sexual health for men over fifty.* New York: Holt Rinehart & Winston.

Schover, L.R., & Jensen, S. (1988). *Sexuality and chronic illness: A comprehensive approach.* New York: Guilford Press.

Schuler, G., Hambrecht, J.R., Schlierf, G., Grunze, M., Methfessel, S., Hayer, K., & Kublen, W. (1992). Myocardial perfusion and regression of coronary artery disease in patients on a regimen of intensive physical exercise and low fat diet. *Journal of the American College of Cardiology, 19,* 34-42.

Schutz, W. (1976). *MATE: A Firo awareness scale* (rev. ed.). Palo Alto, CA: Consulting Psychologists Press.

Seeman, T.E., & Syme, S.L. (1987). Social networks and coronary artery disease: A comparison of the structure and function of social relations as predictors of disease. *Psychosomatic Medicine, 49,* 340-353.

Seligman, M. (1990). *Learned optimism.* New York: Knopf.

Selvini-Palazzoli, M., Cecchin, G., Prata, G., & Boscolo, L. (1978). *Paradox and counter-paradox.* New York: Jason Aronson.

Selye, H. (1974). *Stress without distress.* Philadelphia: Lippincott.

Selye, H. (1976). *The stress of life.* New York: McGraw-Hill.

Selzer, M.L. (1971). The Michigan Alcoholism Screening Test: The quest for a new diagnostic instrument. *American Journal of Psychiatry, 127,* 1653-1658.

Semmens, J.P., & Wagner, G. (1982). Estrogen deprivation and vaginal function in postmenopausal women. *Journal of the American Medical Association, 248,* 445-448.

Semmlow, J.L., & Lubowsky, J. (1983). Sexual instrumentation. *IEEE Transactions on Biomedical Engineering, 6,* 309-319.

Semple, P.D., Beastall, G.H., Watson, W.S., & Hume, R. (1980). Serum testosterone depression associated with hypoxia in respiratory failure. *Clinical Science, 58,* 105.

Seraganian, P., Roskies, E., Hanley, J.A., Oseasohn, R., & Collu, R. (1987). Failure to alter psychophysiological reactivity in Type A men with physical exercise or stress management programs. *Psychological Health, 1,* 195-213.

Sexton, D.L. (1987). Relaxation techniques and biofeedback. In J.E. Hogkin & T.L. Petty (Eds.), *Chronic obstructive pulmonary disease: Current concepts* (pp. 99-112). Philadelphia: Saunders.

Shaffer, J.L. (1991). Spiritual distress and critical illness. *Critical Care Nurse, 11*(1), 42-46.

Shanas, E. (1979). The family as a social support in old age. *The Gerontologist, 19*(2), 169-174.

Shanfield, S.B. (1990). Myocardial infarction and patients' wives. *Psychosomatics, 31,* 138-145.

Shaw, R., Cohen, F., Doyle, B., & Palesky, J. (1985). The impact of denial and repressive style on information gain and rehabilitation outcomes in myocardial infarction patients. *Psychosomatic Medicine, 47,* 262-273.

Sheehan, D.V. (1984). *The anxiety disease and how to overcome it.* New York: Scribners.

Shekelle, R.B., Gale, M., Ostfeld, A., & Paul, O. (1983). Hostility, risk of coronary heart disease and mortality. *Psychosomatic Medicine, 45,* 109-114.

Shekelle, R.B., Hulley, S.B., Neaton, J.D., Billings, J.H., Borhani, N.O., Gerace, T.A., Jacobs, D.R., Lasser, N.L., Mittlemark, M.B., & Stamler, J. (1985a). Incidence of coronary heart disease. *American Journal of Epidemiology, 122*(4), 559-570.

Shekelle, R.B., Hulley, S.B., Neaton, J.D., Billings, J.H., Borhani, N.O., Gerace, T.A., Jacobs, D.R., Lasser, N.L., Mittlemark, M.B., & Stamler, J. (1985b). The MRFIT behavior pattern study: II. Type A behavior pattern and risk of coronary death in MRFIT. *American Journal of Epidemiology, 122,* 559-570.

Shumaker, S.A., & Czajkowski, S.M. (Eds.) (1994). *Social support and cardiovascular disease.* New York: Plenum Press.

Sickbert, S.F. (1989). Coronary care unit visitation and summary of the literature. *American Geriatric Society, 37*(7), 655-657.

Siegman, A.W. (1989). The role of hostility, neuroticism, and speech style in coronary artery disease. In A.W. Siegman & T.M. Dembroski (Eds.), *In search of coronary-prone behavior* (pp. 65-89). Hillsdale, NJ: Erlbaum.

Siegrist, J., Siegrist, K., & Weber, I. (1986). Sociological concepts in the etiology of chronic disease: The case of ischemic heart disease. *Social Science & Medicine, 22,* 247-253.

Sikes, W.W., & Rodenhauser, P. (1987). Rehabilitation programs for myocardial infarction patients: A national survey. *General Hospital Psychiatry, 9,* 182-186.

Sikorski, J.M. (1985). Knowledge, concerns and questions of wives of convalescent coronary artery bypass graft surgery patients. *Journal of Cardiac Rehabilitation, 5,* 74-85.

Simmons, D., & Tiley, K. (1990). Aging population and their families need sensitive consultation by family therapists. *Family Therapy News, 21*(1), 8-9.

Simpson, T. (1991). Critical care patients' perceptions of visits. *Heart and Lung, 20*(6), 681-688.

Sirles, A.T., & Selleck, C.S. (1989). Cardiac disease and the family: Impact, assessment, and implications. *Journal of Cardiovascular Nursing, 3*(2), 23-32.

Sivarajan, E.S., Bruce, R.A., Almes, M.J., Green, B., Belanger, L., Lindskog, B.D., Newton, K.M., & Mansfield, L.W. (1981). In-hospital exercise after myocardial infarction does not improve treadmill performance. *New England Journal of Medicine, 305*(7), 357-362.

Sivarajan, E.S., & Newton, K.M. (1984). Exercise, education, and counseling for patients with coronary artery disease. *Clinics in Sports Medicine, 3,* 349-369.

Sjogren, K. (1983). Sexuality after stroke with hemiplegia: II. With special regard to partnership adjustment and to fulfillment. *Scandinavian Journal of Rehabilitation Medicine, 15,* 63-69.

Skelton, M., & Dominian, J. (1973). Psychological stress in wives of patients with myocardial infarction. *British Medical Journal, 1,* 101-103.

Skinner, H.A., Steinhauer, P.D., & Santa-Barbara, J. (1983). The family assessment measure. *Canadian Journal of Community Mental Health, 2,* 91-105.

Smith, D.A.F., & Coyne, J.C. (1988). Coping with a myocardial infarction: Determinants of patient self-efficacy. Symposium presentation at the 96th annual convention of the American Psychological Association, Atlanta.

Smith, G.R., Jr., Monson, R.A., & Ray, D.C. (1986). Psychiatric consultation in somatization disorder: A randomized controlled study. *New England Journal of Medicine, 314,* 1407-1413.

Smith, G.R., & O'Rourke, D.F. (1988). Return to work after myocardial infarction: A test of multiple hypotheses. *Journal of the American Medical Association, 259,* 1673-1677.

Smith, T.W. (1992). Hostility and health: Current status of a psychosomatic hypothesis. *Health Psychology, 11*(3), 139-150.

Smith, T.W., & Anderson, N.B. (1986). Models of personality and disease: An interactional approach to Type A behavior and cardiovascular risk. *Journal of Personality and Social Psychology, 50,* 1166-1173.

Smith, T.W., & Brown, P. (1991). Cynical hostility, attempts to exert social control, and cardiovascular reactivity in married couples. *Journal of Behavioral Medicine, 14,* 579-590.

Smith, T.W., & Pope, M.K. (1990). Cynical hostility as a health risk: Current status and future directions. *Journal of Social Behavior and Personality, 5,* 77-88.

Smith, T.W., & Rhodewalt, F. (1986). On states, traits and processes: A transactional alternative to individual difference assumptions in Type A behavior and physiological reactivity. *Journal of Research in Personality, 20,* 229-251.

Smith, T.W., & Sanders, J.D. (1986). Type A behavior, marriage, and the heart: Person-by-situation interactions and the risk of coronary disease. *Behavioral Medicine Abstracts, 7,* 59-62.

Soloff, P.H. (1977). Denial and rehabilitation of the post-infarction patient. *International Journal of Psychiatry Medicine, 8,* 125-130.

Sotile, W.M. (1979a). The penile prosthesis: A review. *Journal of Sex and Marital Therapy, 5,* 90-102.

Sotile, W.M. (1979b). The penile prosthesis and diabetic impotence: Some caveats. *Diabetes Care, 2*(1), 26-30.

Sotile, W.M. (1991, December). Using marital therapy techniques with Type A's: How to harness the storm. The Psychology of Health, Immunity and Disease, Third National Conference, The National Institute for the Clinical Application of Behavioral Medicine, Orlando, FL.

Sotile, W.M. (1992). *Heart illness and intimacy: How caring relationships aid recovery.* Baltimore: Johns Hopkins University Press.

Sotile, W.M. (1995). *Coping With Heart Illness.* Champaign, IL: Human Kinetics.

Sotile, W.M., Julian, A., Henry, S.E., & Sotile, M.O. (1990). *Family apperception test manual.* Los Angeles: Western Psychological Services.

Sotile, W.M., & Kilmann, P.R. (1977). Treatments of psychogenic female sexual dysfunctions. *Psychological Bulletin, 84*(4), 619-633.

Sotile, W.M., & Kilmann, P.R. (1978). The effects of group systematic desensitization on female orgasmic dysfunction. *Archives of Sexual Behavior, 7*(5), 61-68.

Sotile, W.M., Kilmann, P.R., & Follingstad, D.R. (1977). A sexual enhancement workshop: Beyond group systematic desensitization for women's sexual anxiety. *Journal of Sex and Marital Therapy, 3*(4), 249-255.

Sotile, W.M., Kilmann, P.R., & Scovern, A.W. (1977). Definitions and classifications of psychogenic female sexual dysfunctions. *Journal of Sex Education and Therapy, 3*(1), 21-27.

Sotile, W.M., Sotile, M.O., Ewen, G.S., & Sotile, L.J. (1993). Marriage and family factors relevant to effective cardiac rehabilitation: A review of risk factor literature. *Sports Medicine Training and Rehabilitation, 4,* 115-128.

Southard, D.R., & Broyden, R. (1990). Psychosocial services in cardiac rehabilitation: A status report. *Journal of Cardiopulmonary Rehabilitation, 10,* 255-263.

Spanier, B.B. (1976). Measuring dyadic adjustment: New scales for assessing the quality of marriage and similar dyads. *Journal of Marriage and Family, 38*, 15-25.

Speedling, E.F. (1982). *Heart attack: The family response at home and in the hospital.* New York: Tavistock.

Speilberger, C.E., Gorsuch, R.L., & Luschene, R.E. (1970). *Manual for the state trait anxiety inventory.* Palo Alto, CA: Consulting Psychologists Press.

Spiegel, D., Bloom, H.C., Kraemer, J.R., & Gottheil, E. (1989, October 14). Effect of psychosocial treatment on survival of patients with metastatic breast cancer. *The Lancet*, 888-901.

Squires, R.W., Allison, T.G., Miller, T.D., & Gan, G.T. (1991). Cardiopulmonary exercise testing after unilateral lung transplantation: A case report. *Journal of Cardiopulmonary Rehabilitation, 11*, 192-196.

Stackl, W., Hasun, R., & Marberger, M. (1988). Intracavernous injection of prostaglandin E1 in impotent men. *Journal of Urology, 140*, 66-68.

Stalonas, P.M., Johnson, W.G., & Christ, M. (1978). Behavior modification for obesity: The evaluation of exercise, contingency management and program adherence. *Journal of Consulting and Clinical Psychology, 46*, 463-469.

Stanton, B., Jenkins, C.D., Savageau, J.A., Harken, D.E., & Aucoin, R. (1984). Perceived adequacy of patient education and fears and adjustments after cardiac surgery. *Heart and Lung, 13*, 525-531.

Stein, E.H., Murdaugh, J., & MacLeod, J.A. (1969). Brief psychotherapy of psychiatric reactions to physical illness. *American Journal of Psychiatry, 8*, 1040-1047.

Stein, H.F., & Pontious, J.M. (1985). Family and beyond: The larger context of noncompliance. *Family Systems Medicine, 3*, 179-189.

Stein, R. (1975). The effects of exercise training on peak coital heart rate in post-myocardial infarction males. *Circulation, 51*(Suppl. 11), 456.

Stern, M.J., Pascale, L., & Ackerman, A. (1977). Life adjustment postmyocardial infarction. *Archives of Internal Medicine, 137*, 623-633.

Stewart, A., Hays, R., & Ware, J.J. (1988). The MOS short-form general health survey: Reliability and validity in a patient population. *Medical Care, 26*, 724-735.

Stewart, I., & Joines, V. (1987). *TA today: A new introduction to transactional analysis.* Nottingham, England: Lifespace.

Stimson, G.V. (1974). Obeying doctor's orders: A view from the other side. *Social Sciences $ Medicine, 8*, 97-104.

Stoll, R. (1979). Guidelines for spiritual assessment. *American Journal of Nursing, 11*(1), 1574-1577.

Storer, J.H., Frate, D.A., Johnson, S.A., & Greenberg, A.M. (1987). When the cure seems worse than the disease: Helping families adapt to hypertension treatment. *Family Relations, 36*, 311-315.

Strachan, J.R., & Pryor, J.P. (1987). Diagnostic intracorporeal papaverine and erectile dysfunction. *British Journal of Urology, 59*, 264-266.

Strijbos, J.H., Koeter, G.H., & Meinesz, A.F. (1990). Home care rehabilitation and perception of dyspnea in chronic obstructive pulmonary disease (COPD) patients. *Chest, 97*, 109s-110s.

Strodtbeck, F.L. (1951). The family as a three-person group. *American Social Review, 19*, 23.

Stuart, R.B., & Davis, B. (1972). *Slim chance in a fat world: Behavioral control of obesity.* Chicago: Research Press.

Suinn, R.M. (1974). Behavior therapy for cardiac patients. *Behavior Therapy, 5*, 569-571.

Suinn, R.M. (1975). The cardiac stress management program for Type A patients. *Cardiac Rehabilitation, 5,* 13-15.

Suinn, R.M. (1977). Type A behavior pattern. In R.B. Williams & W.D. Gentry (Eds.), *Behavior approaches to medical treatment* (pp. 55-65). Boston: Ballinger.

Suinn, R.M., & Bloom, L.J. (1978). Anxiety management training for pattern A behavior. *Journal of Behavior Medicine, 1,* 25-35.

Suls, J., Gastorf, J.W., & Witenburg, S.H. (1979). Life events, psychological distress and the Type A coronary-prone behavior pattern. *Journal of Psychosomatic Research, 23,* 315-319.

Suls, J., & Sanders, G.S. (1989). Why do some behavioral styles place people at coronary risk? In A.W. Siegman & T.M. Dembroski (Eds.), *In search of coronary-prone behavior: Beyond Type A.* Hillsdale, NJ: Erlbaum.

Swan, G.E., Carmelli, D., & Rosenman, R.H. (1990). Cook and medley hostility and the Type A behavior pattern: Psychological correlates of two coronary-prone behaviors. *Journal of Social Behavior and Personality, 5*(1), 89-106.

Swenson, J.R., & Abbey, S.E. (1993). Management of depression and anxiety disorders in the cardiac patient. In F.J. Pashkow & W.A. Dafoe (Eds.), *Clinical cardiac rehabilitation: A cardiologist's guide* (pp. 263-286). Baltimore: Williams & Wilkins.

Tandon, M.K. (1978). Adjunct treatment with yoga in chronic severe airways obstruction. *Thorax, 33,* 514-517.

Tarlov, A., Ware, J., Greenfield, S., Nelson, E.C., Perrin, E., & Zubkoff, M. (1989). The medical outcomes study: An application of methods for monitoring the results of medical care. *Journal of the American Medical Association, 262,* 925-930.

Taylor, C.B. (1987). Discuss work, stress, sex to avert psychological problems. *Consultant, 27,* 45-58.

Taylor, C.B., & Arnow, B. (1985). *The nature and treatment of anxiety disorders* (pp. 313-314). New York: Free Press.

Taylor, C.B., Bandura, A., Ewart, C.K., Miller, N.H., & DeBusk, F. (1985). Exercise testing to enhance wives' confidence in their husbands' cardiac capability soon after clinically uncomplicated acute myocardial infarction. *American Journal of Cardiology, 55,* 635-638.

Taylor, C.B., DeBusk, R.F., Davidson, D.M., Houston, N., & Burnett, K.F. (1981). Optimal methods for identifying depression following hospitalization for myocardial infarction. *Journal of Chronic Disease, 34,* 127-133.

Taylor, C.B., Houston-Miller, N., Kilen, J.D., & DeBusk, R.F. (1990). Smoking cessation after acute myocardial infarction: Effects of a nurse-managed intervention. *Annals of Internal Medicine, 113*(2), 118-123.

Taylor, C.B., Miller, N.H., Haskell, W.L., & DeBusk, R.F. (1988). Smoking cessation after acute myocardial infarction: The effects of exercise training. *Addictive Behavior, 13,* 331-335.

Taylor, C.B., Sheikh, J., Argras, W.S., Roth, W.T., Margraf, J., Ehleys, A., Maddock, R.J., & Gossard, D. (1986). Ambulatory heart rate changes in patients with panic attacks. *American Journal of Psychiatry, 143,* 479-482.

Thockcloth, R.M., So, S.O., & Wright, W. (1973). Is cardiac rehabilitation necessary. *Medical Journal of Australia, 2,* 669-674.

Thomas, S.A., Sappington, E., Gross, H.S., Nector, M., Friedman, E., & Lynch, J.J. (1983). Denial in coronary care patients—an objective assessment. *Heart and Lung, 12,* 74-80.

Thompson, D.R., & Cordle, C.J. (1988). Support of wives of myocardial infarction patients. *Journal of Advanced Nursing, 13*(2), 223-228.

Thompson, D.R., & Meddis, R. (1990). Wives' responses to counselling early after myocardial infarction. *Journal of Psychosomatic Research, 34*(3), 249-258.

Thompson, W.L., & Thompson, T.L. (1984). Treating depression in asthmatic patients. *Psychosomatics, 25*, 809-812.

Thoresen, C.E., Friedman, M., Powell, L.H., Ulman, D., Thompson, L., Price, V.A., Rabin, D.D., Breall, W.S., & Dixon, T. (1985). Altering the type A behavior pattern in postinfarction patients. *Journal of Cardiopulmonary Rehabilitation, 5*, 258-266.

Thoresen, C.E., & Low, K.G. (1990). Women and Type A behavior pattern: Review and commentary. *Journal of Social Behavior and Personality, 5*(1) [Special issue], 117-133.

Thoresen, C.E., & Pattillo, J.R. (1988). Exploring the Type A behavior pattern in children and adolescents. In B.K. Houston & C.R. Snyder (Eds.), *Type A behavior pattern: Research, theory and intervention* (pp. 98-145). New York: Wiley.

Thurman, C.W. (1985). Effectiveness of cognitive-behavioral treatments in reducing Type A behavior among university faculty. *Journal of Counseling Psychology, 32*, 74-83.

Tiep, B.L. (1993). Biofeedback and respiratory muscle training. In J.E. Hodgkin, G.L. Connors, & C.W. Bell (Eds.), *Pulmonary rehabilitation: Guidelines to success* (2nd ed.) (pp. 403-421). Philadelphia: Lippincott.

Toshima, M.T., Kaplan, R.M., & Ries, A.L. (1992). Self-efficacy expectations in chronic obstructive pulmonary disease rehabilitation. In R. Schwazer (Ed.), *Self-efficacy: Thought control of action* (pp. 325-354). New York: Hemisphere.

Trieber, F.A., Mabe, P.A., Riley, W.T., McDuffie, M., Strong, W.B., & Levy, M. (1990). Children's Type A behavior: The role of parental hostility and family history of cardiovascular disease. In M.J. Strube (Ed.), Type A Behavior [Special issue], *Journal of Social Behavior and Personality, 5*(1), 183-199.

Tuttle, W.B., Cook, W.L., & Fitch, E. (1964). Sexual behavior in post-myocardial infarction patients. *American Journal of Cardiology, 13*, 140-153.

Ueno, M. (1963). The so-called coital coition death. *Japanese Journal of Legal Medicine, 17*, 333-340.

Ulmer, D. (1990, December). How to help Type A's enhance their self-esteem within the therapy group setting. Paper presented at the Healing the Heart 4th National Multidisciplinary Conference, Orlando, FL.

Ulrich, R.S. (1984). View through a window may influence recovery from surgery. *Science, 224*, 420-421.

U.S. Department of Health and Human Services. (1993). *Depression in Primary Care: Detection and Diagnosis.* (Publication No. 93-0550). Rockville, MD: Agency for Health Care Policy and Research.

U.S. Government Task Force. (1979). *Epidemiology of respiratory diseases: Task force report on state of knowledge, problems, needs* (NIH Publication No. 81-2019). Washington, D.C.: National Institutes of Health.

Usui, W.M., Feil, T.J., & Durig, K.R. (1985). Socioeconomic comparisons and life satisfaction of elderly adults. *Journal of Gerontology, 40*, 110-114.

Vaillant, G.E. (1977). *Adaptation to life.* Boston: Little, Brown.

van Der Veen, F., Huebner, B.J., Jurgens, B., & Beja, P. (1964). Relationships between the parents' concept of the family and family adjustment. *American Journal of Orthopsychiatry, 34*, 45-55.

van Dixhoorn, J., Duivenvoorden, H.J., & Staal, H.A. (1989). Physical training and relaxation therapy in cardiac rehabilitation assessed through a composite criterion for training outcome. *American Heart Journal, 119*(3), 545-552.

van Dixhoorn, J., Duivenvoorden, H.J., Stall, J.A., Pool, J., & Varghag, F. (1987). Cardiac events after myocardial infarction: Possible effect of relaxation therapy. *European Heart Journal, 8,* 1210-1214.

VanEgeren, L.F. (1979). Social interactions, communications, and the coronary-prone behavior pattern: A psychophysiological study. *Psychosomatic Medicine, 41,* 2-18.

VanEgeren, L.F., Abelson, J.L., & Sniderman, L.D. (1983). Interpersonal and electro-cardiographic responses of Type A's and Type B's in competitive socioeconomic games. *Journal of Psychosomatic Research, 27,* 53-59.

Veith, R.C., Raskind, M.A., Caldwell, J.H., Barnes, R.F., Gumbrecht, G., & Ritchie, J.L. (1982). Cardiovascular effects of tricyclic antidepressants in depressed patients with chronic heart disease. *New England Journal of Medicine, 306,* 954-959.

Vermeulen, A., Lie, K., & Burrer, D. (1983). Effects of cardiac rehabilitation after myocardial infarction: Changes in coronary risk factors and long-term prognosis. *American Heart Journal, 105,* 798-801.

Verwoerdt, A., & Dovenmuhle, R.H. (1964). Heart disease and depression. *Geriatrics, 19,* 856-863.

Vieweg, B.W., & Hedlund, J.L. (1983). The general health questionnaire (GHQ): A comprehensive review. *Journal Of Psychiatry, 14,* 74-81.

Vlay, S.C., & Fricchione, G.L. (1985). Psychosocial aspects of surviving sudden cardiac death. *Clinical Cardiology, 8,* 237-243.

Volow, M.R. (1972). Delirium, dementia, and other organic mental syndromes. In J.O. Cavenar & H.K.H. Brodie (Eds.), *Signs and symptoms in psychiatry* (pp. 511-517). Philadelphia: Lippincott.

von Bertalanffy, L. (1968). *General systems theory.* New York: Braziller.

Wabrek, A.J., & Burchell, R.C. (1980). Male sexual dysfunction associated with coronary heart disease. *Archives of Sexual Behavior, 9,* 69-75.

Wadden, T.A. (1983). Predicting treatment response to relaxation therapy for essential hypertension. *Journal of Nervous and Mental Disorders, 171,* 683-689.

Wakim, K. (1980). Physiologic effects of massage. In J. Rogoff (Ed.), *Manipulation, traction and massage.* Baltimore: Williams & Wilkins.

Walbroehl, G.S. (1992). Sexual concerns of the patient with pulmonary disease. *Postgraduate Medicine, 91*(5), 455-460.

Waldron, I., Zyzanski, S.J., Shekelle, R., Jenkins, C.D., & Tannenbaum, S. (1977). The coronary prone behavior pattern in employed men and women. *Journal of Human Stress, 3,* 2-18.

Wallace, N., & Wallace, D.C. (1977). Group education after myocardial infarction. *Medical Journal of Australia, 2,* 245-247.

Walter, R. (1985). *Return to work after coronary artery bypass surgery: Psychosocial and economic aspects.* Berlin, Germany: Springer.

Waltz, M. (1986). A longitudinal study on environmental and dispositional determinants of life quality: Social support and coping with physical illness. *Social Indicators Research, 18,* 71-93.

Waltz, M., & Badura, B. (1988). Subjective health, intimacy and perceived self-efficacy after a heart attack: Predicting life quality five years afterwards. *Social Industrial Research, 20,* 303-332.

Waltz, M., Badura, B., Pfaff, H., & Schott, T. (1988). Marriage and the psychological consequences of a heart attack: A longitudinal study of adaptation to chronic illness after 3 years. *Social Science & Medicine, 27*, 149-158.

Waring, E.M. (1983). Marriages of patients with psychosomatic illness. *General Hospital Psychiatry, 5*, 49-53.

Weaver, T., & Narsavage, G. (1992). Physiological and psychological variables related to functional status in chronic obstructive pulmonary disease. *Nursing Research, 41*, 286-291.

Wechsler, D. (1981). *Wechsler Adult Intelligence Scale—revised.* New York: The Psychological Corporation, Harcourt Brace Jovanovich.

Wechsler, D. (1987). *Wechsler Memory Scale—revised.* New York: The Psychological Corporation, Harcourt Brace Jovanovich.

Weinberger, D.A., Schwartz, G.E., & Davidson, J.R. (1979). Low anxious and depressive coping styles: Psychometric patterns and behavioral physiological responses to stress. *Journal of Abnormal Psychology, 88*, 369-380.

Weisberger, C.L. (1985). Sexual counseling for the patient following coronary artery surgery. *Medical Aspects & Human Sexuality, 19*, 137-141.

Weiss, R.J. (1991). Effects of antihypertensive agents on sexual function. *American Family Practice Physician, 44*(6), 2075-2082.

Weiss, S.J. (1990). Effects of differential touch on nervous system arousal of patients recovering from cardiac disease. *Heart and Lung, 19*(5), 474-480.

Wengel, S.P., Burke, W.J., Ranno, A.E., & Roccoforte, W.H. (1993). Use of benzodiazepines in the elderly. *Psychiatric Annals, 23*(6), 325-331.

Wenger, N.K. (1987, summer). Impairment, disability, and the cardiac patient (editorial). *Quality of Life and Cardiovascular Care, 37.*

Werko, L. (1971). Can we prevent heart disease? *Annals of Internal Medicine, 74*, 278-288.

Wespes, E., Delcour, C., Struyven, J., & Schulman, C.C. (1984). Cavernometry-cavernography: Its role in organic impotence. *European Urology, 10*, 229-232.

Wethington, E., & Kessler, R.C. (1986). Perceived support, received support, and adjustment to stressful life events. *Journal of Health and Social Behavior, 27*, 78-89.

White, K.L., Grant, J.L., & Chambis, W.N. (1955). Angina pectoris and angina innocens. *Psychosomatic Medicine, 17*, 128-135.

Wickramasekera, I. (1974). Heart rate feedback and the management of cardiac neurosis. *Journal of Abnormal Psychology, 83*, 578-580.

Williams, M.A. (1994). *Exercise testing and training in the elderly cardiac patient.* Champaign, IL: Human Kinetics.

Williams, M.A., Maresh, C.M., Esterbrook, D.J., Harbrecht, J.J., & Sketch, M.H. (1985). Early exercise training in patients older than age 65 years compared with that in younger patients after acute myocardial infarction or coronary artery bypass grafting. *American Journal of Cardiology, 55*, 263-266.

Williams, R.B., Jr., Barefoot, J.C., & Schekelle, R.B. (1985). The health consequences of hostility. In M.A. Chesney & R.H. Rosenman (Eds.), *Anger and hostility in cardiovascular and behavioral disorders* (pp. 173-185). Washington, D.C.: Hemisphere.

Williams, R.B., Haney, T.L., Lee, K.L., Kang, V., Blumenthal, J.A., & Whalen, R.E. (1980). Type A behavior, hostility, and coronary atherosclerosis. *Psychosomatic Medicine, 42*, 529-538.

Williams, R.W., & Williams, V. (1993). *Anger kills.* New York: Harper Collins.

Williams, S.J. (1989). Chronic respiratory illness and disability: A critical review of the psychosocial literature. *Social Science & Medicine, 28,* 791-803.

Wilson, R. (1987). *Don't panic.* New York: Harper & Row Perennial Library.

Wishnie, H., Hackett, T., & Cassem, N. (1971). Psychological hazards of convalescence following myocardial infarction. *Journal of the American Medical Association, 215,* 1292-1296.

Wolinsky, M.A. (1990). *A heart of wisdom: Marital counseling with older and elderly couples.* New York: Brunner/Mazel.

Worby, C.M., Altrocchi, J., Veach, T.L., & Crosby, R. (1991). Early identification of symptomatic post-MI families. *Family Systems Medicine, 9,* 127-136.

Wortman, C.B., & Brehm, J. (1975). Responses to uncontrollable outcomes: An integration of reactance theory and the learned helplessness model. In L. Berkowitz (Ed.), *Advances in experimental social psychology* (Vol. 8). New York: Academic Press.

Wright, L., & Leahey, M. (1984). *Nurses and families: A guide to family assessment and intervention.* Philadelphia: Davis.

Yellowlees, P.M. (1987). The treatment of psychiatric disorders in patients with chronic airways obstruction. *The Medical Journal of Australia, 147,* 349-352.

Yesavage, J.A., & Brink, T.L. (1983). Development and validation of the geriatric depression screening scale: A preliminary report. *Journal of Psychiatry Research, 17,* 37-49.

Yesavage, J.A., & Karasu, T.B. (1982). Psychotherapy with elderly patients. *American Journal of Psychotherapy, XXXVI*(1), 41-55.

Zilbergeld, B. (1992). *The new male sexuality.* New York: Bantam.

Zuckerman, D.M. (1984). Psychosocial predictors of mentality among the elderly poor. *American Journal of Epidemiology, 119,* 410-423.

Zurawski, R.M., Smith, T.W., & Houston, B.K. (1987). Stress management for essential hypertension: Comparison with a minimally effective treatment, predictors of response to treatment, and effects on reactivity. *Journal of Psychosomatic Research, 31,* 453-462.

■ INDEX ■

■ ABOUT THE AUTHOR ■

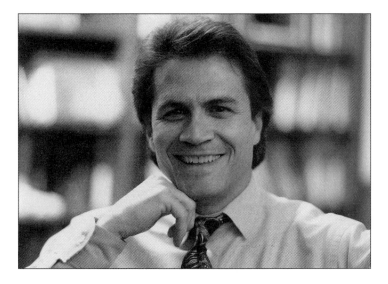

Wayne Sotile, PhD, has been director of psychological services for the Wake Forest University Cardiac Rehabilitation Program and codirector of Sotile Psychological Associates in Winston-Salem, North Carolina, since 1979. A licensed, practicing psychologist, Dr. Sotile has also served as the behavioral science representative to the board of directors of the American Association of Cardiovascular and Pulmonary Rehabilitation (AACVPR). He is a Fellow in AACVPR and an approved supervisor in the American Association for Marriage and Family Therapy.

The author of three books, Dr. Sotile has published numerous professional articles. His practical approaches to managing psychosocial issues have led to international recognition as a speaker (including national television appearances), author, and consultant on stress management, health psychology, and marriage and family life.

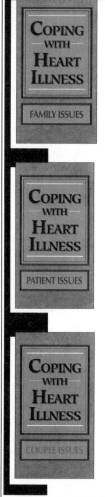